Vocational Rehabilitation of Persons
with Prolonged Psychiatric Disorders

The Johns Hopkins Series in Contemporary Medicine and Public Health

consulting editors

Martin D. Abeloff, M.D.   Edmond A. Murphy, M.D.
Samuel H. Boyer IV, M.D.   Edyth H. Schoenrich, M.D., M.P.H.
Gareth M. Green, M.D.   Jerry L. Spivak, M.D.
Richard T. Johnson, M.D.   Barbara H. Starfield, M.D., M.P.H.
Paul R. McHugh, M.D.

also of interest in this series:

Work and Mental Illness: Transitions to Employment,
Bertram J. Black

Family Management of Schizophrenia:
A Study of Clinical, Social, Family, and Economic Benefits,
by Ian R. H. Falloon and Others

Neuropsychological Rehabilitation after Brain Injury
George P. Prigatano and Others

Vocational Rehabilitation of Persons with Prolonged Psychiatric Disorders

edited by

JEAN A. CIARDIELLO
University of Medicine and Dentistry of New Jersey–
Robert Wood Johnson Medical School
and

MORRIS D. BELL
Yale University School of Medicine

THE JOHNS HOPKINS UNIVERSITY PRESS

Baltimore and London

The Johns Hopkins University Press
701 West 40th Street
Baltimore, Maryland 21211
The Johns Hopkins Press Ltd., London

∞ The paper used in this publication meets
the minimum requirements of American
National Standard for Information
Sciences—Permanence of Paper for Printed
Library Materials, ANSI Z39.48-1984.

Library of Congress Cataloging-in-Publication Data

Vocational rehabilitation of persons with prolonged
  psychiatric disorders.

  (The Johns Hopkins series in contemporary medicine
and public health)
  Includes index.
  1. Vocational rehabilitation. 2. Mentally ill—
Rehabilitation. I. Ciardiello, Jean A., 1948–   .
II. Bell, Morris D. III. Series. [DNLM: 1. Mental
Disorders—rehabilitation. 2. Rehabilitation, Vocational.
WM 29.1 V872]
HD7255.V595   1988   362.2'0425   87-26082
ISBN 0-8018-3635-2 (alk. paper)

For all those who have helped us to love and to work—
   our parents,
   our friends,
   and our patients.

Contents

Tables

Acknowledgments

This book was made possible through the combined efforts of many of our friends and colleagues. We would like to take this opportunity to offer our thanks.

First, we must thank Gary Lamson, Vice-President of Mental Health Services, University of Medicine and Dentistry of New Jersey, whose support and encouragement over the last two years made this project possible. There are many who have influenced our thinking and professional development over the years. In particular we would like to thank those who have inspired us in the area of prolonged psychiatric disorders: Lisbeth Haines, Courtenay Harding, Edward Ryan, John Strauss, and the members of the Continuing Care Leadership Group—Thomas Johnson, Christopher Kosseff, Sherrie Schwab, Margaret Van Horn, and John Woods. Our thanks to the many patients who have shared themselves with us and taught us a great deal about mental illness. For their editorial help in the publication process, we are indebted to Wendy Harris and Carolyn Moser. Special thanks to Sharon Smith and Roberta Waller for their skill and patience in typing and retyping countless drafts. Last, we would like to thank the contributors, whose willingness to share their ideas has given us a great deal to think about.

Vocational Rehabilitation of Persons
with Prolonged Psychiatric Disorders

Introduction

MORRIS D. BELL

From the title to the last page, our volume makes this statement: persons with prolonged psychiatric disorders can lead productive lives. It is a hopeful message based on the experience of our authors in applying the principles of rehabilitation to psychiatric populations. This relatively new professional endeavor draws upon many domains of knowledge in psychiatry, rehabilitation medicine, psychology, social work, sociology, and nursing. The main purpose of this volume has been to identify the boundaries of this interdisciplinary field and to explore the territory within it. We also hope to convey the great social significance of the work and the considerable intellectual and personal challenges to be found in professional commitment to the long-term care and rehabilitation of persons with prolonged psychiatric disorders.

This volume presents for the first time a comprehensive set of readings on the vocational rehabilitation of psychiatric patients. The overview chapters orient the reader to social and scientific developments that created this field, to current conceptual controversies, to the problems of defining the target population, and to the significance of psychiatric rehabilitation for public policy. The second section offers the theoretical background and clinical implications of six different approaches to vocational rehabilitation for psychiatric populations. The chapters in the third section examine processes common to all the approaches: assessment, medication management, ego functioning, and the formation and maintenance of therapeutic alliance in the rehabilitation relationship. The final segment of our volume offers the most comprehensive critique of relevant outcome research to date and maps out directions for further inquiry.

These chapters are testimonies of professional dedication to the many intellectual and clinical problems inherent in the task of aiding persons with prolonged psychiatric disorders to live more productive and satisfying lives. Understanding the biopsychosocial interactions that create the context of our work confronts the thoughtful professional with the myriad dilemmas and paradoxes of individual existence and social participation.

The rehabilitation professional should come to possess a sophisticated understanding of the nature of severe psychopathology and a recognition of the limitations of our scientific knowledge in this regard. Schizophrenia, affective disorders, severe personality disorders, substance abuse, and neurotic dysfunction are disorders of uncertain aetiology, pathogenesis, and prognosis. Assessments of ego deficits reveal unexpected diversity of strengths and weaknesses within and across diagnostic categories. Longitudinal studies now suggest that long-held assumptions about the degenerative course of schizophrenia are not accurate, while other diagnoses, such as personality disorders, that were thought to be less catastrophic are proving to be associated with severe social dysfunction, particularly among younger patients. Facing the daily personal and intellectual demands of rehabilitation work provides opportunities to ask new questions about the nature of the problem and to explore new methods for helping people make meaningful changes in the way they conduct their daily lives.

In this volume, the recipients of our services are described as persons, patients, clients, residents, the chronically mentally ill, the psychiatrically impaired, handicapped, or disabled. The choice of appellation reflects the author's background, professed method of intervention, or current understanding of the nature of the problem. Our preference for using the descriptive term *prolonged disorders* (for which we are indebted to John Strauss and Courtenay Harding) rather than *chronic disorders* is to emphasize the likelihood of sustained recovery while acknowledging the lengthy disruption in adjustment these disorders may cause. The reader will find in these chapters an accumulation of evidence to suggest that rehabilitation can significantly alter the course of psychiatric disorders, resulting in fewer episodes of relapse, more productivity, and a better quality of life. We believe that the groundbreaking clinical and research work presented here can provide the foundation for new advances in understanding the social dysfunction that accompanies psychiatric disorders and lead to progress toward more effective methods of vocational rehabilitation.

I

OVERVIEW

Vocational rehabilitation in the United States has had a short and fragmented history. In the first chapter Neff describes the historical development of rehabilitation and discusses the meanings of work and mental illness. He points to many of the difficult conceptual issues confronting vocational rehabilitation today which are elaborated in Chapter 4. Strauss, Harding, Silverman, Eichler, and Lieberman view work as treatment from nine different perspectives. Although these models have different and often conflicting assumptions, these authors' thoughtful consideration of the conceptual issues offer an important theoretical base for the reading of the rest of this book, as well as for vocational rehabilitation in general.

In Chapter 2 Goldman, Rosenberg, and Manderscheid give further conceptual clarity by defining the target groups for vocational rehabilitation services in terms of diagnosis, disability, and duration. They also discuss the implication of their thinking for national policy. Jansen also discusses public policy issues as they relate to the problems confronting chronically mentally ill individuals in their efforts to work. In addition to system issues, she outlines the many psychological and social difficulties which interact to create substantial obstacles to employment.

1

Vocational Rehabilitation in Perspective

WALTER S. NEFF

Neff describes the historical trends which converged to augment the development of vocational rehabilitation in the United States. He also summarizes the important conceptual issues concerning the nature of mental illness and the meanings of work and rehabilitation. The effects of deinstitutionalization and the community mental health movement are related to the past and present issues confronting psychiatric rehabilitation.

It is now some forty-five years since the enabling federal legislation in the area of vocational rehabilitation was amended to include services to the mentally and emotionally disabled. Prior to that date, 1943, the research and support efforts of the former Office of Vocational Rehabilitation (OVR, a section of the U.S. Department of Health, Education and Welfare) were focused exclusively on the physically disabled. It is probably fair to say that the bulk of another decade had to pass before the state and local arms of the federal office were able to begin effective implementation of the 1943 legislation. In any practical sense, therefore, the history of vocational rehabilitation for psychiatric disability covers a span from the middle 1950s to the present.

A number of trends converged to bring about this shift in federal legislation and service practice. First, the entry of the United States into World War II led to two observations that began to alarm both governmental and military authorities: (1) the large number of potential recruits turned down at the point of conscription because of mental and emotional handicaps, and (2) the large number of serving military men who had to be hospitalized or discharged because of mental "breakdowns" during their service in the armed forces. Second, it was becoming increasingly evident in the late forties and early fifties that our mental hospitals had become desperately overcrowded, and massive deterioration of the quality of care had become the rule; the consequence was a powerful movement for mental hospital reform, involving pressures for intensive treatment and rapid discharge. A third factor was the increasing readiness of sectors of the educated public to accept what might be called "psychological" explanations of deviant behavior. Here, the impact of the psychoanalytic movement and the rise of what came to be called psychosomatic medicine (cf. Wittkower and Cleghorn 1954; Dunbar 1954) have played important roles. Together, these trends had two major consequences: the identification of stress-related mental illnesses which could bring about massive disruptions of the person's capability of functioning (disruptions of the ability to work came to be seen as one of the most serious outcomes of mental illness), and, ultimately, the discharge into the community of thousands of long-term mental patients, for whom the procurement of some kind of gainful employment came to be seen as a prime social necessity. In the present chapter, we shall examine the ways in which the professional community tried to face up to these issues.

Some Conceptual Issues

Before we enter upon our effort to present a history of psychiatric rehabilitation, we need to clarify some conceptual ambiguities, which have troubled the helping professions since their beginnings.

Mental Illness

The very use of the term *mental illness* implies that there must be important differences between *mental* and *physical* illnesses, but what are these differences?

We must take note of the fact that the so-called diseases of the mind are quite unlike the diseases of the body in a number of important respects. Certain of these differences are so basic that some psychiatrists and social scientists have questioned whether the mental disorders are diseases at all, at least in the stricter biological sense of the term *disease*. It is, of course, generally agreed that if there is an impaired organ in question, that organ must be the central nervous system (loosely, the brain), but a century of research has been unable to determine the causes of impaired brain functioning, or even the precise nature of the impairments in question. A number of investigators are firmly convinced that hereditary and constitutional factors play a role in the genesis of the more severe mental disorders (e.g., schizophrenia) but the evidence remains inconclusive. Similarly, certain biochemical substances (the psychotropic medications, such as phenothiazines and lithium carbonate) can ameliorate some manifest psychotic behaviors, but it remains uncertain as to whether these drugs are actually *curative* or merely control certain of the *sequelae* of a mental disorder, such as the anxiety, confusion, and depression generated in a person who is seriously misperceiving the world and people around him or her.

Above all, the mental disorders appear to have very powerful consequences for the general social adjustment of the affected individual. In fact, it is a central feature of the more severe mental disorders (the psychoses) that they massively disrupt the social arrangements and basic social attitudes that underlie the ability to live and function within ordinary society. The best studies of treatment outcome (e.g., Strauss and Carpenter 1974; Strauss 1983) use as criteria of recovery not only eradication of the more florid psychotic symptoms (delusions, hallucinations, thought disorders, etc.), but also such criteria as to whether the "recovered" patient can live outside the walls of the mental hospital, whether he or she can maintain a marriage or relationship without disruption, and whether the person can find and maintain some kind of gainful employment.

All this has led some authorities to argue that the mental disorders are not diseases at all (not, at least, in terms of the primary medical definition of disease) but must be thought of as massive "social breakdown syndromes"—failures or impairments of the complex networks of socialization processes which enable the child to take his or her place in society. Whether or not the mental disorders are "true" diseases in the biological sense of this term, it remains a fact that these disorders typically have massive social consequences, both for the afflicted person and for society at large. The enterprise of psychiatric rehabilitation focuses on efforts to ameliorate some of these consequences.

Rehabilitation

Although the term *rehabilitation* lacks precise definition, modern practice has endowed it with a number of associated meanings. The first of these has to do with the fact that there are many kinds of physical, mental, or emotional disorders that in the present state of medical practice leave behind them some kind of chronic or permanent residual impairment. In this sense, the objective of rehabilitative procedures is not so much "curative" as "ameliorative," with the aim of bringing the person to a maximal level of functioning *within the limits* of a continuing deficiency of some kind. In one of the pioneering texts on rehabilitation medicine Rusk and Taylor (1953), state that since many chronic diseases cannot be cured, medicine must rely on rehabilitation to help those who are disabled to live and work as effectively as possible.

A second meaning of the term has specifically to do with facilitation of the ability to work, involving procedures designed to prepare the individual for gainful employment. A very strong emphasis on vocational objectives has permeated the field of rehabilitation and presents one of the clearest distinctions from the therapeutic goals of other helping professionals. Here we must note the powerful influence of federal agencies, in particular the Rehabilitation Services Administration (the successor to the Office of Vocational Rehabilitation); this agency reports its successes in terms of entry into gainful employment. The consequence has been that the re-search and service professionals involved with the handicapped have been obliged to learn a great deal more about human work than they otherwise may have done (cf. Neff 1985).

A third important connotation of the term *rehabilitation* arises from a recognition that the disabled person appears to face some of the same problems encountered by disfavored minority groups. The rehabilitative process, therefore, must often concern itself with overcoming social bar-riers, related both to attitudes of others toward the disabled person and to the disabled person's self-perception. In this sense, the problems of the dis-abled person are seen to have a strong sociopsychological component.

With these accreted meanings, the term *rehabilitation* has come to im-ply a many-sided and multidisciplinary service which follows upon relief of the acute phases of an illness or a disorder. The typical rehabilitation service center employs a wide range of professionals: physicians, nurses, medical technicians, psychologists, social workers, occupational special-ists, and so on. The objectives of rehabilitation efforts are essentially ame-liorative or adjustive. The goal is an "optimal life adjustment," within the limits of a continued impairment.

Disability versus Handicap

In ordinary usage, *disability* and *handicap* tend to be treated as synonyms. In the field of rehabilitation, however, it is often essential to distinguish clearly between them. The term *disability* is reserved for some sort of diag-nosable or ascertainable condition or impairment, whether physical, men-tal, or emotional. On the other hand, the term *handicap* implies that the disabled person finds himself (or is found) to be disadvantaged in relation to some desired life objective. It follows that not all disabilities, nor all levels of intensity of a given disability, are handicapping. Similarly, it is possible to be handicapped in relation to some vital life objective, without being disabled. An example of the latter might be a deficiency of education or training required for some desired occupation.

The matter is not merely a semantic quibble. Hamilton (1950) makes the point that a disability is an objective condition, while a handicap is the result of the obstacles which the disability puts between the individual and his or her maximum level of functioning. Wright (1960) states that a handicap can be meaningfully appraised only in terms of the cultural set-ting within which a person lives, including the social goals for which the individual strives. When we use the term *handicap* we are in the realm of interpersonal relations and social consequences. In rehabilitation prac-tice, attention has become increasingly focused on the characteristics of the person who "has" the disability. Whitehouse (1962) points out the individual's usual response to threat is perhaps the most significant clue to the nature of his reactions to heart disease. Research on the so-called type

A and type B personality syndromes in relation to the risk of heart disease (Rosenman et al. 1964, 1970) lend additional support to this basic approach. What is implied here is that people display differing reactions to a given disability and it is this differential response pattern which dictates the degree to which a stated disability is handicapping.

In summary, then, the term *disability* in rehabilitation practice is seen to refer to a permanent, residual limitation or impairment, that may or may not interfere with an optimal life adjustment. The objective of the rehabilitative process is to overcome or minimize the possible handicapping effects of a disabling condition. When we speak of *vocational* rehabilitation, we are interested in those aspects of disabling conditions that, depending upon the case, appear to have negative effects upon the ability to work.

Work and Its Meanings

As I have indicated above, a number of historical reasons have induced the rehabilitation movement to accept the ability to work as a primary criterion of rehabilitation success. This has forced investigators in the field to pay attention to the nature and requirements of the human work process, both in the general working population and, in particular, among disabled persons. Elsewhere, I have examined these matters in some depth (Neff 1965, 1968, 1985), and I shall attempt here to summarize my basic findings.

Work is commonly examined in relation to its customary antithesis— play. As we shall see, however, we need also to examine work in terms of the degree to which it departs from or relates to another great sphere of human behavior—the sphere of love. When we contrast work with play, we seem to be on rather safe ground. Work appears to be bound by necessity, whereas play is essentially a free activity. Second, there is a strong element of "pretending" in play. The games of children often include simulation of adult work roles, but everyone is aware, as are the children, that they are "only pretending." Similarly, in the organized play of adults we find many of the characteristics of combat and war, but it remains obvious that we are dealing with a simulation, not an identity. If a competitive game spills over into a free fight among the players, the game is stopped. Again, the games of children may be described as important preparatory activities for adult life, but they are still regarded as play, not work. In play, we attempt to master the environment for the sheer pleasure of doing so; in work, we struggle with the environment for pressing material reasons. Play is not really an instrumental activity at all; it is performed for its own sake.

While it is not, perhaps, customary to juxtapose the terms *work* and *love,* or even to examine their relationships, there are compelling reasons for doing so. One of Freud's greatest contributions to our understanding was to focus on the development of the ability to love as a consequence of the vicissitudes of relationships during infancy and childhood. Following this model, I believe it is possible to find certain important similarities (as well as certain crucial differences) between the ability to love and the ability to work. Like adult love, adult work appears to be the outcome of a long process of individual development, starting in childhood and passing through many stages, many setbacks and advances. The experiences and demands which influence the ability to work are not necessarily identical with those that influence the ability to love (as we shall see below), but both involve the development of distinctive styles of coping which carry over into adult behavior.

Another aspect of the analogy between work and love is that the individual may be entirely or partly unconscious of the motives which influence his behavior. When we ask people why they work, the most ready answer is couched in terms of material reward. But more intensive analysis reveals motives related to self-esteem, to identity, to needs related to activity and mastery. Some or all of these motives may be hidden from the individual's awareness and may serve to continue forms of behavior at work that are counterproductive.

Like love, work also engages the human emotions, the affective sides of human behavior. The workplace is a small society, and work may engage almost any human passion. The rehabilitation worker needs to know the manner in which work arouses both negative and positive affects: fear, guilt, anxiety, and hostility in some persons (in some situations), restlessness and uneasiness in others, satisfaction and enthusiasm in still others. An important diagnostic aim in rehabilitation is to discover the kinds of emotions which work generates in particular individuals and to relate these entanglements to particular forms of work pathology.

This analogy between love and work should not, of course, be pressed too far. The dynamics of love appear to be strongly influenced by transactions with which the individual is involved in infancy and early childhood and which make up the family drama. On the other hand, the habitual modes of response that later coalesce into adult work behavior can be shown to relate to events of later periods of childhood and adolescence, when the individual starts to move out of the family setting into larger social arenas: the school, the peer group, the world of work. In learning to deal with work disabilities, it is important to accept that work, like love, engages the affects, is made up of irrational as well as rational components, and is formed by events of which the person may be unaware as well as those which he can recall. It is equally important to be aware that the conditions which form the ability to work are not identical with those that form the ability to love and that disturbances in either sphere are not traceable to the same causes.

The ability to work is a product of a long period of social learning, which typically takes place from middle childhood to young adulthood. The arena for the acquisition of effective or ineffective work behavior is that of the school, or of whatever process of education and training is characteristic of a given society. The very early experiences of children within the nuclear family are not predictive of later work behavior (cf. Roe 1964; Neff 1965), although these interactions may be clearly related to the behaviors of love and intimacy. On the other hand, it is when children are taken off to school that they are confronted with a number of demands that become important for later work behavior. Children must learn how to relate to strangers in ways that are different from those they have experienced within the family. They must work out their reactions to the demands of time and of alien spaces. It is in school also that children are, for the first time, required to produce something, to execute a given set of tasks. Most important, it is in school that they develop a set of patterns of reaction to persons in authority, as well as to peers and subordinates. In sum, we regard work as a highly complex and socialized activity, the conditions of which are internalized during a long period of education and training; these internalized requirements then operate largely unconsciously as determinants of adult work behavior. It goes without saying that the complexity of this process provides many opportunities in which things can go wrong.

One important aspect of work is that it appears to be an exclusively *human* activity. The important distinction has to do with *planned alteration* of the physical environment. While many animals make certain changes in the world around them—insects and birds build nests, beavers build dams, chimpanzees use twigs to explore anthills—animals other than *Homo sapiens* generally tend to live in the world as they find it. Only man, by virtue of certain physical assets not available to the other species— a hyperdeveloped nervous system, upright posture, opposing thumbs, binocular vision—can massively intervene to change the structure and function of the physical world. Archaeologists accept that this is true when, in trying to decide whether particular fossilized bones are humanoid or anthropoid, they are happy to find artifacts (worked stones along with skeletal remains), which are seen as exclusively human products.

Another important aspect of work is that it is an *instrumental* activity. Work is not merely a given expenditure of activity, but an activity that is purposive, planned, and goal-directed. What is aimed at is some alteration of the physical environment in the service of subsistence. Very early in their tenure on earth, human beings learned to make snares and traps, to dig pits, to trim branches into clubs and spears, and to sharpen stones. The early instances of technology have the appearance of prosthetic devices, that is, instruments designed to make up for man's relative weakness and lack of bodily specialization. Thus, what *Homo* could not run down or seize by mere exercise of speed and agility, he learned to trap or snare; what he could not kill or dismember by sheer strength or the sharpness of fang or claw, he learned to club or spear.

This conceptualization of the meaning of work comprises at least four main elements. First, work is an essentially human activity; other animals, of course, expend directed energy in staying alive, but only human beings work. Second, work is an instrumental activity; it is performed not as an end in itself (as play apparently is) but in order to procure something else. Third, work is self-preservative; it is carried out in order to sustain life. Fourth, work transforms nature; the objective is to alter or change some aspect of the environment. To sum up: Work is an instrumental activity carried out by human beings, the object of which is to preserve and maintain life, which is directed at a planned alteration of certain features of our environment.

Work and Mental Health

For the purposes of this volume, I shall restrict my examination of the relations of work and mental health to the domain of the more severe mental disorders, that is, the psychoses. Here, there are two aspects of interest. The first has to do with the movement for deinstitutionalization, a major shift in treatment philosophy that is currently confronting the mental health establishment with some crucial problems. The second concerns the rise of a new subspecialty, psychiatric rehabilitation.

Deinstitutionalization

The establishment of the mental hospital was a great step forward in the late eighteenth and early nineteenth centuries, but, by the middle of our present century, it began to look like an institution that had outlived its usefulness. Originally established as refuges and intensive care centers (Bockoven 1963), mental hospitals had, through public indifferences and overcrowding, become more like prisons (Goffman 1961), isolated and self-contained small societies (Stanton and Schwartz 1954; Caudill 1958) and, in the long run, warehouses for the unwanted. The deteriorated conditions in what had become largely custodial institutions became a public scandal during the 1940s (Deutsch 1948), led ultimately to a major congressional investigation (Joint Commission on Mental Illness and Health 1961), and culminated in a massive effort to change the structure of the modern management of the psychoses (the Kennedy Mental Health Act of 1963).

Efforts to reform the custodial mental hospital began in the early 1940s, with the movement to "unlock the door" and involve the patient in self-care and self-management, and the establishment of intensive-treatment wards (Jones 1972; Paul and Lentz 1977). The background for these structural changes *within* the mental hospital was a developing conviction that the mental hospital itself (because of its impoverished and dilapidated atmosphere) was a major factor in the production and maintenance of such psychotic behaviors as withdrawal, disorganization, and deterioration (Wing and Brown 1970; Honigfeld and Gillis 1966). The apparently favorable outcomes of these early hospital reforms created the impetus for reduced admission rates, early discharge, and, finally, an active search for alternatives to hospitalization.

The most succinct definition of this movement has been offered by Bachrach (1976; see also Bachrach 1983): Deinstitutionalization involves two elements—(1) a reduction in the use of traditional institutional settings, such as state hospitals, for the care of the chronically mentally ill, and (2) an increased use of community-based services for the treatment of these persons. During the past two or three decades, massive changes have taken place. The resident patient populations in the custodial mental hospitals have been sharply reduced in size (from over 560,000 in 1955—the high point—to less than 180,000 today). A few of the most dilapidated facilities were closed and new, smaller ones established. The total number of public mental hospitals remains about the same (about 330), but many stand more than half-empty, and their internal functioning is greatly altered. Increased barriers to admission and decreased length of stay are now the rule. These policy changes resulted in high rates of readmission. Thirty to forty percent of discharges are back within twelve months and, if we extend the period of follow-up to four or five years, the return rate rises to over 50 percent.

For several reasons, however, it has not been possible to abolish the state hospital system entirely. Although the resident population has been reduced by two-thirds and the average stay dramatically shortened, there remain a residue of mentally disturbed persons for whom commitment to a state hospital appears to be the only available treatment recourse. In most of our fifty states, upwards of 70 percent of funds available for the treatment of the severely disturbed are still locked up in maintenance of the mental hospital system, with very little left over for treatment and/or maintenance in other settings. At the same time, even the most enthusiastic advocates of deinstitutionalization are beginning to recognize that at least one function of the mental hospital might be worth preserving, that is, its function as a refuge for people who, temporarily or permanently, seem unable to cope with the pressures of the outside society. It should be emphasized, however, that the mental hospital is now seen as only one element in a wide spectrum of services, to be utilized only for certain restricted populations and for specific and limited phases of some of the more severe mental disorders. The basic aim of the deinstitutionalization movement has been to shift treatment emphasis from the hospital to the community and to develop community facilities to serve the patient who is deemed insufficiently ill to merit state hospital commitment or who has received early discharge. Correspondingly, the explicit aims of increasing numbers of specialists have begun to shift from an emphasis on "cure" (the causes and cure of the psychoses remain elusive) to a concern for amelioration and adaptation—that is, from treatment to rehabilitation. We shall examine these trends below.

Psychiatric Rehabilitation: A New Specialty

Psychiatric rehabilitation is the child of a somewhat uneasy alliance between institutional psychiatry and vocational rehabilitation. It came into existence in the early 1950s, as a result of the shift in mental hospital policies toward rapid and early discharge. The psychiatrists in charge of the public mental hospitals believed—correctly as it turned out—that many of their charges were too traumatized or too desocialized to be able to survive outside the walls of the mental hospital without some expert assistance. Moreover, the medically trained psychiatrists within the mental hospitals—and their nonmedical auxiliaries such as psychiatric nurses and psychiatric social workers—tended to see their area of expertise as lying in the eradication of psychiatric symptoms, not in what was seen as a (mere) process of social adjustment. Another type of professional had to be recruited to deal with the posthospital careers of discharged mental patients. The new professionals turned out largely to be vocational rehabilitation specialists, who, up to the 1950s, had been concerned exclusively with physical disability. This is a somewhat unexpected outcome, and we need to account for it.

The ideological underpinnings of modern social psychiatry can be traced to the work of the Joint Commission on Mental Illness and Health (set up by act of Congress in 1955); its legal basis is the Kennedy Mental Health Act of 1963. The Joint Commission was made up of leading representatives of psychiatry, psychology, social work, and a number of social science disciplines. It summarized its final recommendations under five headings: research, manpower, services, public education, and costs. The central theme was that the mental disorders—whatever their persistent ambiguities in nature and etiology—were marked by diverse social ramifications and consequences. Thus, under the heading of manpower, the commission's report stressed the need not only for more and better trained psychiatrists and biochemists, but also for the training and recruitment of many kinds of nonmedical personnel: psychologists, rehabilitation specialists, employment counselors, and a variety of less-well-trained paraprofessional "mental health workers."

The recommendations of the Joint Commission with respect to services were very far-reaching. The commission called for a major structural shift from the state mental hospital (then the primary means of management of the severe mental disorders) to "community care." The instrument was to be a newly created facility—the community mental health center—based on population catchment areas. Although this was the core recommendation, it was not all. Summing up their convictions that "after-care and rehabilitation are essential parts of all services to mental patients" and that "the objective of modern treatment of persons with major mental illness is to enable the patients to maintain themselves in the community" (Joint Commission 1961, p. xvii), commission members recommended the following essential services: night hospitals, day hospitals, aftercare clinics, public health nursing services, foster-family care, halfway houses, rehabilitation centers, work-training and employment services, and ex-patient social groups.

Although these proposals seem eminently sound, they have not been easy to implement. In effect, one half of the task (reform of the mental hospital) has been relatively well carried out, but the other half (the development of community-based treatment facilities) is still very weak, so that the average person with a severe mental disorder may actually be in a worse position than he was a generation ago. This is a strong statement and needs some documentation.

The facts are that the mental health industry was ill-prepared to implement those aspects of the recommendations of the Joint Commission that focus upon psychiatric rehabilitation—and has been slow to change. The training of the basic mental health professionals—clinical psychiatrists, clinical psychologists, and psychiatric social workers—is still focused primarily on the traditional techniques of diagnosis and treatment, with little attention to procedures required to restore the disturbed person to some adequate level of social competency. The bulk of these professionals still appear to believe that their tasks are limited to symptom reduction, through one or another form of psychotropic medication or psychotherapy, and that restoration of the patient to an adequate level of social functioning is someone else's problem—assuming it is seen to be a problem at all. By default, the mental health workers who have tried to deal with these "other" problems have largely been people who have some connection with the field of vocational rehabilitation, principally because one of the main problems of many state hospital discharges has been the difficulty of acquiring and maintaining some kind of gainful employment. On the federal institutional level, the National Institute of Mental Health—the chief funding agency for training and research in mental health matters—still focuses its primary attention upon "treatment," while the Office of Vocational Rehabilitation has begun to commit resources to the rehabilitation of patients with mental, as well as physical disabilities. Most of the present corps of professionals working in psychiatric rehabilitation have drifted into the field almost by accident and have received no formal training for the work they are now expected to perform. Formal training programs for work in this field are extremely rare; a notable example of a well-designed program is directed by William Anthony at Boston University, but one is hard put to find many others.

It is difficult to assess the efficacy of psychiatric rehabilitation practice, since the entire field is new and the programs are few, limited in capacity, and have still largely a "demonstration project" character. It has been reported (Anthony et al. 1972) that these projects have demonstrated a moderate effect on the employability of former hospital patients but little influence on the frequency of readmission. In part these meager results may be attributed to the fact that the typical rehabilitation project is directed toward the solution of one small aspect of a multisided problem.

The Present Situation

The deinstitutionalization movement has brought about major shifts both in the manner in which the severe mental disorders are conceptualized and the ways in which these disorders are managed. One of the consequences is a renewed interest in the relations of work and mental disorder.

The chief outcome of the mental hospital policies of reduced admission and early discharge is that the mental health professions are now confronted with relatively large numbers of people who find it extremely difficult to adjust to life outside the walls of the hospital. Not only are community services distinguished more by their paucity than by their adequacy; they also tend to feature short-term treatment and time-limited rehabilitation. However desirable these measures may be for many mentally disordered persons, they are simply not appropriate for the substantial subgroup we call "chronic." It is these people who swell the readmission rolls, who live highly marginal lives in boarding homes and welfare hotels, and whose odd, bizarre, disheveled public appearance has often led to community outcry.

We can already specify some things that are needed. Many discharged patients (and some of those currently denied admission) need to live in benign residential units, under the supervision of people trained to play the roles of surrogate parent and surrogate friend. There is a need also for a widespread network of sheltered and semisheltered work programs, on the assumption that some (many?) former psychotics cannot meet the personal and performance demands of ordinary unprotected employment. We require a host of new facilities, ranging from almost total sheltering at one extreme, to programs that are transitional at the other.

In other chapters in this volume, these new requirements are explored in detail. Many of these efforts to deal with the problems of severe mental disorder are wholly innovative. Some are intensive continuations of earlier conceptualization and research. It can safely be said that if these research and service activities receive the kind of wide support they merit, the basic difficulties of persons with severe mental disorder will, at long last, be ameliorated.

References

Anthony, W. A.; Buell, G. C.; Sharrett, S.; and Althoff, M. E. 1972. Efficacy of psychiatric rehabilitation. *Psychological Bulletin, 78,* 447–56.

Bachrach, L. J. 1976. *Deinstitutionalization: An analytical review and sociological perspective.* Mental Health Statistics, Series D, no. 4, DHEW (ADM 79-351). Washington, D.C.: U.S. Government Printing Office.

———, ed. 1983. *Deinstitutionalization.* San Francisco: Jossey-Bass.

Bockoven, J. 1963. *Moral treatment in American society.* New York: Springer.

Caudill, W. 1958. *The psychiatric hospital as a small society.* Cambridge: Harvard University Press.

Deutsch, A. 1948. *The shame of the states.* New York: Harcourt Brace.

Dunbar, F. 1954. *Emotions and bodily changes.* New York: Columbia University Press.

Goffman, E. 1961. *Asylums.* New York: Doubleday.

Hamilton, K. W. 1950. *Counseling the handicapped in the rehabilitation process.* New York: Ronald Press.

Honigfeld, G., and Gillis, R. 1966. The role of institutionalization in the natural history of schizophrenia. *Central Neuropsychiatric Record Library,* Report no. 64. Perry Point, Md.

Joint Commission on Mental Illness and Health. 1961. *Action for mental health.* New York: Basic Books.

Jones, K. 1972. *A history of mental health services.* Boston: Routledge & Kegan Paul.

Neff, W. S. 1965. Psychoanalytic conceptions of the meaning of work. *Psychiatry, 28,* 323–33.

———. 1968. *Changes in the meaning of work during psychiatric rehabilitation.* Final Report, RD 1603-P. Washington, D.C.: Social and Rehabilitation Service.

———. 1985. *Work and human behavior.* 3d ed. Hawthorne, N.Y.: Aldine.

Paul, G. L., and Lentz, R. L. 1977. *Psychosocial treatment of chronic mental patients.* Cambridge: Harvard University Press.

Roe, A. 1964. Personality structure and occupational behavior. In *Man in the world of work,* ed. H. Borow. Boston: Houghton Mifflin.

Rosenman, R. H.; Friedman, M.; Strauss, R.; Wurm, M.; Kositchek, R.; Hahn, W.; and Werthessen, N. T. 1964. Predictive study of coronary heart disease: The Western Collaborative Group Study. *Journal of the American Medical Association, 189,* 15022.

———. 1970. Coronary heart disease in the Western Collaborative Group study: A follow-up experience of 4½ years. *Journal of Chronic Disease, 23,* 173–90.

Rusk, H. A., and Taylor, E. J. 1953. *Living with a disability.* Garden City, N.Y.: Blakiston Press.

Stanton, A. H., and Schwartz, M. S. 1954. *The mental hospital.* New York: Basic Books.

Strauss, J. S. 1983. The course of psychiatric disorder: A model for understanding treatment. Paper presented at the annual meeting of the American Psychiatric Association.

Strauss, J. S., and Carpenter, W. T. 1974. The predication of outcome in schizophrenia. *Archives of General Psychiatry, 31,* 37–42.

Whitehouse, F. A. 1962. Cardiovascular disability. In *Psychological practices with the physically disabled,* ed. J. F. Garrett and E. S. Levine. New York: Columbia University Press.

Wing, J. K., and Brown, G. W. 1970. *Institutionalization and schizophrenia*. Cambridge: Cambridge University Press.

Wittkower, E. D., and Cleghorn, R. A., eds. 1954. *Recent developments in psychosomatic medicine*. Philadelphia: Lippincott.

Wright, B. A. 1960. *Physical disability: A psychological approach*. New York: Harper and Row.

2

Defining the Target Population
For Vocational Rehabilitation

HOWARD GOLDMAN, JACQUELINE ROSENBERG, and
RONALD W. MANDERSCHEID

Continuing to elaborate the conceptual issues in vocational rehabilitation, Goldman, Rosenberg, and Manderscheid define the target population in terms of diagnosis, disability, and duration. The problems with this definition are discussed with particular attention to the needs of subgroups like the "young adult" or "new" chronic patient. The authors conclude with implications of these conceptualizations for national policy. Specifically, recent changes in the Social Security Administration's standards for determining mental impairment and disability are discussed.

During the last decade, the chronic mental patient has emerged as a major concern of the nation's mental health care policymakers. Significant documents have been written which detail the complex issues associated with the characteristics, care, and treatment of the population, as well as the financial impact of meeting their needs. Notable among these are *The Report of the President's Commission on Mental Health, The Chronic Mental Patient*, and *Toward a National Plan for the Chronically Mentally Ill (NP/CMI)*.

The last document, which grew out of the President's Commission, developed an operational definition of the adult population disabled by chronic mental illness and provided an unduplicated count of those included in the definition. The first section of this chapter provides an overview of the epidemiology of chronic mental disorder, including factors affecting the definition, location, count, and characteristics of the population. The material presented in this section is based on the conceptual model proposed in the *NP/CMI* (see also Goldman, Gattozzi, and Taube 1981) and draws extensively from Goldman and Manderscheid 1987a, which augments and supplements the text of the *NP/CMI* and Goldman, Gattozzi, and Taube (1981) with data from more recent studies.

The second section notes some of the emerging issues related to the conceptualization of the population and discusses the limitations on the availability of rehabilitation services and financial support for this target group. Specifically, the heterogeneity of the population is described, including the characteristics, treatment, and financial and other supports for the subgroup of chronic mental patients often referred to in the literature as the "young adult" or "new" chronic patient (Pepper et al. 1981; Bachrach 1982).

The final section describes recent national policy actions related to the definition of mental impairment and disability. In particular, revisions to the Social Security Administration's standards for determining disability due to mental impairments under the Social Security Disability Insurance (SSDI) and Supplemental Security Income (SSI) programs are described (Goldman and Manderscheid 1987a; Goldman and Runck, 1985; Jansen 1985; Koyanagi 1985).

An Overview of the Chronically Mentally Ill Population

Approximately 1.7 to 2.4 million adults living in the United States are thought to be "chronically mentally ill" (U.S. Department of Health and Human Services 1980). The term encompasses a mix of persons who, like the general population, need housing, food, clothing, medical and dental care, income, recreation, and education. In a similar fashion, they also need a support system comprised of family and friends. Unlike the general public, however, they are disabled by severe and persistent mental illness. For varying periods during their lives, they are often unable to work, go to school, cook, tend to personal health, establish interpersonal relationships, cope with stress, or—in short—function independently.

Prior to 1955, when state mental hospitals in the United States reached their maximum census of 559,000, most chronically mentally ill adults in treatment resided in state mental hospitals (Talbott 1978; U.S. Department of Health and Human Services 1980; GAO 1977; Goldman and Morrissey 1985). These institutions were nearly the exclusive domain for mental health treatment to this population; the hospitals also provided for their health, welfare, housing, and social service needs. As a result of this centralized locus of care, locating and counting the segment of chronically mentally ill persons in treatment was relatively easy. With the advent of deinstitutionalization, however, the pattern and locus of mental health care for this long-term population extended beyond mental hospital walls (President's Commission 1978; Talbott 1978; U.S. Department of Health and Human Services 1980; GAO 1977; Goldman, Adams, and Taube 1983; Goldman, Taube, Regier, and Witkin 1983).

One particular consequence of this dramatic change was, and continues to be, the absence of precise information on the scope of the problem of chronic mental illness. Sources of data, like the affected individuals and their services, have been dispersed. The difficulty is exacerbated by the lack of a consensually validated definition which would accurately delimit the population.

Delimiting the Target Population

In general, a chronic condition is characterized by a long duration of illness, which may include periods of seeming wellness interrupted by flareups of acute symptoms, and secondary disabilities. However, this definition is not easily applied to chronic mental illness, and therefore, the task of identifying persons who are chronically mentally ill is not a simple one. Assessing the prevalence of chronic mental illness is complicated by the dynamic, episodic course of severe mental disorders. Some individuals recover; some have histories marked by exacerbations and remissions; others have a persistent, deteriorating course.

Chronic mental illness encompasses more than an episodic disorder; it implies impairment and disability. One recent attempt to define the chronically mentally ill distinguishes persons who are severely *mentally ill* (defined by diagnosis), those who are *mentally disabled* (defined by level of disability), and those who are *chronic mental patients* (defined by duration of hospitalization) (Minkoff 1978).

These three dimensions—diagnosis, disability, and duration—are sufficiently operationalizable to serve as criteria for delimiting the target population. Applying these three operational dimensions can also be used in generating an initial description of the chronically mentally ill. This population encompasses persons who suffer from severe and persistent emotional disorders that interfere with their functional capacities in relation to such primary aspects of daily life as self-care, interpersonal relationships, and work or schooling, and that often necessitate prolonged mental health care and social support.

Diagnosis

General agreement exists that the psychotic and other major disorders predominate among the chronically mentally ill. These include organic mental disorders, schizophrenic disorders, major affective disorders, paranoid disorders, and other psychotic disorders (American Psychiatric Association 1980). However, other disorders may also result in chronic mental disability. Recently proposed changes in the listings of mental impairments for disability programs of the Social Security Administration also include the anxiety disorders, somatoform disorders, and personality disorders. Furthermore, alcohol and drug-abuse disorders and mental retardation may complicate the course of severe mental disorders (occasionally becoming designated as the primary diagnosis) or may become chronically disabling conditions themselves. Nonpsychotic organic mental disorders, or "senility without psychosis" (as designated in U.S. Department of Health, Education, and Welfare 1966) among the elderly may also lead to chronic disability.

Disability

Most definitions of disability center on the concept of functional incapacity, for example, "partial or total impairment of instrumental (usually vocational or homemaking) role performance" (Minkoff 1978, p. 12). One statutory definition refers to a condition that "results in substantial functional limitations in three or more of the following areas of major life activity: (i) self-care, (ii) receptive and expressive language, (iii) learning, (iv) mobility, (v) self-sufficiency" (Public Law 95-602). However, objective measures of these "functional limitations" are not now in widespread use, although progress is being made in measurement methodologies (Grusky et al. 1985; McCarrick, Manderscheid, and Bertolucci 1985).

Chronicity of disability may be operationally defined by SSDI and SSI eligibility in terms of receipt of SSDI or SSI payments. Eligibility implies that the beneficiary has been unable to "engage in any substantial gainful activity" (P.L. 98-640 1984) because of a disorder "which has lasted or can be expected to last for a continuous period of not less than 12 months." General agreement exists that approval of SSI or SSDI eligibility is a measure of chronic disability for noninstitutionalized persons. Similar vocational criteria are common to other definitions of disability, such as those used in the Survey of Disabled Adults (Social Security Administration) and the Survey of Income and Education (U.S. Bureau of the Census). Chronicity also may be inferred from the need for extended hospitalization or other forms of supervised residence or sheltered work.

Duration

To infer disability from the need for extended hospitalization or supervised residential care requires specifying some duration of residence. Most would agree that one year of continuous institutionalization in a state mental hospital or of residence in a nursing home would qualify as a measure of chronic mental disability. However, at least half of the population of chronically mentally ill are not continuously institutionalized. Although these latter individuals reside in the community, many of them were hospitalized in the past or are hospitalized sporadically during the course of the year. Some formula is necessary for determining what duration of hospitalization to use as a criterion for chronicity for the chronically mentally ill living in the community.

Treated prevalence estimates may be obtained by reference to the National Reporting Program of the National Institute of Mental Health (NIMH), which uses a three-month period of follow-up for providing data on extended hospitalization. Eighty percent of all patients admitted to psychiatric hospitals and general hospital psychiatric units are discharged within ninety days (Goldman, Adams, and Taube 1983; Goldman, Taube, Regier, and Witkin 1983). Likelihood of release diminishes after this point; hence, these unreleased patients represent an intermediate-stay (3–12 months) population of the chronically mentally ill.

It should be noted that some persons with characteristics fitting the diagnosis and disability criteria have received short-term (less than 90 days) inpatient care, or solely outpatient care from a medical or mental health professional, or no care other than what their families or other natural support groups have provided. Although it is not possible to definitely locate or enumerate such individuals, they are included in the target population. For the purposes of defining and delimiting the population, prolonged functional disability caused or aggravated by severe mental disorders, not prior hospitalization, is the chief distinguishing characteristic of chronic mental illness.

The Chronically Mentally Ill

There have been several recent attempts to operationally define the chronically mentally ill. The definitions reviewed here were developed to provide estimates of the size of the population. They are not conceptual definitions; they are practical definitions designed to identify mentally disabled individuals who are eligible for services and to estimate the scope of the problem of chronic mental illness.

In 1978, the Community Support Program (CSP) of NIMH developed the following parameters for eligibility for its target population of noninstitutionalized chronically mentally ill: "Severe mental disability (must satisfy at least one of the following): A single episode of hospitalization in the last five years of at least six months duration; or two or more hospitalizations within a 12-month period" (U.S. Department of Health and Human Services 1980, p. 2-8). This definition included individuals with nonchronic conditions who may have required two brief hospitalizations in one year and excluded multiple-admission chronic patients who have not been hospitalized more than once in any twelve-month period.

The CSP changed its definition of program eligibility to ameliorate problems associated with earlier definitions. The current definition focuses on assessing functional disabilities and minimizes reliance on a history of prior institutionalization. This opens eligibility to the mentally disabled who may not have been hospitalized because of current state mental health policies. Unfortunately, preliminary field tests of the reliability of these new eligibility criteria were disappointing (Naierman 1982). Moreover, a 1981 CSP study conducted by Macro Systems, Inc., found that definitions of the chronically mentally ill vary from state to state (Ben-Dashan, Morrison, and Kotler 1981). A number of recent studies report on methodologies for estimating the prevalence of the chronically mentally ill in the community (Ashbaugh and Manderscheid 1985; Ashbaugh 1982; Ashbaugh, Hoff, and Bradley 1980; Szymanski et al. 1982; Warheit et al. 1977).

The NP/CMI adopted the following definition of its target population based on the dimensions of diagnosis, disability, and duration:

The chronically mentally ill population encompasses persons who suffer certain mental or emotional disorders (organic brain syndrome, schizophrenia, recurrent depressive and manic-depressive disorders, paranoid and other psychoses, plus other disorders that may become chronic) that erode or prevent the development of their functional capacities in relation to (three or more of) such primary aspects of daily life as personal hygiene and self-care, self-direction, interpersonal relationships, social transactions, learning, and recreation, and that erode or prevent the development of their economic self-sufficiency. Most such individuals have required institutional care of extended duration, including intermediate-term hospitalization (90 days to one year in a single year), long-term hospitalization (one year or longer in the preceding five years), nursing home placement on account of a diagnosed mental condition or diagnosis of senility without psychosis. Some such individuals have required short-term hospitalization (less than 90 days), other have received treatment from a medical or mental health professional solely on an outpatient basis, or despite their needs, have received no treatment in the professional-care service system. Thus, included in the target population are persons who are or were formerly "residents" of institutions (public and private psychiatric hospitals and nursing homes), and persons who are at high risk of institutionalization because of persistent mental disability. (U.S. Department of Health and Human Services 1980, p. 2-11).

This definition facilitates the identification and enumeration of the chronically mentally ill. Bearing in mind the caveat concerning the dynamic nature of any definition of the population, the paragraphs that follow outline a series of separate segments of the population of the chronically mentally ill population. The numbers of chronically mentally ill persons in each of these segments may be determined by several methods. Over time, these numbers are subject to change because of the movement of people from one location to another (Goldman and Manderscheid 1987b). For purposes of this chapter, the institutionalized chronically mentally ill are those individuals with any psychiatric diagnosis in mental hospitals for more than one year and those individuals in nursing homes (as defined by the National Center for Health Statistics) with a diagnosed mental condition or a diagnosis of senility without psychosis. The latter are included because simple senility, either alone or in a combination with other chronic medical conditions, was a reason for admission to a state mental hospital prior to policies encouraging deinstitutionalization and the transfer or diversion of the elderly into nursing homes.

Within communities, the chronically mentally ill are those individuals residing in a variety of settings (e.g., with families, in boarding homes, in community residential facilities, in single-occupancy hotel rooms, in the street, or in correctional facilities) who are considered to be disabled by any one of several criteria (e.g., SSI/SSDI eligibility, episodic or prolonged hospitalization, inability to work). This community-dwelling segment may be subdivided into several groups on the basis of their location, their utilization of mental health services, and the level and type of their disability.

Counting the Chronic Population

Defining the target population in terms of diagnosis, duration, disability, and location permits specification of the number in the population. As Table 2.1 indicates, estimates of the number of the chronically mentally ill range from 1.7 million to 2.4 million, including 900,000 who are institutionalized. Table 2.2 presents estimates of the degree of disability suffered

Table 2.1
Estimates of the Number of the Chronically Mentally Ill, United States, 1975–1977

Institutionalized population	
Location (unduplicated count)	
Mental health facilities[a]	150,000
Nursing homes[b]	
Residents with mental disorder[c]	350,000
Residents with senility without psychosis[d]	400,000
Subtotal	900,000
Community population	
Level of disability (unduplicated count)	
Severe[e]	800,000
Moderate[f] and severe	1,500,000
Subtotal (as a range)	800,000–1,500,000
Total[g]	1,700,000–2,400,000

aResidents for one year or more in the following facility types: state and county hospitals, Veterans Administration inpatient facilities, private psychiatric hospitals, residential treatment centers, community mental health centers. (Source of estimates: Division of Biometry and Epidemiology, NIMH, 1975.)

bUniverse of 1.3 million residents of skilled nursing and intermediate care facilities sampled by National Center for Health Statistics, National Nursing Home Survey, 1977.

cResidents with a diagnosis (primary or nonprimary) from Section V of the International Classification of Diseases-9. (Source: National Nursing Home Survey, 1977.)

dResidents with diagnosed condition (primary or nonprimary) coded 797 in the International Classification of Diseases-9. (Source: National Nursing Home Survey, 1977.)

eIncludes individuals with a mental disorder unable to work at all for one year and those who could work only occasionally or irregularly. (Source of estimates: Urban Institute, Comprehensive Needs Survey, 1973, and Social Security Administration, Survey of Disabled Adults, 1966.)

fIncludes so-called "partially disabled" individuals whose work (including housework) was limited by a mental disorder. (Source of estimates: Urban Institute, Comprehensive Needs Survey, 1973.)

gFor purposes of the National Plan, the lower figure (1.7 million), representing the severely disabled chronically mentally ill, will be used as the size of the target population.

Table 2.2

Estimates of the Number of the Chronically Mentally Ill by Type of Disability and Utilization of Mental Health Facilities (duplicated counts), United States, 1975–1977

Type of disability	
Receiving SSI/SSDI	225,000–425,000[a]
Complete work disability[b]	350,000
Activity limitation[c]	700,000
Utilization of mental health facilities[d]	
Admissions (length of stay ≥ 90 days)	150,000
Readmissions[e]	650,000

[a]This prevalence range is based on two separate estimates of the percentage of individuals who are disabled by mental disorders multiplied by the approximately 2 million individual recipients of SSI/SSDI. (Source: Kathryn H. Allan and Mildred E. Cinsky, *General Characteristics of the Disabled Population,* Social Security Survey of the Disabled, 1966, Report no. 19, [Washington, D.C.: DHEW, 1972], and the *Social and Rehabilitation Services, National Center for Social Statistics, Findings of the 1970 APTD Study* [Washington, D.C.: DHEW, 1972].)

[b]Prevalence of disability in population aged 18–64. (Source: Digest of Data on Persons with Disabilities, Bureau of the Census, Survey of Income and Education, 1976, DHEW, 1979.)

[c]Prevalence of disability in population 3 years or older. (Source: Digest of Data on Persons with Disabilities, Bureau of the Census, Survey of Income and Education, 1976, DHEW, 1979.)

[d]Facilities include state and county mental hospitals, private psychiatric hospitals, psychiatric units in general hospitals, and residential treatment centers. (Source: Division of Biometry and Epidemiology, NIMH, 1975.)

[e]Readmission counts will overestimate chronic patients. Some patients with less severe disorders are admitted many times for brief admissions. (Source: Division of Biometry and Epidemiology, NIMH, 1975.)

by persons with chronic psychiatric illness and their utilization of mental health facilities. These estimates of the total number of chronically mentally ill are derived from a number of sources, including true prevalence estimates of chronic mental disability and treated prevalence data on chronic mental patients (Goldman and Manderscheid 1987b).

Emerging Issues

Despite progress made during the past decade in defining, delimiting, locating, and counting the population labeled as suffering from severe, chronic, and disabling mental illness, a number of problems have emerged which point out the limitations of our current knowledge, and which call for shifts in our conceptualization of the population and its treatment and support needs. These problems include the accurate definition, identification, treatment, and support of the "young adult" or "new" chronic patient, and the homeless chronically mentally ill (Pepper, Kirshner, and Ryglewicz 1981; Schwartz and Goldfinger 1981; Bachrach 1982; Bassuk 1984; Goldman and Morrissey 1985; Segal and Baumohl 1982; Goldman and Manderscheid 1987b).

The young adult chronic patient has been described in the literature as more likely to have multiple problems, more likely to be transient, more difficult to treat, and less likely to have had continuous contact with the mental health care system (Pepper, Kirshner, and Ryglewicz 1981;

Schwartz and Goldfinger 1981; Bachrach 1982). Although the rates of disorder may be no different in this age group (typically 18–35) than in other age cohorts, the number of persons with chronic disorders is likely to be substantial because of the size of the baby-boom generation born between 1946 and 1964. NIMH data suggest that a segment of this population is replacing the elderly in state hospitals (Taube et al. 1983). Projections of current trends in this service setting anticipate an expansion of state hospitals in the future; this would revise the downward trend in resident population that has occurred since 1955 (Stroup and Manderscheid 1984). Among the young adult chronic patients participating in the CSP, results show that young chronics tended to receive nonpsychotic diagnoses, exhibit deviant and disruptive behaviors, and use mental health and other services at higher rates than older chronic patients. Clinical histories varied by age group in expected ways, while demographic characteristics and degree of psychiatric disability tended to be similar across age groups (Woy, Goldstrom, and Manderscheid 1983). Development of effective services for this chronic population will be a major challenge in the coming decade.

The homeless chronically mentally ill represent an equal challenge (Goldman and Morrissey 1985; Bassuk 1984). Estimates of the entire homeless population range from a daily count of 250,000–550,000 (Department of Housing and Urban Development) to an annual total of 2.5 million (National Coalition for the Homeless). Based on a review of available local studies, Goldman and Manderscheid (1987b) have found that deinstitutionalized chronically mentally ill persons appear to represent about 25 percent of the homeless population in urban areas. When combined with a second subgroup—chronically or acutely mentally ill persons who have been diverted from inpatient care or who have rejected psychiatric treatment—the mentally ill appear to comprise one-third to two-thirds of the homeless population in urban areas. These estimates may be conservative, since most local studies are based on shelter users, and the mentally ill are less likely to use shelters. Thus, the number of chronically mentally ill individuals who are homeless cannot be clearly specified at the present time. However, estimated most conservatively, the number would be considerable.

An ancillary problem is the use of correctional facilities by the mentally ill homeless. As with the homeless population, little factual information is available on the number of mentally ill persons in correctional facilities on a given day or during an entire year. The National Coalition for Jail Reform has estimated that approximately 700,000 incarcerations of mentally ill persons occur each year in local and county jails. Given the significant representation of chronically mentally ill persons in the homeless population, it is reasonable to assume that they are also represented among the mentally ill incarcerated in criminal justice settings.

Problems with the Standard Definition

Reviewing our conceptual model, the condition of chronic mental illness is characterized by the dimensions of diagnosis, disability, and duration. These three dimensions allow us to describe and delimit the population. However, the imprecision of these criteria has resulted in their inappropriate use and, ultimately, in the target population's exclusion from benefits essential to their access of services necessary for rehabilitation.

In particular, under the standards used by SSA in 1981 and 1982 to review cases of eligibility for SSI and SSDI, a disproportionate number of chronically mentally ill among the disabled population were disallowed benefits (Goldman and Runck 1985; Anthony and Jansen 1984). Jansen (1985) reports that although only 11 percent of those on the disability rolls are mentally disabled, 28.6 percent of those terminated the first year were those with mental disorders. This exclusion was due in part to existing SSA rules which did not reflect current knowledge on the episodic nature and course of chronic mental illness (Goldman and Runck 1985; Jansen 1985; Koyanagi 1985; Anthony and Jansen 1984). Anthony and Jansen (1984) note in their excellent review of the literature on the predictability of vocational functioning of the target population that a central aspect of rehabilitation "is whether or not psychiatrically disabled persons can qualify for disability benefits and maintain those benefits throughout a lengthy rehabilitation process" (p. 537).

A number of critical issues are raised by the benefits question. One issue is that of the duration and course of chronic mental illness. Chronicity implies an episodic, erratic, and evolutionary course of severe and disabling mental illness. Persons suffering from chronic mental illness experience periods of remission and exacerbation of their overt symptomatology, and fluctuations in their levels of functioning (U.S. Department of Health and Human Services 1980; Anthony and Jansen 1984; Strauss et al. 1985).

One unfortunate consequence of the lack of understanding about the nature of this illness was the denial in 1981 of SSI and SSDI benefits to approximately 45,000 mentally ill persons (Koyanagi 1985). A disproportionate number of these people were young adult chronic mental patients, many of whom were unable to work despite amelioration of the symptoms of their illnesses. The old SSA rules were so vague that they allowed widely varying interpretations. When applied strictly, as they were in the 1981 case reviews, many chronic mental patients were judged able to work and were thus dropped from the disability roles. The old rules did not incorporate the precise characteristics and nature of chronic disabling mental illness discussed above (Koyanagi 1985).

Research findings of the past decade confirm the ability of many adults disabled by chronic mental illness to function at varying levels of independence during periods of their illness, given adequate treatment, rehabilitation, and support (U.S. Department of Health and Human Services 1980; Strauss et al. 1985; Turner and TenHoor 1978; Harding et al. 1984; Stein and Test 1980; Tessler and Goldman 1982). Yet despite, and even during, these periods of higher social functioning, many chronically mentally ill persons are unable to engage in competitive employment (Anthony and Jansen 1984; Tessler and Goldman 1982; Summers 1981).

Anthony and Jansen (1984) enumerate nine significant research findings which are critical to the accurate determination of vocational functioning for chronically mentally ill adults. These findings, listed below, are quite relevant to conceptualization and definition of persons disabled by chronic and severe mental illness and have implications for the young chronically mentally ill adult and, concomitantly, for the new SSA "listings," or criteria.

1. Psychiatric symptomatology is a poor predictor of future work performance.
2. Diagnostic category is a poor predictor of future work performance.
3. Intelligence, aptitude, and personality tests are poor predictors of future work performance.
4. A person's ability to function in one environment (e.g., a community setting) is not predictive of a person's ability to function in a different type of environment (e.g., a work setting).
5. There is little or no correlation between a person's symptomatology and most measures of functional skills.
6. The best clinical predictors of future work performance are ratings of a person's work adjustment skills made in a workshop setting or sheltered job site.
7. The best demographic predictor of future work performance is the person's prior employment history.
8. A significant predictor of future work performance is a person's ability to get along or function socially with others.
9. The best paper-and-pencil predictors of future vocational performance are tests that measure a person's ego strength or self-concept in the role of worker. (Pp. 538–42)

Federal regulations require that a person's capacity to work be assessed quite apart from overt psychiatric symptomatology (U.S. Department of Health and Human Services 1981). Despite these requirements, SSA concluded that if a person did not meet the criteria for overt psychiatric symptomatology, he or she was in fact able to work. Thus, many chronically mentally ill persons with few overt psychiatric symptoms were disqualified from receiving benefits and yet remained functionally unable to hold a competitive job.

In response to the public's outcry against the termination of benefits, Congress mandated that new standards be developed for determining disability due to mental impairments under the SSDI and SSI programs. The new standards, proposed in February 1985, were developed by a work group jointly sponsored by SSA and the American Psychiatric Association. Also represented were the American Psychological Association, the Mental Health Law Project, the National Association of Social Workers, the American Nurses' Association, state disability determination services, and the Department of Health and Human Services, including NIMH (Goldman and Runck 1985). Compared to the old standards, the new ones give more weight to chronicity and the limitation of available treatments. The new criteria, using diagnostic categories based on DSM-III, are better defined and more easily observable than the old criteria. Four criteria pertaining to restrictions or limitations in four areas of functioning have been developed. They are

1. Performance in activities of daily living, including adaptive activities such as cleaning, shopping, grooming, paying bills, and maintaining a residence. The quality of the patient's activities is judged by the independence, appropriateness, and effectiveness with which he or she carries them out, and the patient's ability to initiate and participate in activities without supervision or direction.

2. Social functioning, which refers to one's capacity to interact appropriately and communicate effectively with other individuals both at work and in one's personal life. Impairments are demonstrated by a history of altercations, evictions, firings, social isolation, and the like.

3. Performance in terms of concentration, task persistence, and pace, or the ability to focus attention long enough to permit the timely completion of tasks commonly done as part of work activities.

4. Deterioration or decompensation in work or worklike situations, which refers to repeated failure to adapt to stressful circumstances such as making decisions, meeting schedules, maintaining regular attendance, or interacting with supervisors and peers. These demands cause the individual either to withdraw from the situation or to experience exacerbation of signs and symptoms of illness, with accompanying difficulties in daily activities, social relationships, or concentration and persistence (U.S. Social Security Act Regulation 1985).

In general, the new functional criteria address many of the findings enumerated by Anthony and Jansen (1984), in that they emphasize work-related limitations, adding difficulties with concentration, task persistence, and adaptability to the old criteria that focused exclusively on activities of daily living and social functioning. In addition, the new criteria do not require that a person have limitations in all areas of functioning to qualify, as the old ones did.

The new preface to the standards emphasizes the importance of evidence of the person's condition over the course of a mental disorder rather than relying on an evaluation done at one point in time. It also requires that the individual's past experience with work and the circumstances surrounding work termination be evaluated. The preface points out that medication, hospitalization, or highly structured living situations may minimize overt indications of severe disorders without improving a person's ability to work. Medication side effects that interfere with the ability to work are also noted (U.S. Department of Health and Human Services 1985).

Challenge for the Future

The chronically mentally ill population includes persons whose clinical conditions and functional disabilities vary widely at any point in time and, moreover, change over time. This variability makes an accurate determination of the size and nature of the population extremely difficult. Although the definition proposed above encompasses persons with prolonged moderate-to-severe disability, a significant proportion possess the capacity to live in relative independence if adequate community-based services, social supports, and life opportunities are provided (Tessler and Goldman 1982; Stein and Test 1980; Strauss et al. 1985; U.S. Department of Health and Human Services 1980; Harding et al. 1984). The probability that adults disabled by severe, persistent, and disabling mental illness can participate in rehabilitation programs and achieve their full functional potential increases significantly as we continue to refine our ability to accurately and precisely describe, define, locate, and delimit the population and incorporate that knowledge in federal policy decisions. The new rules for determining eligibility under SSI and SSDI offer greater opportunity to young adults disabled by chronic mental illness for participation in appropriate vocational rehabilitation programs. The technical criteria for defining the chronically mentally ill establish the objective boundaries of the target population which are vital to the activities of planners and policy-makers. But they do no more than hint at the clinical, socioeconomic, ethnic, and cultural heterogeneity of this population. They cannot convey any sense of the individual people referred to, their families, their hope and their striving, however falteringly, for normalcy.

Recent research indicates that a segment of the population with severe and chronic mental illness can experience partial and even full rehabilitation (Harding et al. 1984; Tessler and Goldman 1982; Stein and Test 1980; Strauss et al. 1985). Yet we know little regarding the course of their illness, the unique characteristics of the more "successfully" rehabilitated amongst them, or the characteristics of their environments. As the population of chronically mentally ill patients ages, our conceptualization and knowledge of their characteristics and needs must also mature to promote an improved quality of life for persons suffering from chronic mental illness.

References

American Psychiatric Association. 1980. *Diagnostic and statistical manual of mental disorders.* 3d ed. Washington, D.C.: American Psychiatric Association.

Anthony, W. A., and Jansen, M. A. 1984. Predicting the vocational capacity of the chronically mentally ill: Research and policy implications. *American Psychologist, 39,* 537–44.

Ashbaugh, J. W. 1982. Assessing the need for community supports. In Tessler and Goldman 1982, pp. 141–58.

Ashbaugh, J. W.; Hoff, M. K.; and Bradley, V. 1980. *Community support program needs assessment project: A review of the findings in the state CSP reports and literature.* Boston: Human Services Research Institute.

Ashbaugh, J. W., and Manderscheid, R. W. 1985. A method for estimating the chronically mentally ill in state and local areas, *Journal of Hospital and Community Psychiatry, 36,* 389–93.

Bachrach, L. L. 1982. Young adult chronic patients: An analytical review of the literature. *Hospital and Community Psychiatry, 33,* 189–97.

Bassuk, E. 1984. The homeless problem. *Scientific American, 251,* 40–45.

Ben-Dashan, T.; Morrison, L.; and Kotler, M. 1981. *Community support program performance measurement system development and short-term evaluation: Final report.* Silver Spring, Md.: Macro Systems.

Community Support Program. 1977. Guidelines. Rockville, Md.: National Institute of Mental Health. Mimeographed.

GAO. 1977. See U.S. Government Accounting Office 1977.

Goldman, H. H.; Adams, N.; and Taube, C. A. 1983. Deinstitutionalization data demythologized. *Hospital and Community Psychiatry, 34,* 129–34.

Goldman, H. H.; Gattlozzi, A. A.; and Taube, C. A. 1981. Counting and defining the chronically mentally ill. *Hospital and Community Psychiatry, 32,* 21–27.

Goldman, H. H., and Manderscheid, R. 1987a. Epidemology of psychiatric disability. In *Psychiatric disability,* ed. A. Meyerson and T. Fine. Washington, D.C.: American Psychiatric Association Press.

Goldman, H. H., and Manderscheid, R. 1987b. Chronic mental disorder in the United States. In *Mental Health, United States, 1987,* ed. R. W. Manderscheid and S. A. Barrett. DHHS Pub. No. (ADM) 87-1518. Washington, D.C.: Supt. of Docs., U.S. Government Printing Office.

Goldman, H. H., and Morrissey, J. P. 1985. The alchemy of mental heatlth policy: Homelessness and the fourth cycle of reform. *American Journal of Public Health, 75,* 727–31.

Goldman, H. H., and Runck, B. 1985. Social Security Administration revises mental disability rules. *Hospital and Community Psychiatry, 36,* 343–45.

Goldman, H. H.; Taube, C. A.; Regier, D. A.; and Witkin, M. 1983. Multiple functions of the state mental hospital. *American Journal of Psychiatry, 140* (3), 296–300.

Grusky, O.; Tierney, K.; Manderscheid, R. W.; and Grusky, D. 1985. Social bonding and community adjustment of chronically mentally ill adults. *Journal of Health and Social Behavior, 26,* 49–63.

Harding, C. M.; Brooks, G. W.; Ashikaga, T.; and Strauss, J. S. 1984. The Vermont longitudinal study of persons with severe mental illness, I: Methodology, study sample, and overall current status. *American Journal of Psychiatry, 144,* 718–26.

Jansen, M. A. 1985. Introduction to the series of articles on Social Security disability reform. *Psychosocial Rehabilitation Journal, 9,* 3–7.

Koyanagi, C. 1985. Social Security Disability Benefits Reform Act of 1984: Implications for those disabled by mental illness. *Psychosocial Rehabilitation Journal, 9,* 21–31.

McCarrick, A. K.; Manderscheid, R. W.; and Bertolucci, D. E. 1985. Correlates of acting-out behavior among the chronically mentally ill. *Hospital and Community Psychiatry, 36,* 848–53.

Minkoff, K. 1978. A map of chronic mental patients. In Talbott 1978.

Naierman, N. 1982. *The chronically mentally ill in community mental health centers.* Washington, D.C.: Abt Associates, January 29. Mimeographed.

Pepper, B.; Kirshner, M. C.; and Ryglewicz, H. 1981. The young adult chronic patient: Overview of a population. *Hospital and Community Psychiatry, 32,* 463–69.

President's Commission. 1978. Report on mental health. Vol. 1. Washington, D.C.: U.S. Government Printing Office.

Public Law 95-602. Rehabilitation, Comprehensive Services, and Developmental Disabilities Amendments of 1978.

Public Law 98-640. The Social Security Reform Act of 1984.

Schwartz, S. R., and Goldfinger, S. M. 1981. The new chronic patient: Clinical characteristics of an emerging subgroup. *Hospital and Community Psychiatry, 32,* 470–74.

Segal, S. P., and Baumohl, J. 1982. The new chronic patient: The creation of an underserved population. In *Reaching the underserved: Mental health needs of neglected populations,* ed. L. R. Snowden, pp. 95–113. Beverly Hills, Calif.: Sage Annual Reviews of Community Mental Health.

Stein, L. I., and Test, M. D. 1980. Alternative to mental hospital treatment. *Archives of General Psychiatry, 37,* 392–97.

Strauss, J. S.; Hafez, H.; Lieberman, P.; and Harding, C. 1985. The course of psychiatric disorder, III: Longitudinal principles. *American Journal of Psychiatry, 142,* 289–96.

Stroup, A. L., and Manderscheid, R. W. 1984. The development of the state mental hospital system in the United States, 1840–1980. Unpublished paper.

Summers, F. 1981. The effects of aftercare after one year. *Journal of Psychiatric Treatment and Evaluation, 3,* 405–9.

Szymanski, H. V.; Schulberg, H. C.; Salter, V.; and Gutterman, N. 1982. Estimating the local prevalence of persons needing community support programs. *Hospital and Community Psychiatry, 33,* 370–73.

Talbott, J. A. 1978. *The chronic mental patient.* Washington, D.C.: American Psychiatric Association.

Taube, C. A.; Thompson, J. W.; Rosenstein, M. J.; Rosen, B. M.; and Goldman, H. H. The chronic mental hospital patient. *Hospital and Community Psychiatry, 34,* 611–15.

Tessler, R. C., and Goldman, H. H. 1982. *The chronically mentally ill: Assessing community support programs.* Cambridge, MA: Ballinger.

Turner, J. C., and TenHoor, W. J. 1978. The NIMH community support program: Pilot approach to needed social reform. *Schizophrenia Bulletin, 4,* 319–48.

U.S. Department of Health and Human Services. 1980. *Toward a national plan for the chronically mentally ill.* Final draft report to the Secretary of Health and Human Services. Washington, D.C.: U.S. Government Printing Office.

U.S. Department of Health and Human Services. 1981. *Social Security regulations: Rules for determining disability and blindness.* SSA Publication no. 64–104. Washington, D.C.: U.S. Government Printing Office.

U.S. Department of Health and Human Services. 1985. Determination of disability in cases of mental impairment, listing of impairments: Mental disorder. *Federal Register,* February 4.

U.S. Department of Health, Education and Welfare. 1966. *International classification of disease.* 8th ed. Washington, D.C.: U.S. Government Printing Office.

U.S. Government Accounting Office. 1977. *Returning the mentally disabled to the community: Government needs to do more.* Washington, D.C.: U.S. Government Printing Office.

Warheit, G. J.; Buhl, J. M.; and Schwab, J. J. 1977. *Need-assessment approaches: Concepts and methods.* Department of Health, Education, and Welfare Publication no. (ADM) 79-472. Rockville, Md.: Public Health Service, National Institute of Mental Health.

Woy, J. R.; Goldstrom, I. D.; and Manderscheid, R. W. 1983. The young chronic mental patient: Report of a national survey. Unpublished paper.

3

The Psychological and Vocational Problems of Persons with Chronic Mental Illness

MARY A. JANSEN

Turning from the conceptual issues, Jansen gives a general introduction to many of the problems confronting the person with a prolonged psychiatric disorder who tries to enter the work force. She describes how these problems interact with each other and the environment and offers solutions to assist the practitioner in helping the client deal more effectively with these dilemmas. Topics included are ego deficits (i.e., low self-esteem, poor anxiety and frustration tolerance, and inadequate social supports and skills); vocational immaturity characterized by unrealistic aspirations; the disincentives of the Social Security disability system; and the lack of a coordinated network of community services.

Persons with chronic mental illness face many problems as they attempt to overcome residuals of the illness and develop social and vocational skills which will allow them to become functioning and productive members of society. These problems can be categorized as those which are psychological and directly related to the illness, those which are social and vocational and confront the individual at work and at home, and those which are systemic, arising from public policies which have not provided effective support mechanisms for this population. These problems often interact in ways that cause clients to be caught in a "catch-22" where repeated failure seems almost inevitable. With proper understanding of the nature and scope of these problems, rehabilitation practitioners can design intervention strategies that will assist clients with chronic mental illness in achieving successful rehabilitation. This chapter presents an overview of some of the psychological, vocational, and systemic problems experienced by persons with chronic mental illness and offers suggestions for more effective rehabilitation plans for this population.

The Scope of the Problem

The importance of establishing effective rehabilitation programs for persons with chronic mental illness is apparent when one considers the number of persons affected. A report from the International Labor Office has noted that "mental illness constitutes one of the world's most critical social and health problems. It affects more human lives and wastes more human resources than any other disabling condition" (International Labor Office 1979, p. 1). The World Health Organization has estimated that up to two-fifths of all disability in the world is related to psychiatric conditions (Canavan et al. 1984). It has been estimated that in the United States "three million people suffer severe mental disorder annually. Of these 2.4 million people become moderately to severely disabled on account of the disorder. And of these, 1.7 million people suffer prolonged severe disability; they constitute the chronically mentally ill population" (U.S. Department of Health and Human Services 1980, p. 2-1). Recently the plight of the homeless, chronically mentally ill has gained national attention (U.S. Congress 1984), and this challenge is likely to grow as the large cohort of young, acute, and chronic patients in the system continues to increase (Lamb 1984).

Despite recognition that persons with chronic mental illness constitute one of the most severely disabled populations, as a nation we have been reluctant to provide adequate resources to help these individuals overcome the problems they face in their attempt to achieve a successful rehabilitation outcome. These problems include psychological and emotional deficits, vocational and social skills deficits, and problems imposed by an environment which is hostile and fearful of persons with chronic mental illness. Overcoming these problems frequently involves long-term rehabilitation efforts aimed at utilizing whatever residual capacity remains. Although this challenge is not an easy one, the scope of the problem demands serious attention by those concerned with rehabilitation of these individuals.

An Overview of Problems Faced by Persons with Chronic Mental Illness

Psychological Problems

Ego deficits play a critical role in the inability of persons with chronic mental illness to function effectively and maintain employment. Lack of self-esteem and self-confidence, an inability to tolerate frustration, a fear of failure manifested as poor motivation, and overarching anxiety and inability to get along with others have all been identified as factors which contribute to poor rehabilitation outcomes for persons with chronic mental illness (Berry and Miskimins 1969; Greco and Stein 1980; Griffiths 1974; Griffiths 1977; Watts and Po-Kwan 1976). Because of repeated failures and the inability to separate their own sense of self-worth from their illness, persons who are chronically mentally ill are unable to bounce back from repeated failures in attempts at maintaining sanity, employment, good relations with others, and successful independent living. Lack of self-confidence leads to fear of failure and rejection and gives rise to internal terror. The person with chronic mental illness deals with this terror by withdrawing from the stimulus environment (usually other people or a work situation); without proper understanding and support, the cycle begins again. When an inhospitable work or social environment is added, the person may regress to the point of never wanting to try to work or socialize again. These deficits are not easily overcome, and traditional psychotherapy has not proven effective with this population. This is why long-term psychosocial and vocational rehabilitation programs which provide support are essential as the safety net to avoid devastating failures and severe regression.

Social and Vocational Problems

Vocational immaturity, a lack of successful vocational experiences, an inability to live independently, and lack of an adequate personal and social support network constitute a second set of problems encountered in rehabilitation efforts. Although the best predictor of future vocational success is previous successful employment (Anthony and Jansen 1984), persons with chronic mental illness frequently do not have successful vocational experiences to look back on and to build future efforts upon. This lack of realistic work experience can contribute to the vocational immaturity often seen in clients with chronic mental illness (Ciardiello and Bingham 1982). Vocational immaturity, frequently manifested by unrealistic expectations, can be frustrating for the practitioner unless it can be viewed as another manifestation of the client's fear of acknowledging failure. It is difficult enough for most healthy persons to acknowledge that they will never set the world on fire; how much more difficult for someone who has failed at the most basic tasks of socialization. Thus, the idealized and immature vocational goals often verbalized by persons with chronic mental illness are logical when viewed in the context of frequent failures. Yet, these clients seldom really believe that attainment of these goals is possible; hence the fear of failure, manifested as lack of motivation, which accompanies their attempts at rehabilitation.

Successful rehabilitation efforts are made more difficult by the interactive and circular effect which the psychological, social, and vocational deficits have on each other. Each time an individual with chronic mental illness attempts to make friends, live independently and work, and then fails, he or she experiences a further assault on self-worth and heightened fears of future attempts. The increased anxiety and lessened motivation which result make future attempts at such activities less likely and increase the chance that future attempts will fail.

Problems Created by the Public Policy System

A third category of problems which persons with chronic mental illness face consists of those which have been created by our system of providing health and social support services. Several years ago the United States instituted a deinstitutionalization policy but did so without providing an adequate community-based system of care. The problems of deinstitutionalization have been well documented (Larsen 1983; Miller 1981, Schwartz and Goldfinger 1981), and it is because of these problems and the lack of an adequate system of community-based care that many persons with chronic mental illness are unable to secure appropriate treatment services. This lack of an integrated community support system is best reflected in our growing homeless population and in the large number of young adult chronic patients. Further, our treatment and rehabilitation system, although cognizant of the importance of long-term psychosocial and vocational methods, has not adequately responded to this need. There are few facilities which provide the kinds of long-term psychosocial and vocational treatment which has been demonstrated to be effective, and there is inadequate funding maintaining persons with chronic mental illness in these programs for long periods of time. Additionally, research designed to determine the best ways of identifying those individuals with chronic mental illness who are most likely to succeed in various kinds of rehabilitation programs has been poorly funded, and we know little about the most efficient means for rehabilitating people with varying degrees of chronic mental illness. Moreover, stigmatization of persons with chronic mental illness is great and many employers have been unwilling to risk involvement in long-term vocational rehabilitation programs for this population, especially in times of high unemployment.

Finally, the Social Security disability system, designed to provide financial support for persons in all categories of disability, has itself been responsible for impeding rehabilitation of persons with chronic mental illness. This has happened in two ways. First, the Social Security system does not provide incentives for long-term psychosocial and vocational rehabilitation, so necessary for this population, but instead has built in disincentives which often preclude persons with chronic mental illness from working in transitional employment programs. Yet, these transitional employment programs have demonstrated the most success in rehabilitation of persons with chronic mental illness. Secondly, the trauma experienced by many persons with chronic mental illness during the recent reform of the Social Security disability system graphically demonstrated our nation's insensitivity to the fragile hold which persons with chronic mental illness have on economic and emotional security (Anthony and Jansen 1984; Jansen 1985). By denying benefits to thousands of persons with chronic mental illness, the Social Security disability system not only violated the law but caused irreparable harm to many of our most vulnerable citizens (Mental Health Association of Minnesota v. Schweiker 1982). Yet, experts in other countries have recognized that providing economic security is important and can have a major positive impact on the course of disability (Canavan et al. 1984). With specific respect to the issue of economic stability and chronic mental illness, the potential negative impact has been succinctly stated: "The combination of impairment and disadvantage is deadly" (Wing and Olsen 1979, p. 173). This is precisely what happened when the Social Security Administration targeted persons with chronic mental illness for benefit cessation (U.S. House of Representatives 1982). Although the Social Security disability system has now been revised and these policies changed, the basic system, with its disincentives for appropriate rehabilitation, remains.

An additional problem is that it is frequently too difficult for persons with chronic mental illness to comply with the necessary formalities inherent in our bureaucratic system. Frequently the structures for obtaining employment and benefits such as Social Security are so complex and overwhelming that chronically mentally ill persons cannot cope with the anxiety these structures engender (Amiel 1975).

The Practitioner's Role in Establishing Rehabilitation Programs

Overcoming Psychological, Social, and Vocational Problems

Several elements are important if the basic psychological, social, and vocational deficits are to be dealt with, paving the way for successful rehabilitation efforts. Perhaps most importantly, practitioners must assist their clients to gain insight into the psychological consequences of their mental illness so that the anxiety and fear of failing again can be dealt with realistically. Next, practitioners must help the individual gain insight into unrealistic and immature vocational aspirations so that the tendency to set overly demanding goals which ultimately lead to failure and regression can be overcome. The practitioner can do this by emphasizing short-term goals that will lead to successful experiences and by working with clients and employers to anticipate and tolerate short-term failures. One outcome of rehabilitation efforts with clients who have chronic mental illness is that clients can increase their ability to use appropriate support systems when needed and avoid unnecessary failures.

Once these issues are addressed, clients with chronic mental illness may be more willing to view rehabilitation efforts more positively and more realistically and participate more fully in the rehabilitation process. Then the rehabilitation practitioner and the client can begin to realistically assess the client's skills, values, and preferences along with social and vocational skill deficits. Once these have been identified, a plan can be drawn up which accounts for these findings and addresses ways to overcome skill deficits. The plan must account for factors which will produce increased stress during the entire rehabilitation process, and additional support must be built in to help the client deal with these added stressors. Since some regression should be anticipated, the rehabilitation plan should be flexible enough to allow the client to progress slowly or to take time off if needed. Easy return to the program is essential, and continued contact must be maintained by the practitioner.

Next, the practitioner can look for environments which will facilitate the client's development of skills needed to succeed in the rehabilitation effort. A structured environment which provides stimulation but is not overly stimulating is important, as is access to a supportive network of persons with whom the client can relate. The value of work which is "real" but not overly pressured has also been identified (Affleck 1971), and this is why transitional employment settings have proven effective. One study has shown that persons with mental illness are more likely to remain employed when employment situations are characterized by (a) opportunity to learn on the job, (b) freedom to organize work, (c) clear supervision, (d) a trusting social climate, and (e) work which requires a working relationship with other workers—that is, not isolated work (Floyd 1982). The same study also found that persons with mental illness work better when they have the opportunity to evaluate their own performance in relation to their co-workers as well as to receive feedback from supervisors. It may be that the need to make self-evaluations in relation to other workers is why nonisolated work fared better, in contrast to some earlier thinking which stressed the need for isolated work opportunities. In addition, clients doing more skilled work have been shown to remain employed for longer periods of time (Floyd 1982). Since more skilled positions can produce added stress, the practitioner will need to identify just what elements constitute a stressful situation for a given client. Clearly, a good relationship among colleagues and supervisors is important.

In addition, several authors have emphasized the importance of a skills-building approach, which reduces opportunities for failure and thus enhances self-esteem and motivation (Anthony 1977; Anthony 1980; Anthony and Margules 1974; Dincin 1975). Inherent in this approach is the requirement of a consistent, clearly identified set of criteria. The skills-building approach to developing good work behavior can also help to build frustration tolerance, assist the client in learning about his or her strengths and limitations, and help to establish social skills that go along with successful work experiences (Kunce 1970).

Acquisition of skills may also be therapeutic in itself. Recent research has also shown that providing an accelerated program of transitional employment, especially for work-experienced clients, may produce better rehabilitation results than the traditional approach, which very gradually readies the client for employment experiences (Bond and Dincin 1986). It may be that allowing work-experienced clients to remain away from work for too long enhances their fears of failure and allows them to become too dependent on the support system. Clearly, additional research is needed to identify which clients, under which sets of conditions, will do best in which programs, but if an accelerated approach proves to be best, the need for long-term psychosocial support networks will still be critical, and the rehabilitation practitioner can help to ensure provision of these support networks by working closely with employers, psychosocial agencies, community mental health centers, and housing authorities to ensure integration of community support systems.

Although establishment of appropriate social skills and work behaviors increases self-confidence, frustration tolerance, motivation, and self-esteem, and reduces anxiety, these changes do not occur quickly. This process can be a lengthy one for persons with chronic mental illness (International Labor Office 1974; Watts and Bennett 1983) and one which requires adequate planning for the individual, the family, and the rehabilitation system, including prospective employers.

A second critical element is that of client involvement in the rehabilitation process (Danley 1987). The client's chances of success are maximized when he or she is responsible for making the process work and actively involved in making the decisions which will affect his or her future life. Client investment is facilitated when fear of failure is reduced and motivation to succeed enhanced. Thus, clients should be actively involved in all stages of the rehabilitation process from evaluation of the impact of psychological problems, to identification of social and vocational skill deficits, to planning treatment interventions and vocational strategies, to evaluation of each step in the process.

In all cases, the practitioner must attempt to identify with the client those events which are likely to produce increased stress in the client's home life and at work. Once identified, these can be planned for and increased supports can be made available to help the client cope with these higher levels of stress.

Although employers have traditionally resisted rehabilitation partnerships for persons with chronic mental illness, recently there has been a trend toward greater cooperation between industry and the mental health and rehabilitation systems. Innovations have begun to occur in large organizations as well as small ones, and employers are beginning to recognize the benefits of mental health programs (Goldbeck 1982). As recently as 1984, 609 employers reported providing over one thousand positions in transitional employment programs for persons with mentally disabling

conditions (Fountain House 1984). Although the number is small compared to the number of employers nationwide, it represents increased recognition and a dramatic step forward on the part of employers. Credit
must be given to proponents of the psychosocial rehabilitation system
who worked to enhance employer awareness in bringing about these
changes. Many more agreements with industry are needed, however, if
needed services are to reach those with chronic mental illness. Rehabilitation practitioners can facilitate this effort by designing programs with local businesses to provide flexible transitional employment programs and
long-term psychosocial support methods for their clients with chronic
mental illness.

Overcoming Systemic Problems and Defining Public Policy

Rehabilitation practitioners can play an important part in helping to
shape public policies which directly affect rehabilitation outcomes of persons with chronic mental illness. Practitioners must become aware of the
issues facing policy makers vis-à-vis the mental health and rehabilitation
systems and must become involved in the process whereby public policy
decisions are made. One very easy and logical way to begin this process is
to join national and state associations such as the International Association of Psychosocial Rehabilitation Services (IAPSRS), whose mission is to
enhance treatment and rehabilitation opportunities for persons with
chronic mental illness.

Under ideal conditions, persons with chronic mental illness would be
afforded a treatment and rehabilitation system which met their needs and
did so in an efficacious and cost-effective manner. Under such a system,
treatment services designed to remedy ego deficits inherent in the illness
would be provided and would be coordinated with other community-
based services designed to remedy the social and vocational problems
which result. In this model, direct-treatment services would be interlinked
with community-based services designed to address the psychosocial and
vocational ramifications of the disability. Included would be long-term
psychosocial and vocational services such as adequately staffed and
funded patient clubs, appropriate living arrangements, treatment programs in close proximity to patients' homes, and sheltered employment
and transitional employment programs. There would also be coordination between mental health treatment facilities, vocational rehabilitation
agencies, Social Security disability offices, psychosocial patient clubs, independent living facilities, and employers which provide sheltered and
transitional employment. Joint funding capabilities would exist to coordinate provision of health, rehabilitation, and social services. Although
comprehensive community-based rehabilitation services are costly, available data from the Rehabilitation Services Administration indicate that
the vocational rehabilitation system is the only social program in the

United States which has shown an effective return for costs incurred. Additionally, the literature supports the notion that a combined program of community-based mental health services and social welfare and rehabilitation services designed to provide the necessary elements of financial security, access to community-based treatment, and long-term psychosocial support and vocational rehabilitation including transitional employment, will assist persons with chronic mental illness to achieve productive employment and lower treatment costs, including those incurred by hospital readmission. Although up-front costs are higher, the economic return for this investment is greater both in humanitarian terms and in real dollars when measured by return to productive employment. But this model can succeed only when there is a sense of community responsibility and an adequate understanding and acceptance of chronic mental illness. While it is naive to believe that attitudinal differences can be imparted overnight, we must increase efforts to lessen the stigmatization of persons with disabilities of all kinds, including persons with chronic mental illness. Without this basic attitudinal change, funding priorities will not be shifted, and a commitment to providing an integrated and coordinated system of community-based care will not occur.

Summary

Although the importance of an integrated system of care for persons with chronic mental illness has been identified by policy-makers in this country and abroad (Council of Europe 1985; International Labor Office 1979; National Institute of Mental Health 1983; World Health Organization 1980), we have not made a commitment to adequate planning for a comprehensive and integrated system of mental health care, social support services, and rehabilitation.

Adequate funding, effective rehabilitation research, adequate rehabilitation programming, recognition of the necessity for long-term Social Security support, and an integrated mechanism of social support services are necessary if persons with chronic mental illness are to achieve successful employment and maximize their full residual capacity.

In addition to recognizing that long-term psychosocial and vocational rehabilitation services are necessary for persons with chronic mental illness, we must ensure provisions for comprehensive community-based services for this population. Mental health treatment services should be in close proximity to the individual's home, and there should be close cooperation between the mental health treatment system, the rehabilitation system, and the social service network which provides housing, Social Security benefits, and other community support services. Employers must become allies through efforts to remove the stigma attached to chronic mental illness. A recognition that regression to previous functional levels frequently occurs must be built into financing structures, employment contracts, psychosocial and support systems, and treatment strategies. Without this recognition and acceptance, those who need to take several steps backwards before going ahead will experience rejection, loss of self-esteem and confidence, and the sense of having failed again. When potential regression is accepted as a part of the rehabilitation process, it can be dealt with developmentally so that the individual can proceed to the next step with a renewed sense of confidence. Clearly, however, additional research is needed to identify the best rehabilitation approach for persons with different degrees of mental illness. For some, especially those with previous employment history, an accelerated approach to transitional employment will work best. For others, longer-term approaches which offer a more gradual approach to building basic vocational skills are needed. In all cases, more research is needed to identify the parameters around which decisions can be made about types of program, ultimate rehabilitation potential, and feasibility of various demand schedules. In all cases, one issue is very clear: a comprehensive and integrated system of social support services is necessary, over a long period of time, in order to ensure the safety net so necessary for continued support.

Given the economics of health care and the rapid escalation of health care costs, we cannot afford to waste resources on a significant segment of our population. Therefore, we must formulate comprehensive national policies designed to facilitate the effective rehabilitation of our chronically mentally ill citizens. It is only through the effective rehabilitation of these citizens that we will begin to harness their potential resources in the community, in the workplace, and in the home. From both an economic and a social perspective, this becomes especially important when we consider the potential for decreased dependence on the health care system, Social Security programs, and our national welfare system, and the potential for increased self-reliance and independence.

References

Affleck, J. 1971. Emotional factors in resocialization. *Occupational Mental Health, 1*, 18–20.

Amiel, R. 1975. *Health insurance and mental illness.* Copenhagen: WHO Regional Office for Europe.

Anthony, W. 1977. Psychological rehabilitation: A concept in need of a method. *American Psychologist, 32*, 658–62.

———. 1980. *The principles of psychiatric rehabilitation.* Baltimore: University Park Press.

Anthony, W., and Jansen, M. 1984. Predicting the vocational capacity of the chronically mentally ill: Research and policy implications. *American Psychologist, 39*, 537–44.

Anthony, W., and Margules, A. 1974. Toward improving the efficacy of psychiatric rehabilitation: A skills building approach. *Rehabilitation Psychology, 21*, 101–5.

Berry, K., and Miskimins, R. 1969. Concept of self and posthospital vocational adjustment. *Journal of Consulting and Clinical Psychology, 33*, 101–8.

Bond, G., and Dincin, J. 1986. Accelerating entry into transitional employment in a psychosocial rehabilitation agency. *Rehabilitation Psychology, 31,* 143–55.

Canavan, K.; Schwarz, R.; Wiersma, D.; Jablensky, A.; and Biehl, H. 1984. Assessment and reduction of psychiatric disability. *International Digest of Health Legislation, 35,* 509–49.

Ciardiello, J., and Bingham, W. 1982. The career maturity of schizophrenic clients. *Rehabilitation Counseling Bulletin, 26,* 3–9.

Council of Europe. 1985. *Second conference of European health ministers: Report, list of participants, and final text.* Strasbourg: Council of Europe.

Danley, K. S. 1987. Improving vocational rehabilitation for persons with psychiatric disabilities. In *Advances in clinical rehabilitation,* ed. M. G. Eisenberg and R. C. Grzesiak, vol. 2. New York: Springer.

Dincin, J. 1975. Psychiatric rehabilitation. *Schizophrenia Bulletin, 13,* 131–47.

Floyd, M. 1982. Employment problems of expsychiatric patients. *Employment Gazette, 90,* 21–27.

Fountain House. 1984. Transitional employment. Survey Memorandum 271. New York: Fountain House.

Goldbeck, W. 1982. Psychiatry and industry: A business view. *The Psychiatric Hospital, 13,* 95–98.

Greco, M., and Stein, L. 1980. An alternative to hospitalization program: The contributions of a rehabilitation approach. *Rehabilitation Counseling Bulletin, 24,* 85–93.

Griffiths, R. 1974. Rehabilitation of chronic psychotic patients: An assessment of their psychological handicap, and evaluation of the effectiveness of rehabilitation and observations of the factors which predict outcome. *Psychological Medicine, 4,* 316–25.

———. 1977. The prediction of psychiatric patients' work adjustment in the community. *British Journal of Social Clinical Psychology, 16,* 165–73.

International Labor Office. 1974. Rehabilitation of the mentally ill and disabled: ILO paper for ad hoc interagency meeting on rehabilitation of the disabled. Geneva: International Labor Office.

———. 1979. *Vocational rehabilitation of the mentally restored.* Geneva: International Labor Office.

Jansen, M. 1985. A chronicle of a major health policy of the 1980s: Social Security disability reform—reasons for optimism and caution. *Psychosocial Rehabilitation Journal, 9,* 3–48.

Kunce, J. 1970. Is work really therapeutic? *Rehabilitation Literature, 31,* 297–99, 320.

Lamb, H., ed. 1984. *The homeless mentally ill.* Washington, D.C.: American Psychiatric Association.

Larsen, R. 1983. The deinstitutionalized environment: A case for better planning. *Quality Review Bulletin, 9,* 126–30.

Mental Health Association of Minnesota v. Schweiker, 554 F. Supp. 157 (D. Minn. 1982), *appeal docketed,* No. 83-1263-MN (8th cir. Feb. 24, 1983).

Miller, R. 1981. Deinstitutionalization and other fairy tales. *Psychiatric Quarterly, 53,* 53–59.

National Institute of Mental Health. 1983. *NIMH definition and guiding principles for community support systems.* Rockville, Md.: National Institute of Mental Health.

Schwarz, S., and Goldfinger, S. 1981. The new chronic patient: Clinical characteristics of an emerging subgroup. *Hospital and Community Psychiatry, 32,* 470–74.

U.S. Congress. 1984. *House and Senate conference report.* Washington, D.C.: U.S. Government Printing Office.

U.S. Department of Health and Human Services. 1980. *Toward a national plan for the chronically mentally ill.* Washington, D.C.: U.S. Government Printing Office.

U.S. House of Representatives. 1982. *Report of the Select Committee on Aging.* Washington, D.C.: U.S. Government Printing Office.

Watts, F., and Bennett, D. 1983. *Theory and practice of psychiatric rehabilitation.* Winchester, England: John Wiley and Sons.

Watts, F., and Po-Kwan, Y. 1976. The structure of attitudes in psychiatric rehabilitation. *Journal of Occupational Psychology, 49,* 39–44.

Wing, J., and Olsen, R. 1979. Principles of the new community care. In *Community care for the mentally disabled,* ed. J. Wing and R. Olsen. Oxford: Oxford University Press.

World Health Organization. 1980. *Changing patterns in mental health care.* EURO Reports and Studies, no. 25. Copenhagen: WHO Regional Office for Europe.

4

Work as Treatment for Psychiatric Disorder: A Puzzle in Pieces

JOHN S. STRAUSS, COURTENAY M. HARDING, MORTON SILVERMAN,
ANITA EICHLER, and MAURY LIEBERMAN

In their consideration of work as treatment, Strauss, Harding, Silverman, Eichler, and Lieberman identify nine models which were brought together by representatives at a conference on work. Despite attempts at synthesis, they are unable to come to a unified perspective; however, by articulating the nature of the conceptual problems, they make an important contribution toward integration. Using these models as a conceptual base, they outline some of the implications of work for treatment, service delivery, and public policy.

In the story of the blind men and the elephant, each person describes to the others the feel of a different part of the animal and thus presents a different perspective. In understanding the role of work as a potential contributor to the treatment of mental illness, people from various disciplines are at an even earlier stage than were the blind men with the elephant: many of those interested in work and mental illness have not even been communicating. Although industrial psychologists for years have studied topics such as person-environment fit as it applies to the work situation, the perspectives and methods of this group have not been applied to the problems of work and mental illness. Contributors to the field of vocational rehabilitation and occupational therapy often view their orientation as somehow parallel to but not interacting specifically with the details of psychopathology. The finding that diagnosis and work functioning are poorly correlated is often given as a rationale for this separate but equal approach. And clinicians such as psychiatrists, psychologists, and even many social workers tend to be trained so exclusively with a focus on pathology when dealing with mental disorders that careful attention to the issues of competence that are so central to rehabilitation programs is rare. Furthermore, the literature, the training, and the work settings for each of these disci-

This chapter was funded in part by the Scottish Rite Schizophrenia Research Program, N.M.J. USA and by NIMH Grants MH 34365, MH 00340, and MH 29575.

plines tend to be so sequestered that in many instances there is almost no contact with or even consideration of cross-disciplinary issues, with the possible exception of the common irritations that develop when the needs of a client bring one group in contact with another.

In order to deal with the isolation of these various groups that potentially have so much to contribute to each other in considering the role of work in treating mental disorders, a conference was organized by the authors and sponsored by the Center for Prevention Research at NIMH.* The goal of the conference was to involve participants from diverse backgrounds and orientations in a review of the current status of the field of work as treatment for mental disorders. This report was developed from that conference. Given the nature of the issues and the size of the chasms that separate the various orientations, unfortunately it has not been possible either in the conference or in this report to synthesize the orientations into a final common elephant. This brief report, therefore, is presented as a description of some of the different orientations as they relate to various key issues in the topic of work as a contributor to treatment for mental disorders. Our hope is, first, that this report will serve as a thorn to any who feel they can deal with the issues from any single perspective while ignoring the others and, second, that it will provide a basic description of the various orientations and the contributions each makes to provide the impetus for eventual synthesis in a creative way.

There are three major issues central to understanding how these various disciplines contribute to considering work as treatment of mental illness. The first of these issues is the conceptual orientation with which the topic is approached. It is the orientation that determines what kind of information is considered relevant to understanding, the way in which the information is combined, and how the information influences treatment and research. The basic conceptualization even determines whether work is considered relevant in treatment programs, merely ancillary, or without value. The other two issues are each discipline's contribution to applying work as treatment and their perspective on service delivery and policy.

For the purposes of this report, "work" will be defined somewhat arbitrarily as activity for which one receives pay. "Treatment" will be defined as a process for promoting the improvement of a disorder. Whether this improvement must produce change in the basic disorder itself or can be limited to improving functioning will be left as an open issue. It is just one of many basic questions determined by the conceptual model selected.

---

*Participants in the conference "Work as Treatment for Psychiatric Disorder," September 12–13, 1983: Dr. Sheila H. Akabas, Dr. William Anthony, Dr. Mary Cerney, Dr. Rene Dawis, Ms. Anita Eichler, Dr. Courtenay M. Harding, Dr. Robert Kahn, Dr. Sam Keith, Mr. Robert Lagor, Dr. Robert Liberman, Mr. Maury Lieberman, Dr. Elliott Liebow, Dr. Dennis J. McCrory, Dr. Walter Neff, Dr. James Schmidt, Ms. Beth Silverman, Dr. Morton Silverman, Dr. Sam Silverstein, Dr. John S. Strauss, Dr. Herbert H. Vreelan.

Conceptual Models

In the course of the conference nine models were identified for considering work as a treatment for mental disorder. Although the models overlap somewhat, each has different basic underlying assumptions. Each has different implications regarding the role of work for treatment, service delivery, and public policy. The models can be placed on a rough continuum from narrow versions of the medical model at one pole to models focused on social competence at the other. In addition, there were some integrative models presented which include both poles.

1. *The natural history model* for mental illness has inevitability as its hallmark. This model utilizes a narrow and familiar version of the general medical model of illness. It states that a disorder has its natural history, its inherent evolution. Thus, for example, before more systematic data became available, schizophrenia was portrayed as a basic disease process with an inevitable deteriorating course (Kraeplin 1915). A common, although not necessarily warranted, implication of the natural history model is that few factors other than the disease itself, have an impact on changing the natural history of the disorder. Further, this model often implies that the person with the illness is passive in determining its evolution. The natural history model, for all these reasons, suggests that work is irrelevant to the treatment of psychiatric disorder, discourages work research, and deemphasizes work programs other than as ancillary or palliative.

2. *The diathesis-stress model* of mental illness emphasizes both a basic, underlying, and (usually) immutable vulnerability for a disease and a role for environment as a trigger for manifest illness (Zubin and Spring 1977). This model views the underlying vulnerability to disorder as psychological and/or biological in nature. Stress converts this vulnerability into the illness. Although this model has certain advantages—for example, a basis for considering environmental impact (such as stress)—it also has certain serious shortcomings. Vulnerability and stress are far more difficult to define adequately than they appear. Work might be a stressor on some occasions for some persons with a given vulnerability and might be a buffer and serve a protective role in other instances for other persons with the same vulnerability. The degree of vulnerability may also be variable within each patient over time.

3. *The stimulus window model* focuses on the restricted range of coping believed to be generated by some diseases. This model, sometimes viewed as especially relevant to schizophrenia, conceptualizes persons with this disorder as requiring a certain limit, or "window," of stimulation. Above that limit, symptoms return; below that limit, dysfunction, such as apathy and withdrawal, may occur. This model combines certain elements of the natural history and diathesis-stress models. Like them, it

pays relatively little attention to the possibility of changing the disorder (and thus the window). This model implies that certain kinds of work, especially low-demand jobs, might be helpful for a person with severe mental illness, but that little can be done to widen the window by changing the work environment or challenging the individual in a new work setting.

4. *The deficit model* implies a notion of basic defect, emphasizing that persons with certain kinds of disorders lack some capacity (Chodoff and Carpenter 1975). The implication is that this is chronic, perhaps even immutable. This model often suggests that all that can be done is to help the person adjust to the deficit. For example, there is an impressive rehabilitation concept of providing a "prosthetic" work environment which compensates for the deficit (Liberman et al. 1985). In this view, certain kinds of work might represent too severe an adjustment or might amplify the impact of the deficit and generate further problems. Work would not be viewed as having any impact on changing the basic disorder.

5. *The conflict model* emphasizes the importance of the meaning of situations in terms of psychological conflicts, such as conflicts around authority, success, or close relationships (Chodoff and Carpenter 1975). This model suggests, for example, that work could generate a conflict for the person (e.g., fear of success), and that such a conflict would have to be resolved (e.g., through psychotherapy), or that the kind of work chosen would have to avoid the conflict issues. This model does not generally imply that work in itself helps to cure basic conflicts, but that conclusion is not logically precluded by this orientation.

6. *The social learning model,* drawn from behaviorist principles, focuses on the reward and/or punishment impacts of various experiences including the effects of symptoms and of functioning competently. This orientation views behaviors of all kinds as being "shaped" by rewards and/or punishments. Applied to work as treatment, this model would view work successes as providing rewards for competent behavior or work failures as providing punishments. Rewards from successful work behavior might counteract any secondary "rewards" that might accrue from psychiatric symptoms.

7. *The rehabilitation model,* a model at the furthest extreme from the narrow version of the medical model with which this list started, focuses on three concepts of functioning—impairment, disability, and handicap —with little attention to possible underlying causes or "diseases" (Anthony 1977; WHO 1980). Impairment is viewed as a basic problem (analogous, e.g., to muscle atrophy in organic illness) which might lead to disability (e.g., a problem in carrying out certain acts) if unresolved. The disability could become a handicap (a disruption in competence to handle the complex activities of daily life). This model focuses on the competencies still left and builds on this base to achieve maximal possible function-

ing. Interventions are seen as improving functional capacities by providing compensating mechanisms and/or shaping the environment so that a person with disability can exist more adequately.

Although this model is compatible with the notion of treatment, the basic concept usually implies that rehabilitation is rehabilitation and treatment is for illness. Impairment and its consequences are seen as not directly affecting the disease process in a feedback loop. In theory, the rehabilitation model appears to be more optimistic than the medical model. In practice, however, the person is often viewed as having a persisting deficit, analogous to an amputated leg, for which compensations need to be made. The illness is not targeted for intervention by a work program but is viewed as a relatively permanent entity resistant to change and therefore maneuvered around.

8. *The person-environment fit model* is a more integrative and flexible model than the others presented so far. This model, developed with particular sophistication in the field of industrial psychology, suggests that optimal functioning is determined by interactions between the person and the environment and that specific characteristics of the person and the environment can be defined in ways which allow a determination of the "fit" (Dawis and Lofquist 1976). The model focuses in relatively microscopic ways on characteristics of both sides of the fit (e.g., it could consider the motor retardation and depressed mood of a person with major depressive disorder and the pace and structure of the work setting, and it leaves open the option of attempting to alter either or both). Although this approach has many methodologic and conceptual implications for work as treatment, it has not yet been systematically applied to this issue.

9. *The interactive-developmental model* is also an integrative model that focuses on interaction between the individual and the environment (Strauss and Carpenter 1981). This model focuses on person/illness/environment interactions, the evolutionary changes in all three, and the active role of the person as an influence on this evolution. According to this model, change occurring in the person or illness could influence the environment which might stimulate further changes in the person or illness. Or an evolution in the environment might begin the sequence of person/illness/environment shifts.

One advantage of the interactive-developmental model is its provision for understanding changes and their complexities. For example, although certain aspects of the individual and the environment may not change over time, others might, so that a fit becomes a "misfit." The factors disrupting fit may involve characteristics that are often not noted in narrowly focused practice or research, such as changes in nonwork life contexts.

A more complex longitudinal view can be built on the interactive-developmental model suggesting that improvement following psychiatric disorder may reflect a kind of helix. McCrory suggests that some patients may improve, worsen slightly, perhaps learn some new skills, improve still further, fall back slightly for a while, and improve further (D. McCrory, verbal report). Such a progression, which represents the clinical experience of many observers, implies that both research and clinical practice involving work and other possible treatments must consider such differentiated phases in the evolution of disorders in the timing of assessments and planning of interventions.

These models have fundamental impacts on the focus of research and programs related to work as treatment for mental illness because they shape how the problem is perceived and the possible courses of action. The models pose critical questions. Does any work really have an impact on the processes and outcomes of disorder? If so, which aspect of work might be crucial for which people with which mental disorders at which stage in the disorder?

Treatment Concerns

The nine models described above have divergent implications for the integration of work into treatment for the patient as well as for the kinds of research most appropriate to study those interventions. Work as a possible treatment juxtaposes areas of concern usually kept separate; it poses particular problems for determining which aspects of the person or of the work situation might be important in a work-treatment situation.

Neither the usual variables dealt with in industrial psychology nor those in psychopathology may be most relevant. Symptoms, for example, may have little direct impact on a person's ability to work or on the way work can serve as a treatment modality. It is known, for example, that symptoms such as hallucinations and delusions do not preclude a person's working effectively at difficult tasks. Even the severity of symptoms, although somewhat related to ability to function in the work setting, may not be definitive in determining who can work or will be helped by work settings.

Rehabilitation agencies, drawing from policies on physical disabilities, often see low motivation in a client as precluding the person's participation in a work program. With mental disorders, however, low motivation may be a key part of the disorder itself, should not be ignored, and may require creative approaches to work settings in order to be resolved.

To make a bridge between psychopathology and work, those functional characteristics directly influencing their association will be more crucial than the traditional variables from either field. Thus, problems with attention, bizarre behavior, withdrawal, apathy, and similar aspects and effects of mental disorders which directly affect social and work functioning may be the most relevant aspects of psychopathology to consider in determining a person's ability to work and respond well to work intervention, rather than symptoms most used for diagnosis. Furthermore, such personal characteristics as self-esteem, courage, motivation, and hope, which are rarely mentioned in psychopathology texts, may also be important, both in assessing the person's ability to work and determining how work may be of assistance. Such complex characteristics as the person's sense of identity as a sick person or as a worker seem likely to be important determinants of the nature of the work-treatment-psychopathology interface.

On the other side of the work-patient equation, the variables in the work situations used traditionally in industrial psychology may not always be the most relevant for determining whether work will be helpful or harmful to a person with mental disorder. Is it the activity, the involvement, the remuneration, the self-esteem, the opportunity for social contact, the structure, or some other characteristics of the work setting that is the most crucial? Small work settings and supervisors with particular kinds of characteristics have been frequently noted by rehabilitation workers to be important for many persons attempting to recover from mental disorders. The longitudinal characteristics of the timing of a work intervention or holding off or starting a job placement also may relate to diverse characteristics of person and work setting. Some people who are acutely symptomatic respond well to working in structured situations. Those same situations, once symptoms have diminished, may lead to boredom and symptom recurrence. Such characteristics need to be the focus of treatment planning and work-treatment research in a far more systematic way than has so far been accomplished.

The issue of what characteristics to note also extends to the selection of a work-treatment program for a patient. Work-treatment programs are often chosen on the basis of a patient's diagnosis instead of taking into account the person's previous experience or lack of experience with employment.

The question of what characteristics of the person and the work situation to notice is reflected not only in the approach to using work as treatment but also in the training of clinicians and rehabilitation workers. Assumptions taught in training programs and then used by clinicians, rehabilitation workers, and agencies about the relevant personal and work situation characteristics are untested and often erroneous. In fact, clinicians rarely have a sense of what characteristics in their patients might relate to the ability to succeed in what kind of a work setting. And, as in the case of motivation problems, rehabilitation workers may not know enough about some of the characteristics of mental disorders that need to be dealt with by rehabilitation efforts.

Program and Social Policy Issues

Just as the various orientations towards work as a possible contribution to the treatment of mental disorders represent scattered pieces of a single puzzle, so too the implications of these orientations for program planning and broader policy issues related to employment and mental illness are dispersed in a confusing way.

Many key assumptions about rehabilitation are involved. For example, it is often stated, in the tandem orientation to work and illness, that vocational rehabilitation programs can be used only *after* the patient's symptomatology has stabilized. Yet there are no data to support this key assumption for program planning. Further, there are clinical experiences suggesting that for some people a work setting can actually have the effect of helping to stabilize symptom status. Another common assumption is that vocational programs should focus primarily on persons with prolonged mental illness and severe work disability. But it appears that many patients with acute disorders may be at high risk for becoming more chronic if problems at work are not resolved rapidly and effectively. For example, the person with an acute disorder who is sent back repeatedly to an extremely difficult work situation may have repeated stresses and failures contribute to recurrent symptoms and perhaps a lowering of motivation.

The orientations toward work as possible treatment for mental disorders have broad policy implications as well. What should be done regarding work-treatment programs during a period of depressed economy when jobs are scarce and marginal employees are fired? For society, it may be more economical, to say nothing of more humane, to make sure that persons with severe mental disorders, even marginal workers, can continue to be employed during such phases of the economy. More often recognized, but still very important, are such unresolved questions as, what is the impact of welfare, how do we tailor disability programs to help people return to work, and, in what ways can we make adjustments in job situations to reflect the changing needs of persons with mental disorders? These questions continue to provide major issues needing attention from multiple perspectives.

Summary

In the consideration of work as a possible treatment for mental disorders, the pieces of the puzzle have been sequestered in various places. We have tried to bring some of the major issues together to put them forth for consideration. Clarifying the role of work as a contributor to treatment for mental disorder requires the combined input of the clinical, rehabilitation, and industrial psychology arenas. The fact that these disciplines have remained so segregated is a historical and social fact, but this segregation does a disservice to persons with mental disorders who might be able to use work as a major key to improvement.

We regret that it has not yet been possible to assemble these pieces into a coherent picture. Nevertheless, at least they are out of their isolated boxes and on the table together for the advances that now need to be made.

References

Anthony, W. A. 1977. Psychological rehabilitation: A concept in need of a method. *American Psychologist, 32,* 658–62.

Chodoff, P., and Carpenter, W. T. 1975. Psychogenic theories of schizophrenia. In *Schizophrenia: Biological and psychological perspectives,* ed. G. Usdin. New York: Brunner/Mazel.

Dawis, R. V., and Lofquist, L. H. 1976. Personality style and the process of work adjustment. *Journal of Consulting Psychology, 23,* 55–59.

Kraepelin, E. 1915. *Clinical psychiatry: A textbook for students and physicians,* 7th ed., trans. A. R. Defendorf. New York: Macmillan.

Liberman, R. P.; Massel, H. K.; Mosk, M. D.; and Wong, S. E. 1985. Social skills training for chronic mental patients. *Hospital and Community Psychiatry, 36,* 396–403.

Strauss, J. S., and Carpenter, W. T., Jr. 1981. *Schizophrenia.* New York: Plenum.

Wing, J. K. 1975. Impairments in schizophrenia. In *Life history research in psychopathology,* vol. 4, ed. R. O. Wirt, G. Winokur, and M. Roff. Minneapolis: University of Minnesota Press.

World Health Organization. 1980. *International classification of impairments, disabilities, and handicaps.* Geneva, Switzerland.

Zubin, J., and Spring, B. 1977. Vulnerability: A new view of schizophrenia. *Journal of Abnormal Psychology, 86,* 103–26.

II

APPROACHES

Because the conceptual basis of vocational rehabilitation has grown out of many diverse perspectives, approaches have also varied widely. This section offers six different ways to understand the vocational rehabilitation process with their respective implications for intervention. In Chapter 5 Anthony, Cohen, and Danley describe how the traditional psychiatric rehabilitation model can be applied to vocational rehabilitation. Many behavioral and social learning techniques are implicit in Anthony's model, and are directly addressed in Chapter 6. Mueser and Liberman give the rationale and several alternate approaches to skills training in a job-finding club. Johnson uses a family-systems approach to suggest several ways of working with the families of chronically mentally ill clients in order to improve vocational functioning. Turning from an interpersonal to an intrapsychic point of view, Munich and Glinberg integrate the ideas of several psychoanalytic theorists to offer a psychodynamic approach to work and its inhibition. Bingham uses the ego-functioning approach described in the previous chapter and combines it with the vocational theories of Super and Holland to offer a vocational psychology perspective. Finally, in their chapter on transitional employment Malamud and McCrory describe a supportive employment approach and the ways it interfaces with a psychosocial program.

5

The Psychiatric Rehabilitation Model as Applied to Vocational Rehabilitation

WILLIAM A. ANTHONY, MIKAL R. COHEN, and KAREN S. DANLEY

Anthony, Cohen, and Danley give a theoretical and empirical rationale for the psychiatric rehabilitation process, which they then apply to vocational rehabilitation. They describe and illustrate the important characteristics of an effective vocational rehabilitation program. These include the program mission, the program structure for delivering diagnosis, planning and interventions, and the network of environments in which programming occurs. The characteristics of the vocational rehabilitation practitioner and the principles of psychiatric rehabilitation are also articulated.

A person discharged from a psychiatric inpatient unit has a better chance of returning to the hospital than of returning to work. It seems that the mental health/rehabilitation system has done a better job teaching persons with psychiatric disabilities how to be patients than teaching them how to be workers.

For the last decade Anthony and his associates (Anthony et al. 1972, 1978, 1984) have reviewed the employment outcomes of psychiatrically disabled persons. They have concluded that after hospital discharge, no more than 20–30 percent will be working competitively at any one time. Studies conducted most recently seem to suggest a 10–15 percent employment figure, with some reported outcomes as low as 0–10 percent.

Clearly, the typical interventions which psychiatrically disabled persons experience have only a minimal impact on employment outcomes. The overwhelming majority of severely psychiatrically disabled persons of employment age are not employed. Unger and Anthony (1983) reported on a nationwide survey of family members of young adult severely psychiatrically disabled persons. This survey found a full- and part-time employment rate of 16 percent for this 18–35-year-old population.

New interventions based on different models are needed. The psychiatric rehabilitation model is a useful model for guiding future developments in the vocational rehabilitation of the psychiatrically disabled.

This chapter describes the conceptual and empirical foundations of the psychiatric rehabilitation model, and illustrates the model's application to vocational rehabilitation. The practitioner and program dimensions necessary to implement the model are identified, and the principles underlying its implementation are described.

The Conceptual Foundation of the Psychiatric Rehabilitation Model

The model underlying physical rehabilitation provides the conceptual foundation for the psychiatric rehabilitation model. The rehabilitation model originally developed by the leaders in physical medicine and rehabilitation (Kessler 1935; Rusk and Taylor 1949; Wright 1960) can be logically extended to serve as the conceptual base for psychiatric rehabilitation.

Anthony (1982) has described how, in spite of the obvious differences between a severe psychiatric disability and a severe physical disability, there are enough similarities to use the practice of physical rehabilitation as a conceptual foundation for the practice of psychiatric rehabilitation. For example, in terms of the clients, both physically disabled persons and psychiatrically disabled persons exhibit handicaps in role performance; both often need a wide range of rehabilitation, medical, and human services, frequently for a long period of time; and both may not experience a total recovery from their disabilities.

Anthony (1982) pointed out that there are a number of advantages in using the physical rehabilitation model as a conceptual foundation for psychiatric rehabilitation. A physical disability is considered to be less stigmatizing than a psychiatric disability. Furthermore, the rehabilitation of the physically disabled appears more credible and understandable to the layperson. Thus, by using the rehabilitation model and philosophy in psychiatric rehabilitation, the concept of psychiatric rehabilitation can be more clearly articulated and made more legitimate and acceptable.

Table 5.1 illustrates the three stages in the rehabilitation model. Historically, rehabilitation professionals have described the stages of impairment, disability, and handicap somewhat differently over the years. However, the integrative work of Wood (1980) and Frey (1984) has brought conceptual clarity to these terms. Most simply, the *impairment* of structure or function can lead to *disability*—that is, decreased ability to perform certain skills and activities—and limit the persons's fulfillment of certain roles—in other words, create a *handicap*.

Typically, mental health treatment has tried to intervene at the impairment stage. Somatic and psychological treatments attempt to alleviate the signs and symptoms of the pathology. Leitner and Drasgow (1972), in analyzing the differences between treatment and rehabilitation, point out that, in general, treatment is directed toward minimizing sickness and rehabilitation is directed toward maximizing health. However, eliminating

Table 5.1
Stages in the Rehabilitation Model

Stages	Definitions	Typical interventions
I. Impairment	Any loss or abnormality of psychological, physiological, or anatomical structure or function	Treatment, focused on alleviating or eliminating pathology
II. Disability	Any restriction or lack (resulting from an impairment) of ability to perform an activity in the manner or within the range considered normal for a human being	Clinical rehabilitation, focused on developing client skills and environmental supports
III. Handicap	A disadvantage for a given individual (resulting from an impairment and/or a disability) that limits or prevents the fulfillment of a role that is normal depending on age, sex, and social/cultural factors for that individual	Societal rehabilitation, focused on changing the system in which the individual lives

or suppressing impairments does not lead automatically to higher functioning. Likewise, a decrease in disability does not lead to reductions in impairment. It is important to note that a chronic or severe impairment (e.g., diabetes, a stroke) does not always mean a chronic disability or handicap. What the impairment does is to increase the risk of chronic disability and handicap.

Anthony (1980) based his descriptions of the clinical practice of psychiatric rehabilitation on the practice of physical rehabilitation. In essence, both physical and psychiatric rehabilitation are comprised of two intervention strategies: (a) client skill development and (b) environmental resource development. These intervention techniques in physical rehabilitation practice are guided by the basic philosophy of rehabilitation, that disabled persons need skills and environmental supports in order to fulfill the role demands of various living, learning, and working environments. Similarly, the assumption of psychiatric rehabilitation practice is that if psychiatrically disabled persons' use of skills and/or the supports in their immediate environments are improved, they will be more able to perform those activities necessary to function in specific roles of their choice, including the role of worker. In other words, interventions designed to lessen the disability are assumed to lead to a decrease in the handicap.

In addition to clinical rehabilitation interventions, psychiatrically disabled persons can be helped to overcome their handicaps through societal rehabilitation interventions (Anthony 1972). Societal rehabilitation is designed to change the system in which psychiatrically disabled persons must function. Unlike clinical rehabilitation, it focuses neither on the skills of specific psychiatrically disabled individuals nor on their unique environments, but rather, on systems changes which can help many psychiatrically disabled persons overcome their handicaps. Examples of this type of systems interventions are the Targeted Job Tax Credit legislation, changes in the length and definition of the trial work period in the Social Security disability program, and the development of a European-type quota system for the employment of disabled workers. These systems interventions support the notion that a handicap may be more a function of a nonaccommodating and discriminating social and economic system than it is the person's impairment and disability.

The Empirical Foundation of the Psychiatric Rehabilitation Model

A number of research studies have supported the empirical basis for psychiatric rehabilitation, and in particular its applicability to improving the client's vocational performance. In general, the research indicates that

1. Measures of psychiatric symptoms do not predict vocational rehabilitation outcome.
2. The psychiatric diagnosis does not predict vocational rehabilitation outcome.
3. Measures of psychiatric symptoms do not correlate with the psychiatrically disabled person's skills.
4. Measures of skills do predict vocational rehabilitation outcome.
5. Training in critical vocational skills improves vocational rehabilitation outcome.

This section of the chapter identifies the research studies which support these conclusions. Collectively, these five conclusions point to the need for an intervention model based on the assessment and improvement of functioning, rather than the typical assessing and treating of symptomology. This research also indicates that functioning or skill performance is an entirely different dimension from pathology or symptoms. In other words, a singular focus on symptom removal will not improve functioning. Typically, a rehabilitation approach is needed to complement treatments aimed at reducing symptoms.

1. *Measures of psychiatric symptoms do not predict vocational rehabilitation outcome.* A number of studies illustrate the lack of a relationship between future work performance and a variety of assessments of psychiatric symptomatology (Berg 1983; Ciardiello, Klein, and Sobkowski 1984; Ellsworth et al. 1968; Green, Miskimins, and Keil 1968; Gurel and Lorei 1972; Moller et al. 1982; Schwartz, Myers, and Astrachan 1975; Strauss and Carpenter 1972, 1974; Wilson, Berry, and Miskimins 1969). There appear to be no symptoms or symptom patterns that are routinely related to individual work performance.

Examples from studies indicating what did *not* correlate with vocational performance include assessments of tension, distress or alienation, antisocial behavior (Lorei 1967); depression, anxiety, paranoid hostility, deteriorated thought (Ellsworth et al. 1968); alertness, orientation, use of defenses (Green, Miskimins, and Keil 1968); anxiety, verbal hostility, depression (Gurel and Lorei 1972); thought disorder, depression, flattened emotion (Strauss and Carpenter 1974); confusion, mania, depression (Schwartz, Myers, and Astrachan 1975); and global psychopathological state (Moller et al. 1982). In a more general statement, Strauss and Carpenter (1972) commented that 30 of 32 measures of signs and symptoms were *not* significantly correlated with unemployment. Similarly, Wilson and co-workers (1969) reported that "very few" of the psychiatric variables used in their investigation were able to differentiate vocational successes from failures, either in the validation or cross-validation groups.

In contrast to the lack of relationship between symptoms and vocational outcome are those studies which have found a relationship between measures of ego strength (of self-concept) and vocational outcome. While the number of studies is small, the findings are consistent. In all studies the measures of self-concept or ego functioning related to vocational outcome (Berry and Miskimins 1969; Bidwell 1969; Ciardiello, Klein, and Sobkowski 1984; Conners et al. 1960; Stotsky and Weinberg 1956). Ciardiello and her associates have done the most integrative and most recent work in this regard, and have suggested that the independence of symptom measures and vocational rehabilitation functioning may be due to the fact that persons use a different set of ego functions in work than are needed to maintain mental health.

2. *The psychiatric diagnosis does not predict vocational rehabilitation outcome.* Given the previous findings of no consistent relationship between symptoms and vocational performance, it would be expected that there would be no relationship between diagnostic labels and future vocational performance. An overwhelming number of studies have confirmed the absence of such a relationship (Distefano and Pryer 1970, Ethridge 1968; Goss and Pate 1967, Hall, Smith, and Skimkunas 1966; Lorei 1967; Moller et al. 1982; Sturm and Lipton 1967; Watts and Bennett 1977).

3. *Measures of psychiatric symptoms do not correlate with the psychiatrically disabled person's skills.* Measures of a psychiatrically disabled person's skills and measures of that person's symptoms show little relationship to one another. This is most apparent in studies that have targeted either skills or symptoms as their diagnostic or treatment focus, but that have not taken measures of both. In terms of diagnosis, Lowell and associates (1985) assessed and clustered inpatients into ten different skill groups. They reported no relationships between primary diagnostic category and skill category. In terms of treatment, it is well known that hospitalization and drug treatment affect symptomatology, yet have little impact on a person's vocational skills (Anthony, Cohen, and Vitalo 1978; Ellsworth et al.

1968; Englehardt and Rosen 1976). Englehardt and Rosen (1976) concluded from their review of drug treatment that although psychotropic medication impacts on symptomatology, "evidence for a direct effect of pharmacotherapy on the work performance of schizophrenic patients is, so far, lacking." Similarly, researchers who have reported increases in skill performance have not found corresponding decreases in symptoms. Vitalo (1971) found that a group of psychiatrically disabled persons who successfully learned interpersonal skills also increased in their level of symptomatology. Other investigators have reported that while hospitalization and/or drug treatment significantly reduces severe psychiatric symptoms, there is no corresponding dramatic increase in role performance (Billings and Moos 1985; Dion 1985; Summers 1981).

4. *Measures of skills do predict vocational rehabilitation outcomes.* In every study in which work-adjustment skills have been assessed, they were found to be significantly related to future performance (Cheadle et al. 1967; Distefano and Pryer 1970; Ethridge 1968; Fortune and Eldridge 1982; Green, Miskimins, and Keil 1968, Griffiths 1973; Miskimins et al. 1969; Watts 1978; Wilson, Berry, and Miskimins 1969). In every instance in which an overall measure of work-adjustment skills was calculated, the total score was predictive of future vocational performance (Cheadle et al. 1967; Cheadle and Morgan 1972; Distefano and Pryer 1970; Ethridge 1968; Griffiths 1973).

A nationwide survey of 281 vocational evaluators who assess psychiatrically disabled persons supported the empirical relationship between work-adjustment skills and vocational rehabilitation outcome (Hursh 1983). The vocational evaluators rated work-adjustment and interpersonal skills as the client characteristics most strongly related to vocational outcome. They also rated psychiatric symptomatology as a poor predictor of future vocational success.

Similar to these data on work-adjustment skills, ratings of social abilities or skills have been found to predict vocational performance (Green, Miskimins, and Keil 1968; Griffiths 1974, Gurel and Lorei 1972; Miskimins et al. 1969; Strauss and Carpenter 1974; Sturm and Lipton 1967). Unfortunately, one of the difficulties in reviewing these studies is that it is not always clear whether those rating social functioning used information about a person's present or past work-related social behavior as part of their overall estimate of social functioning. Nevertheless, the data are once again consistent in suggesting that knowledge of persons' social abilities can be used to make inferences about their future vocational performance.

5. *Training in critical vocational skills improves vocational rehabilitation outcome.* If client skills are related to vocational outcome, it stands to reason that training clients to perform at higher levels of vocational skills should increase vocational rehabilitation outcome. Most of the research on vocational skill development has focused on career placement

and job-seeking skills. Career-placement training, first developed over fourteen years ago by the Minnesota Rehabilitation Center (Anderson 1968), has become a credible rehabilitation intervention. Research conducted throughout the 1970s indicates that training clients in career-placement skills does have a significant impact on vocational outcome (Anderson 1968; Azrin, Flores, and Kaplan 1975; Azrin and Philip 1979; McLure 1972; Stude and Pauls 1977; Ugland 1977; Wesolowski 1980). Evidence of the intense interest in career-placement training is provided in a comparative review of six current career-placement packages (Wesolowski 1981).

An occupational skills/work-adjustment training program conducted at a state hospital was reviewed by Rubin and Roessler (1978). Thirty-seven of the forty patients who entered the program completed it, twenty-two obtained jobs, and six enrolled in further training. The effects of skills training in career decision-making is rarely reported in the literature. However, in a small quasi-experimental study, Kline and Hoisington (1981) did investigate the impact of a work values group which met for 1.5 hours per week for twelve weeks. Over 50 percent of the participants in the work values group obtained employment; in the comparison group, only 10 percent obtained employment. In summary, the data on vocational skills development suggest the potential of skills training for improving the vocational rehabilitation of the severely psychiatrically disabled.

The Psychiatric Rehabilitation Process

The psychiatric rehabilitation process is built on the conceptual and empirical foundations described in the previous sections. The process of psychiatric rehabilitation consists of three phases: diagnosis, planning, and intervention. The vocational rehabilitation process is an application of this three-pronged process to severely psychiatrically disabled persons who want to improve their vocational functioning.

The diagnostic phase lays the groundwork for the development of the rehabilitation plan. In contrast to the traditional psychiatric diagnosis, which describes symptomotology, the rehabilitation diagnosis yields a practical description of the psychiatrically disabled person's current level of skill functioning and environmental supports in relation to the environment in which the client wants to function.

Vocational rehabilitation begins, as does the general psychiatric rehabilitation process, with a diagnosis of whether the client has the skills and supports important for success and satisfaction in the environment in which the client chooses to work. While it seems obvious that the client needs to first choose the environment in which she or he wishes to work and needs then to participate in a vocational evaluation for that chosen environment, it often does not happen that way. Too often it is the practitioner who chooses the environment for the client, or who evaluates the client's potential independent of the client's stated vocational goals.

The diagnostic information enables the rehabilitation practitioner to work with the client in the planning phase to develop a vocational rehabilitation plan. A rehabilitation plan specifies how to change the person's skills and/or the person's work environment to achieve the person's vocational rehabilitation goals. The vocational rehabilitation plan (VRP) is similar to the individualized written rehabilitation plan (IWRP) used by counselors employed by state divisions of vocational rehabilitation in that both specify a vocational outcome, and schedule over time the interventions needed to assist the client in attaining the outcome. In an IWRP, the desired vocational outcome, or vocational objective, is designated as a specific occupation or type of work. However, there are differences. The overall rehabilitation goal on a VRP specifies the specific environment or setting in which the work related to a desired vocational outcome will be performed. Also on a VRP, the interventions listed are always directly related to the individual skills or resources a client will need to function successfully in this specified environment.

In the intervention phase, the vocational rehabilitation plan is carried out to increase the person's skills and/or to make the work environment more supportive of the person's functioning. The skill-development interventions include direct skills teaching and skills programming. Severely psychiatrically disabled clients do not use skills as needed either because they cannot perform the skills or because they have a problem using the skills in the particular work environment. When clients cannot perform skills, they usually need to be taught systematically. When clients have a problem using skills in a particular environment, they need to develop a step-by-step procedure to overcome the specific barriers to skill use. In addition to the two skill development interventions there are two types of resource-development interventions designed to make the environment more supportive of the client; resource coordination, which links the client to a preferred resource, and resource modification, which improves the level of support given by an existing resource.

The Characteristics of a Vocational Rehabilitation Practitioner

The articulation of the three phases of the psychiatric rehabilitation process—rehabilitation diagnosis, rehabilitation planning, and rehabilitation intervention—has made it possible to specify the practitioner skills and program characteristics required for vocational rehabilitation to occur. Vocational rehabilitation practitioners who work with the psychiatrically disabled need certain kinds of knowledge, attitudes, and skills to effectively guide the client through the three phases of rehabilitation. The knowledge required includes knowledge about the client population, psychiatric disabilities, vocational rehabilitation practice, research on vocational rehabilitation with the psychiatrically disabled, and the functions of other disciplines involved with this particular client group. Vocational rehabilitation practitioners also need to know about work settings and their functional requirements (Farkas and Anthony 1980). Attitudinally, practitioners need to be positive about severely psychiatrically disabled clients' potential for employment, as well as believe in their own ability to facilitate vocational rehabilitation through the application of the psychiatric rehabilitation process.

In addition to the basic knowledge and favorable attitudes, the practitioner needs a comprehensive repertoire of skills to increase client success in their chosen work settings. The Center for Psychiatric Rehabilitation has described the critical skills a practitioner needs to assist clients through the three phases of rehabilitation (Center for Rehabilitation Research and Training 1984; Cohen, Danley, and Nemec 1985; Cohen, Farkas, and Cohen 1986). Table 5.2 provides a summary of the major practitioner skill areas categorized by the rehabilitation phase in which they are used.

Skills Needed in Rehabilitation Diagnosis

Practitioners conducting a rehabilitation diagnosis involve clients in coming to an agreement about the environments in which they intend to function in the next six to eighteen months, that is, they must help clients set overall rehabilitation goals—for example, "working in the maintenance program at the alternatives workshop until October of next year." This overall vocational rehabilitation goal is the basis for a subsequent skill and resource assessment.

By means of a functional assessment, the practitioner and client develop an understanding of those work-related skills which the client can and cannot perform related to achieving the client's overall vocational rehabilitation goal. Practitioners work with clients to generate a list of unique skills based on the behavioral requirements of the chosen work setting, as well as based on the behaviors which the clients believe to be important to increasing their satisfaction in the particular settings they have chosen. Usually, the behavioral requirements of work settings focus on three key

Table 5.2
Skills Needed by Psychiatric Rehabilitation Practitioners in Three Areas

Rehabilitation diagnosis	*Rehabilitation interventions*
Setting overall rehabilitation goals	Direct skills teaching
Functional assessment	Skills programming
Resource assessment	Resource coordination
	Resource modification
Rehabilitation planning	
Selecting high-priority objectives	
Assigning interventions	
Monitoring the plan	

areas: doing the job, dependability, and getting along with others. For example, a skill important for getting along with others is the ability to respond to criticism. The use of that skill on the job may be described as follows: "The percentage of times per week the client restates the feelings of her supervisor and reasons for those feelings when the supervisor has told her that her work is not satisfactory." Once use of the skill is described, the client and practitioner evaluate the client's present and needed use of this skill.

A resource assessment evaluates the presence or absence of supports critical to the client's achieving the vocational rehabilitation goal. By means of a resource assessment, the practitioner involves the client in listing those persons, places, or things which are necessary for the client to be successful in the client's chosen work setting. Again, the resources listed are based on both environmental requirements and personal needs. For example, the work setting may require the client to wear a laundered uniform. The resource assessment might evaluate the present and needed "number of days per week the client's uniform is washed and ironed before she leaves home at 4 P.M. to go to work." Table 5.3 presents a sample portion of a completed functional assessment chart, and Table 5.4 presents a sample portion of a resource assessment chart.

Skills Needed in Rehabilitation Planning

On the basis of the diagnosis, the practitioner assigns priorities to the skill and resource development objectives which will be the initial focus of the intervention phase. The practitioner identifies a specific intervention for each skill or resource objective in the plan and organizes the persons responsible for carrying out each intervention. The client and practitioners sign the rehabilitation plan to indicate agreement. Table 5.5 presents a sample portion of a vocational rehabilitation plan.

Skills Needed in Rehabilitation Intervention

The rehabilitation practitioner uses two major types of interventions: skill development and resource development. These interventions improve the client's use of skills and supportive resources. There are two ways to develop skills. The first is direct skills teaching. This intervention is used when the functional assessment indicates that the client has not acquired the skill. Direct skills teaching involves leading the client through a systematic series of instructional activities that will result in the client's competent use of new skills. Direct skills teaching is unique in its use of comprehensive teaching methods.

The second way to develop skills is through skills programming, which prescribes a step-by-step procedure to prepare the client to use an existing skill as needed. Skills programming is designed to help clients overcome barriers to using a skill they *can* do. For example, the practitioner might

Table 5.3
Functional Assessment Chart

Name: _____ Eddie _____

Overall Vocational Rehabilitation Goal: To work at the Comet Supermarket Warehouse through January 1987

			Skill functioning[a]					
			Spontaneous use		Prompted use		Perfor-mance	
+/−	Critical skills	Skill use descriptions	Present	Needed	Yes	No	Yes	No
+	Dressing	No. of days/week Eddie puts on clothing appropriate to his work task in his apartment between 7:00 A.M. and 7:30 A.M. weekdays before leaving for work	5	5				
−	Clarifying directions	% of times/week Eddie requests additional information when he is confused by instructions given by the work supervisor at the job site	0	80%	X			
−	Requesting social contact	% of times/week Eddie asks someone to spend time with him when he is doing nothing during breaks or after work	0	75%	X		X	

[a]The client skill level is evaluated in three different ways. The "spontaneous use" column indicates the client's highest level of use of the skill in the particular environment as compared to the needed level of skill use. The "prompted use" column indicates whether the client can (Yes) or cannot (No) perform the skill when asked to in the particular environment. The "performance" column indicates whether the client can (Yes) or cannot (No) perform the skill outside of the particular environment. If the client's present (p) level of spontaneous skill use is zero, then prompted use is evaluated. Similarly, if the client has been evaluated as unable to use the skill when prompted (No), then skill performance is evaluated.

first help the client develop the skill of Responding to Criticism by first teaching her how to "restate another person's feeling and the reasons for the feeling" in simulated situations in the teaching setting. Then the practitioner, together with the client, would use skills programming to generate a series of action steps to overcome the barriers that prevent her from using this skill in the chosen environment as frequently as needed (i.e.,

Table 5.4
Resource Assessment Chart

Name:	Eddie			

Overall Vocational Rehabilitation Goal: To work at the Comet Supermarket Warehouse through January 1987

+/−	Critical resources	Resource use descriptions	Use	
			Present	Needed
−	Supportive supervisor	No. of times/week job site supervisor praises Eddie for completing tasks	0	1
+	Recreational facility	No. of days/weekend staff open the Recreational Center between 10:00 A.M. and 10:00 P.M.	2	2
−	Social contact	No. of days/week friends phone Eddie to talk for 10 min. or more	1	5

70% of the times per week with her supervisor when supervisor says her work is not satisfactory).

In contrast to skill-development interventions, resource-development interventions are designed to link the client with a new resource (resource coordination) or to develop resources which exist but are not meeting the particular needs of the client (resource modification).

Resource coordination involves selecting a preferred resource, arranging for its use, and supporting the client in following through on using the resource. For example, for the client's resource need of "a uniform laundered daily," the client and her practitioner would work to clarify the important values in making a choice about where to go for laundering (e.g., cost, location, type of service offered). Once the resource was selected, the client would be assisted in connecting with the resource. The practitioner would work with both the launderer and the client to overcome any barriers that might prevent the client from successfully using the resource.

Resource modification is the technique of adapting an existing resource to better fit the values or needs of the client. For example, the client's preferred launderer might be her mother. The mother may fit most of her values except that the mother is unable to launder the uniform daily because of other responsibilities. The practitioner might work with the mother to negotiate an arrangement in which the client handles some of the mother's other responsibilities in exchange for daily laundering of the client's uniform.

In summary, the vocational rehabilitation practitioner has a set of skills which engage clients and significant others in diagnosing, planning, and intervening to develop the skills and resources required by the client to be successful and satisfied in a chosen vocational environment. The practitioner's ability to involve the client is facilitated by the practitioner's abil-

Table 5.5
Vocational Rehabilitation Plan

Name: _____ Eddie _____

Overall Vocational Rehabilitation Goal: To work at the Comet Supermarket Warehouse through January 1987

Development objective			Intervention prescribed	Person(s) responsible	Starting date		Completion date	
Skill	Resource	Name			Projected	Actual	Projected	Actual
X		Clarifying directions	Skills programming	Job coach	Sept. 15		Oct. 15	
	X	Social contact	Resource coordination	Mental health case manager	July 6		Sept. 15	
X		Requesting social contact	Direct skills teaching	Work adjustment counselor	Aug. 1		Sept. 15	
	X	Supportive supervisor	Resource modification	Job coach	July 6		Aug. 15	
Mental health intervention								

Plan Development Date: June 30, 1986   Rehabilitation client: _____
Plan Review Date: October 1, 1986   Plan developer: _____

ity to explain the rehabilitation process to the client and the practitioner's level of interpersonal skills. Rehabilitation is done *with* clients and not *to* them (Anthony 1979), and to that extent they must understand the process and be encouraged to participate.

Characteristics of a Vocational Rehabilitation Program

The major characteristics of a vocational rehabilitation program have been described and defined (Anthony, Cohen, and Farkas 1982, 1986; Farkas, Cohen, and Nemec 1985). These are the program mission; program structure for delivering diagnosis, planning, and interventions; and the network of environments in which the program operates.

The Program Mission

The statement of the program mission gives overall direction and purpose to the program. The psychiatric rehabilitation mission is "to increase a person's ability to function in the environment of that person's choice, given the least amount of intervention necessary" (Anthony 1979). The program's mission is demonstrated by written statements of program purpose and by verbal statements by program leaders and administrators.

Based on the psychiatric rehabilitation mission, an ideal vocational rehabilitation mission statement includes four key concepts: functioning, client choice, environmental specificity, and independence.

The first key mission concept addresses the program's focus on client
functioning. This orientation directs program activitites towards the development of the client's work-related competencies, rather than the reduction of symptoms. The second concept critical to psychiatric rehabilitation stresses the importance of client choice. To the degree possible the
clients are in control of the rehabilitation process, with the right to obtain
practitioner assistance in becoming successful and satisfied in work environments they choose, rather than ones in which they are placed. The
third concept, environmental specificity, emphasizes the need to view the
person's functioning in relationship to the demands of a particular setting.
The last concept basic to the psychiatric rehabilitation program's mission
is independence. The mission of the program is to increase the client's vocational independence progressively rather than to maintain the client in a
vocational setting permanently by providing a high level of support (e.g.,
permanent placement in a sheltered workshop.) The psychiatric rehabilitation mission defines increased independence as "the least amount of
intervention necessary." While the mission puts forth the value of independence, there is also recognition that some support (i.e., relative dependency) may always be needed. In psychiatric rehabilitation, it is expected
that a minimal level of support may always be needed. The goal is to increase client functioning while decreasing professional support.

The Program Structure

The program structure is designed to facilitate the client's movement
through the rehabilitation process of diagnosis, planning, and intervention. The program's structure includes activities, policies, and record-
keeping which reflect the program's mission. Upon client entrance into the
agency, the program structure provides the client the opportunity to explore and define his or her overall vocational rehabilitation goals. A program may organize visits to various work sites to allow clients to begin to
clarify for themselves what work they want and do not want to do. Program activities are also organized to involve clients in (1) an assessment of
their skills and supports in relation to their overall vocational rehabilitation goals; (2) development of rehabilitation plans; (3) skill teaching designed to develop the work-related skills they do not have; and (4) practice
of the skills they need to improve. Such a program structure requires
a flexible policy that designs activities based on the needs of the current
clients.

The program structure also includes time to develop skill-use programs
that assists the clients in using their skills in their chosen work environments. In addition to skill-development interventions, the program struc-

ture also assists the clients in obtaining the resources they lack. Program records based on the psychiatric rehabilitation approach require the practitioner to document evidence for each portion of the rehabilitation process. For instance, the records ask for an overall vocational rehabilitation goal chosen by the clients during the rehabilitation diagnosis; a section of the records asks for an evaluation of the clients' functioning on described skills (i.e., functional assessment).

Practitioners' job descriptions based on the rehabilitation approach include the diagnosis, planning, or intervention activities which are appropriate for them. The intake worker may, for instance, be designated as the staff person who, with the client, identifies the overall vocational rehabilitation goal. Evaluation unit staff may conduct functional assessments on critical skills related to specific work settings; a curriculum developer may develop content outlines and lesson plans, while work skills teachers conduct the classes and work site supervisors develop skill-use programs with clients. The assignment of staff varies greatly from program to program. The total job description reflects the entire process of diagnosis, planning, and intervention.

The Network of Environments

A vocational rehabilitation program is complete only to the extent that it has access to a range of vocational settings for both preparation and placement. The range of settings includes work, educational and training sites that vary to accommodate different vocational interests, the amount of skill required, and the supports offered to accommodate different levels of client functioning.

The vocational settings are a network in that the entry and exit criteria of the different settings are related. Such a network can prepare a client to succeed in an indepedent work setting such as competitive employment by offering a less demanding setting initially (e.g., transitional employment), a setting which requires fewer skills and offers more support in which to work and improve skills.

An ideal network of environments allows clients a variety of options that match their values as well as their functional abilities. Some clients prefer to work with people in service jobs; some prefer to work with computers in information jobs. The types of work settings included in the network of environments vary according to the interests and needs of the specific client population, as well as the types of jobs available in the particular geographic area. Thus, there is not a recommended continuum of standard types of vocational settings; rather, there is an individualized range of integrated settings. An ideal vocational rehabilitation program has access to a sufficient variety of work, educational, and training settings so that the client does not have to "fit" or be placed in a setting simply because it is available.

In summary, the essential ingredients of a vocational rehabilitation program for the psychiatrically disabled include (*a*) a mission which focuses the program on increasing client functioning in a specific vocational environment of choice, while decreasing the amount of long-term professional support; (*b*) a structure which is designed to involve clients in rehabilitation diagnosis, rehabilitation planning, and rehabilitation interventions; and (*c*) a network of environments which allow clients to choose settings that match their abilities and preferences.

Principles of Psychiatric Vocational Rehabilitation

The principles underlying the vocational rehabilitation of the psychiatrically disabled flow from a conceptual and empirical foundation. They are rooted in the psychiatric rehabilitation process and evidenced in the functioning of expert practitioners and model programs.

While there is still much to learn about the vocational rehabilitation of persons with psychiatric disabilities, there is enough knowledge available to formulate some basic principles which should be inherent in effective vocational rehabilitation programs. The following is a delineation of some of the major considerations necessary to the development of effective vocational rehabilitation programs for persons with psychiatric disabilities.

1. *Effective vocational programming acknowledges each client's values and personal strengths.* Although there is an obvious need to consider a client's limitations and to provide interventions to overcome them, it is essential to base vocational rehabilitation on a comprehensive understanding of what the client wants to gain from working and what he or she can contribute as a worker. A vocational goal anchored in understanding of the client is more likely to be a goal in which the client is invested and which he or she is motivated to attain.

2. *Effective vocational rehabilitation programs have access to a network of learning and working environments.* If successful job tenure is to occur, clients must have the opportunity to select work settings which match their occupational values and skills. Also, they may have access to a variety of "learning environments" which can help them develop the knowledge and skills required for desired occupational goals.

In some cases, special learning environments are needed for the development of basic skills associated with appropriate work behavior, such as getting along with co-workers or dependability. In other cases, more formal educational settings are needed in which knowledge, credentials, and specialty skills can be obtained. The number and variety of educational settings will vary with the needs of each client, as will time required in each setting.

Even more important than preparatory settings is the availability of nonstigmatizing work settings which are compatible with client interests, values, and abilities. Presently, psychiatric disabilities are among those which are least understood and most feared by employers. Effective vocational rehabilitation programs contain assertive and supportive job development and placement components which are rooted in a thorough and realistic knowledge of the client. In addition, effective job development and placement programming reflects a detailed understanding of the businesses and industries in which prospective clients may be placed.

For optimal results, interventions may be required with both the client and the employer. These interventions may begin before placement and may be needed for an indefinite length of time throughout the client's work experience. Thus, some clients may be participating simultaneously in learning and work environments for extended time periods so that skill and resource deficits which emerge as a result of work experiences can be identified and eliminated.

3. *Effective vocational rehabilitation programming provides the opportunity for clients to engage in activities designed to increase vocational maturity.* Vocational maturation can be described as the process by which vocational behavior becomes more goal-directed, more realistic, and more independent. The assumption is that those persons with higher levels of vocational maturity will make and implement vocational decisions which result in higher levels of success and satisfaction. Vocational maturity is acquired through implementation of the appropriate vocational development tasks during different life stages (Crites 1961).

For persons with psychiatric illness, the vocational development process is not consistent or smooth. Some lives have been interrupted during adolescence when peers are engaged in high levels of occupational exploration. Others' lives have been disrupted at a later date, so that they must to come to terms with new limitations. Thus, it is necessary to adopt a developmental perspective when doing vocational rehabilitation with persons who have psychiatric disabilities. Vocational immaturity, often expressed as unrealistic goals or inappropriate vocational behavior, may be more a function of "vocational illiteracy" due to inexperience than delusional thinking due to pathology. For many persons in this population, it may be necessary to engage in extensive vocational exploration, so that accurate and current information about themselves and the world of work can be obtained and vocational maturity can be enhanced.

4. *Effective vocational rehabilitation programming provides for activities and environments which enhance self-esteem.* The experience of mental illness often fosters an image of oneself as useless, inadequate, and incompetent. This leads to feelings of hopelessness and helplessness associated with low self-esteem. Since high self-esteem is one of the few personality variables which are somewhat predictive of vocational outcome (Anthony 1979), it is essential for clients to have the opportunity to acquire or regain a positive sense of themselves. One means of enhancing self-esteem

is to provide the opportunity for successful work experience. Many persons with psychiatric disabilities have had little or no work experience. Others have had only bad experiences with work. Still others have previous successful work experiences in which they can no longer engage because of the handicapping nature of their disability. In any case, there is a need to document current levels of function in a real work setting.

Transitional and supported employment settings can provide the opportunity for this documentation (Cohen, Anthony, and Kennard 1986). Such an opportunity contributes to a definition of oneself as a productive person, and additionally can provide the written evidence of successful work experience which is so essential when presenting oneself to a prospective employer.

Throughout the vocational rehabilitation process, care should be taken (1) to demonstrate positive regard and respect for the client, and (2) to provide continuous constructive feedback to reinforce the client's positive behavioral assets. There should be frequent reviews of progress to highlight accomplishments to date and to identify potential problems so that the possible failures can be avoided through advance planning. Vigilant monitoring of the vocational rehabilitation process can promote smooth implementation, a benefit to both the client and the practitioner. Measured achievement during the process of vocational rehabilitation produces concrete evidence of growth and contributes to an improved self-image.

5. *Effective vocational rehabilitation programming applies the psychiatric rehabilitation approach of diagnosis, planning, and intervention.* The process of vocational rehabilitation for psychiatrically disabled clients is a specific application of the psychiatric rehabilitation approach. Each client must be aided to identify, develop, and use the skills and supports needed to succeed and be satisfied in a chosen vocational environment.

During vocational rehabilitation the client participates in a variety of activities in a number of different settings for the purpose of vocational preparation and placement. If a client is to participate successfully in these vocational activities and settings, the rehabilitation practitioner must diagnose, plan, and provide the appropriate skill development and support development interventions to ensure success *in each environment* in which these activities occur. For example, if a client is to spend a period of time in a setting for the purpose of occupational skills training, the client and practitioner should select a setting most compatible with the client's values, identify the skills and supports the client will need to be a full participant in the setting, and engage in a planned series of interventions designed to enable the client to develop the skills and supports needed to be successful in the setting. Later, when the client is ready for an actual work placement, the process of diagnosis, planning, and intervention must be repeated in relation to the relevant work environment. This procedure should be repeated for every educational and work setting in which the client will function, throughout all phases of vocational rehabilitation. Such care in environmental selection and client preparation will improve the client's chances of participating fully and of making progress in each new setting.

Summary

The psychiatric rehabilitation model can guide the practice of vocational rehabilitation for persons who have experienced a severe psychiatric disability. Conceptually, the psychiatric rehabilitation model is based on the philosophy and principles of physical rehabilitation. Empirically, it is grounded in numerous studies of the relationship between vocational functioning, client characteristics and program ingredients.

The process of vocational rehabilitation of persons with psychiatric disabilities is a special application of the psychiatric rehabilitation model. The practitioner and program characteristics relevant to a positive vocational rehabilitation outcome of the severely psychiatrically disabled are observable and can be described in concrete, measurable terms.

References

Anderson, J. A. 1968. The disadvantaged seek work—through their efforts or ours? *Rehabilitation Record*, 9, 5–10.

Anthony, W. A. 1979. *Principles of psychiatric rehabilitation*. Baltimore: University Park Press.

———. 1980. A rehabilitation model for rehabilitating the psychiatrically disabled. *Rehabilitation Counseling Bulletin*, 24, 6–21.

———. 1982. Explaining "psychiatric rehabilitation" by analogy to "physical rehabilitation." *Psychosocial Rehabilitation Journal*, 5, 61–66.

Anthony, W. A.; Buell, G. J.; Sharratt, S.; and Althoff, M. E. 1972. The efficacy of psychiatric rehabilitation. *Psychological Bulletin*, 78, 447–456.

Anthony, W. A.; Cohen, M. R.; and Farkas, M. 1982. A psychiatric rehabilitation treatment program: Can I recognize one if I see one? *Community Mental Health Journal*, 18, 83–96.

———. 1986. Training and technical assistance in psychiatric rehabilitation. In *Psychiatric disability: Clinical administrative and legal aspects*, ed. A. Meyerson. Washington, D.C.: American Psychiatric Association.

Anthony, W. A.; Cohen, M. R.; and Vitalo, R. 1978. The measurement of rehabilitation outcome. *Schizophrenia Bulletin*, 4, 365–83.

Anthony, W. A.; Howell, J.; and Danley, K. 1984. The vocational rehabilitation of the psychiatrically disabled. In *The chronically mentally ill: Research and services*, ed. M. Mirabi. New York: SP Medical and Scientific Books.

Azrin, N. H.; Flores, T.; and Kaplan, S. J. 1975. Job-finding club: A group-assisted program for obtaining employment. *Behavior Research and Therapy*, 13, 17–27.

Azrin, N. H., and Philip, R. A. 1979. The job club method for the job handicapped: A comparative outcome study. *Rehabilitation Counseling Bulletin*, 23, 144–55.

Berg, G. 1983. Locus of control, vocational control, and vocational value as predictors of the post-hospital employment status of psychiatric patients. Ph.D., Diss., New York University.

Berry, K. L., and Miskimins, R. W. 1969. Concept of self and post-hospital vocational adjustment. *Journal of Consulting and Clinical Psychology, 33*, 103–8.

Bidwell, G. 1969. Ego strength, self-knowledge, and vocational planning of schizophrenics. *Journal of Counseling Psychology, 16*, 45–49.

Billings, A. G., and Moos, R. H. 1985. Life stressors and social resources affect post-treatment outcomes among depressed patients. *Journal of Abnormal Psychology, 94*, 140–53.

Center for Rehabilitation Research and Training in Mental Health. 1984. Final Report of National Institute of Handicapped. Research Grant no. G00 800 5486. Washington, D.C.

Cheadle, A. J.; Cushing, D.; Drew, C.; and Morgan, R. 1967. The measurement of the work performance of psychiatric patients. *British Journal of Psychiatry, 113*, 841–46.

Cheadle, A.J., and Morgan, R. 1972. The measurement of work performance of psychiatric patients: A reappraisal. *British Journal of Psychiatry, 120*, 437–41.

Ciardiello, J. A.; Klein, M. E.; and Sobkowski, S. 1984. Ego functioning and the vocational rehabilitation of schizophrenic clients. In *The broad scope of ego function assessment.* ed. L. Bellack and L. Goldsmith. New York: Wiley and Sons.

Cohen, B. F.; Anthony, W. A.; and Kennard, W. A. 1986. Opening the work place to the psychiatrically disabled. *Business and Health,* March, pp. 9–11.

Cohen, M.; Danley, K.; and Nemec, P. 1985. *Psychiatric rehabilitation trainer packages: Direct skills teaching.* Boston: Center for Psychiatric Rehabilitation.

Cohen, M.; Farkas, M.; and Cohen, B. 1986. *Psychiatric rehabilitation trainer packages: Functional assessment.* Boston: Center for Psychiatric Rehabilitation.

Conners, J. E.; Wolkon, G. H.; Haefner, D.; and Stotsky, B. A. 1960. Outcome of post-hospital rehabilitative treatment of mental patients as a function of ego strength. *Journal of Counseling Psychology, 7*, 278–82.

Crites, J. 1961. A model for the measurement of vocational maturity. *Journal of Counseling Psychology, 8*, 255–59.

Dion, G. L. 1985. Parameters and predictors of functional outcome on bipolar patients hospitalized for a manic episode: Results of a two- and six-month follow-up. Ph.D. diss., Boston University.

Distefano, M. K., and Pryer, M. W. 1970. Vocational evaluation and successful placement of psychiatric clients in a vocational rehabilitation program. *American Journal of Occupational Therapy, 24*, 205–7.

Ellsworth, R. B.; Foster, L.; Childers, B.; Arthur, G.; and Kroeker, D. 1968. Hospital and community adjustment as perceived by psychiatric patients, their families, and staff. *Journal of Consulting and Clinical Psychology Monographs, 32* (3), pt. 2.

Englehardt, P. M., and Rosen, B. 1976. Implications of drug treatment for the social rehabilitation of schizophrenic patients. *Schizophrenia Bulletin, 2*, 454–62.

Ethridge, D. A. 1968. Prevocational assessment of the rehabilitation potential of psychiatric patients. *American Journal of Occupational Therapy, 22*, 161–67.

Farkas, M., and Anthony. W. 1980. Training rehabilitation counselors to work in state agencies, rehabilitation and mental health facilities. *Rehabilitation Counseling Bulletin, 24*, 128–44.

Farkas, M., Cohen, M., and Nemec, P. 1985. Psychiatric rehabilitation programs: Putting concepts into practice? Center for Psychiatric Rehabilitation, Boston University, Boston.

Fortune, J., and Eldredge, G. 1982. Predictive validation of the McGarron-Dial evaluation system for psychiatrically disabled sheltered workshop workers. *Vocational Evaluation and Work Adjustment Bulletin,* Winter, pp. 136–41.

Frey, W. 1984. Functional assessment in the '80's. In *Functional assessment in rehabilitation,* ed. A. Halpern and M. Fuhrer. Baltimore: Paul H. Brookes.

Goss, A. M., and Pate, K. D. 1967. Predicting vocational rehabilitation success for psychiatric patients with psychological tests. *Psychological Reports, 21,* 725–30.

Green, H. J.; Miskimins, R. W.; and Keil, E. C. 1968. Selection of psychiatric patients for vocational rehabilitation. *Rehabilitation Counseling Bulletin, 11,* 297–302.

Griffiths, R. 1973. A standardized assessment of the work behavior of psychiatric patients. *British Journal of Psychiatry, 123,* 403–8.

———. Rehabilitation of chronic psychotic patients. *Psychological Medicine, 4,* 316–25.

Gurel, L., and Lorei, T. W. 1972. Hospital and community ratings of psychopathology as predictors of employment and readmission. *Journal of Consulting and Clinical Psychology, 34,* 286–91.

Hall, J. C.; Smith, K.; and Skimkunas, A. 1966. Employment problems of schizophrenic patients. *American Journal of Psychiatry, 123,* 536–40.

Hursh, N. 1983. Diagnostic vocational evaluation with psychiatrically disabled individuals: A national survey. Paper presented at the annual meeting of the American Psychological Association, Anaheim, Calif.

Kessler, H. H. 1935. *The crippled and the disabled: Rehabilitation of the physically handicapped in the United States.* New York: Columbia University Press.

Kline, A., and Hoisington, B. 1981. Placing the psychiatrically disabled: A look at work values. *Rehabilitation Counseling Bulletin, 25,* 365–69.

Leitner, L, and Drasgow, J. 1972. Battling recidivism. *Journal of Rehabilitation,* July–August, pp. 29–31.

Lorei, T. W. 1967. Prediction of community stay and employment for released psychiatric patients. *Journal of Consulting Psychology, 31,* 349–57.

Lowell, W. E.; MacLean, N. V.; and Carrol, M. 1985. The use of cluster analysis in determining patient selection for rehabilitation programs. *Psychosocial Rehabilitation Journal, 8* (3), 15–27.

McLure, D. P. 1972. Placement through improvement of client's job-seeking skills. *Journal of Applied Rehabilitation, 3,* 188–96.

Miskimins, R.; Wilson, L.; Berry, K.; Oetting, E.; and Cole, C. 1969. Person-placement congruence: A framework for vocational counselors. *Personnel and Guidance Journal,* April, pp. 789–93.

Moller, H.; von Zerssen, D.; Werner-Eilert, K.; and Wuschenr-Stockheim, M. 1982. Outcome in schizophrenic and similar paranoid psychoses. *Schizophrenia Bulletin, 8,* 99–108.

Rubin, S. W., and Roessler, R. T. 1978. Guidelines for successful vocational rehabilitation of the psychiatrically disabled. *Rehabilitation Literature, 39,* 70–74.

Rusk, H. A., and Taylor, E. 1949. *New hope for the handicapped: The rehabilitation of the disabled from bed to job.* New York: Harper.

Schwartz, C.; Myers, J.; and Astrachan, B. 1975. Concordance of multiple assessments of the outcome of schizophrenia. *Archives of General Psychiatry, 32,* 1221–27.

Stotsky, B., and Weinberg, H. 1959. The prediction of the psychiatric patient's work adjustment. *Journal of Counseling Psychology, 3,* 3–7.

Strauss, J., and Carpenter, W. 1972. The prediction of outcome in schizophrenia. *Archives of General Psychiatry, 27,* 739–46.

———. The prediction of outcome in schizrenia, 2. *Archives of General Psychiatry, 31,* 37–42.

Stude, E. W., and Pauls, T. 1977. The use of a job-seeking skills group in developing placement readiness. *Journal of Applied Rehabilitation Counseling, 8,* 115–20.

Sturm, I. E., and Lipton, H. 1967. Some social and vocational predictors of psychiatric hospitalization outcome. *Journal of Clinical Psychology, 23,* 301–7.

Summers, F. 1981. The post-acute functioning of the schizophrenic. *Journal of Clinical Psychology, 37,* 705–14.

Ugland, R. P. 1977. Job seekers' aids: A systematic approach for organizing employer contacts. *Rehabilitation Counseling Bulletin, 22,* 107–15.

Unger, K., and Anthony, W. A. 1983. Are families satisfied with resources to young adult chronic patients? A recent survey and proposed alternative. In *Advances in treating the young adult chronic patient*, ed. B. Pepper and H. Ryglewicz. New Directions for Mental Health Services Source Book. San Francisco: Jossey-Bass.

Vitalo, R. L. 1971. Teaching improved interpersonal functioning as a preferred mode of treatment. *Journal of Clinical Psychology, 27,* 166–71.

Watts, F., and Bennett, D. 1977. Previous occupational stability as a predictor of employment after psychiatric rehabilitation. *Psychological Medicine, 7,* 709–12.

Watts, R. 1978. A study of work behavior in a psychiatric rehabilitation unit. *British Journal of Clinical Psychology, 17,* 85–92.

Wesolowski, M. D. 1980. JOBS (job-obtaining behavior strategy) in VR agencies: The effects of attendance and disincentives. *International Journal of Rehabilitation Research, 3,* 531–32.

————. 1981. Self-directed job placement in rehabilitation: A comparative review. *Rehabilitation Counseling Bulletin,* November, pp. 80-89.

Wilson, T. L.; Berry, L. K.; and Miskimins, W. R. 1969. An assessment of characteristics related to vocational success among restored psychiatric patients. *The Vocational Guidance Quarterly, 18,* 110–14.

Wood, P.H.N. 1980. Appreciating the consequences of disease: The classification of impairments, disabilities, and handicaps. *The WHO Chronicle, 34,* 376–80.

Wright, B. A. 1960. *Psychical disability: A psychological approach.* New York: Harper.

6

Skills Training in Vocational Rehabilitation

KIM T. MUESER and ROBERT PAUL LIBERMAN

Many approaches to rehabilitation over the years have been based on behavioral or social learning techniques. In this chapter, Mueser and Liberman describe three models of skill training: the basic model, the problem-
solving model, and the attention-focusing model. The job-finding club is
used as an illustration of the ways in which skills training can be applied to
vocational rehabilitation. Job-search training and job maintenance are
emphasized and applied to a case example.

The huge influx of chronic psychiatric patients into the community as a
result of deinstitutionalization has created a growing awareness among
the public and mental health practitioners that many of these patients have
severe social deficits, often untouched by their psychoactive medications.
Deficits in life skills are revealed in the difficulties psychiatric patients experience securing and maintaining jobs, gaining social acceptance, and
managing interpersonal relationships. The recognition of social deficiencies among psychiatric patients in the community (Sylph, Ross, and Kedward 1978) has changed the goals of treatment from isolation and con-
tainment to the active building of new repertoires of skills. These skills are
imparted to patients through systematic organization of their immediate
environment (e.g., token economy, social learning, recreation programs)
or the use of structured teaching procedures (e.g., social skills training).
What is new about skills-based treatment is the high level of active participation by the patient and the treatment team, and the specificity with
which behaviors and cognitive skills are targeted for modification.

Research suggests that improving psychiatric patients' skill competencies may not only improve the quality of life of psychiatric patients but
may also be a fruitful strategy for lowering symptoms and remediating

Preparation of this chapter was supported, in part, by grant MH39998 from the National
Institute of Mental Health.

vocational skills. Interpersonal skill deficits have been related to poor employment history. The difficulty chronic mental patients have getting and maintaining jobs has been demonstrated to be more often due to their interpersonal deficits than the actual difficulty of performing the job task (Kelly et al. 1979). Job-finding programs and job-maintenance programs aim at improving these social skills. The adequacy of patients' social functioning has also been correlated with their symptomatology (Casey, Tyrer, and Platt 1985), suggesting that socialization may facilitate reality testing and reduce symptoms that impair vocational skill; and social adjustment has consistently been shown to be a potent predictor of symptom relapses, rehospitalization, and long-term outcome (Phillips and Zigler 1961; Linn, Klett, and Coffey 1982).

Research on the relationship between familial stress and psychiatric relapse also suggests the potential benefits of a skills-based treatment approach. High levels of "expressed emotion"—defined as excessively critical, hostile, or emotionally overinvolved attitudes and behavior by a relative—predispose recovering schizophrenic and depressed patients living at home to more frequent symptom relapses and rehospitalizations (Brown, Birley, and Wing 1972; Hooley, Orley, and Teasdale 1986). Improving the social skills of patients living at home could reduce the stress experienced by family members living with an ill relative whose social behavior does not conform to their expectations, as well as the reciprocal stress on the patient as relatives attempt to induce him to conform. Similarly, teaching healthier communication patterns to relatives and patients could lower ambient negative emotion, thus minimizing patients' psychopathology and frequency of rehospitalizations.

In this chapter we review recent psychosocial techniques that teach interpersonal and cognitive skills through procedures based on the principles of human learning. While many treatment programs share the goal of improving social functioning, it is important to distinguish between nonspecific group activities that engage patients in social interactions, and methods which deliberately and systematically utilize behavioral learning techniques in a structured approach to skills building. While activities that facilitate socialization can lead to skills acquisition through incidental learning during spontaneously occurring interactions, they do not harness social learning and reinforcement techniques that may be required to promote the acquisition, generalization, and maintenance of skills needed in interpersonal situations.

The present review first addresses skills-training innovations based on environmental modifications of the therapeutic milieu. Next, recent social skills training techniques are outlined, followed by the use of these techniques in rehabilitation. Finally, we review advances in behavioral skills development in the context of family therapy.

Skills Training in Social-Learning Environments

It has often been observed that the milieu of many psychiatric hospitals reinforces patients' remaining in the hospital and discourages them from becoming active participants in their own recovery (Goffman 1961; Mechanic 1969), thereby perpetuating their "sick role." One alternative to traditional inpatient "milieu therapy" has been to alter the reinforcement structure of the environment, such that prosocial, desirable behaviors are rewarded, and bizarre, "crazy" behaviors are not. Such programs are called "social-learning" or "token-economy" programs, and usually specify in measurable terms those behaviors that are to be increased in frequency, behaviors that are to be decreased, and the precise rewarding consequences given for engaging in these behaviors.

One of the most comprehensive social learning programs was established by Gordon Paul in the early 1970s (Paul and Lentz 1977; Paul, Tobias, and Holly 1972). Paul and his colleagues worked for more than six years in a regional mental health center with 102 chronic, treatment-refractory inpatients, comparing the clinical efficacy of a social-learning program with an equally structured milieu therapy and custodial care at a state mental hospital. The social-learning program was a token economy designed to modify four categories of behaviors which Paul believed were barriers to leaving the hospital and remaining in the community: poor self-help and social skills, poor instrumental role performance, inadequate community support, and high rates of bizarre behavior.

Results clearly favored the social-learning program over milieu therapy and state hospital custodial care. Ninety-seven percent of the social-learning patients improved sufficiently to attain long-term community placement, compared to 71 percent of the milieu therapy patients, and only 45 percent of the state hospital patients. Furthermore, fewer than 25 percent of the patients in either active psychosocial program required neuroleptic medication by the end of the second year of programming, and this proportion declined even more as the programs continued.

This study's rigorous methodology and meticulous attention to detail makes it a landmark in documenting the clinical superiority of the social-learning approach over milieu and custodial care for the chronically mentally ill. Several other hospital-based social-learning programs have replicated the use of reinforcement procedures to teach new behaviors that improve social functioning (Liberman et al. 1974; Liberman 1976; Banzett et al. 1984).

Social-Skills Training

Psychiatric patients' interpersonal behaviors can be improved by using instructional sessions aimed at teaching, generalizing, and maintaining specific behavioral and cognitive skills. The teaching procedures include goal-setting, focused instructions, modeling, behavior rehearsal, prompting, social reinforcement, shaping successive approximations to desired behaviors, *in vivo* practice of skills, and homework assignments. These teaching procedures are combined in a structured teaching format, which has been variously termed social-skills training (Hersen and Eisler 1976), assertion training (Wolpe 1958; Wolpe and Lazarus 1966), structured-learning therapy (Goldstein 1973), and personal effectiveness training (Liberman et al. 1975).

Social skills can be defined as interpersonal behaviors that are (1) instrumental for maintaining and optimizing independence and community survival, and (2) socio-emotional for establishing, maintaining, and deepening supportive personal relationships. While early definitions of social skills were limited strictly to the domain of behavior, cognitive and affective modalities are now included as relevant dimensions of this construct.

Social-skills training resembles a classroom teaching environment more than a traditional therapy setting. Sessions are highly structured and require the active participation of the patient(s) and the therapist(s). Sessions may be conducted with individual patients or in groups, and may be as brief as ten minutes a day or as long as two hours, depending on the attentional capacities of the patients. Massed practice (i.e., multiple training sessions per week) is preferred to learning less intensively over a longer period. Agendas specifying the behavioral goals are planned in advance and implemented using specific procedures following written guidelines derived from a trainers' manual. Role playing (behavior rehearsal) is the main vehicle for assessing and teaching those social skills which are targeted for intervention. Two types of behavior are usually targeted for modification: *response-topography* behaviors, such as voice volume, fluency, eye contact; and *content* behaviors, such as making a positive statement or requesting additional information. Cognitive problem-solving skills (Siegel & Spivak, 1976) may also be targeted for intervention in some populations.

Over the past fifteen years more than fifty studies have been published in social-skills training with psychiatric patients (for reviews see Wallace et al. 1980; Morrison and Bellack 1984; Brady 1984a, 1984b). These studies provided the first evidence that social-skills training was a feasible treatment strategy, and laid the empirical foundation for recent innovations in training techniques. Many of the early studies suffered from methodological shortcomings, including lack of diagnostic assessment, specifying concomitant psychotropic medications, and use of widely accepted outcome measures, such as symptomatology or relapse rate.

The results of these studies can be summarized by three conclusions:

1. Psychiatric patients can be trained in behaviors that will improve their social skills in specific interpersonal situations.

2. Patients show moderate to substantial generalization of trained behaviors to untrained scenes and items (Goldsmith and McFall 1975; Kelly, Urey, and Patterson 1980; Liberman et al. 1984). The problem of behavioral generalization to different and novel situations appears to be greater for complex behaviors (e.g., requests for behavior change) than for simple behaviors such as eye contact (Bellack, Hersen, and Turner 1976; Fredericksen et al. 1976). This presents a special problem for social-skills training with chronic mental patients living in the community, for whom complex social behaviors may be necessary to utilize accessible resources and generate social support.

3. Comprehensive, intensive social-skills training can reduce clinical symptoms and relapse in psychiatric patients. Among neuroleptic-stabilized schizophrenics, social-skills training significantly lowered symptoms and relapses for both inpatients (Liberman, Mueser, and Wallace 1986) and outpatients (Hogarty et al. 1986). Similarly, schizophrenic patients who participated in a day hospital program and concurrently received social-skills training showed symptom reductions that were more durable over a six-month follow-up period than patients who were in the day program but did not receive social-skills training (Bellack et al. 1984). Social-skills training also alleviates depression for unmedicated depressed outpatients (McKnight et al. 1984), has clinical effects equivalent to antidepressant medication, and is associated with a lower rate of dropout from treatment (Bellack, Hersen and Himmelhoch 1981, 1983).

Many psychiatric patients manifest learning disabilities that require highly directive behavioral techniques for teaching social skills. Chronic patients often have information-processing and attentional deficits and show hyperarousal or hypoarousal during psychophysiological testing. These patients may experience overstimulation from emotional stressors or even from therapy sessions that are not adequately structured and modulated. Chronic patients often fail to be motivated by customary forms of social and tangible rewards available in traditional therapy. The acquisition of other social skills is impaired by their lack of conversational skills, an important building block to the attainment of social competence. Patients with schizophrenia often have deficiencies in their social perception and their ability to generate response alternatives for coping with everyday problems such as making an appointment or getting help with annoying drug effects. Patients with verbal dysfluencies, minimal vocal intonation, and poor eye contact may be further impaired in their social learning.

Psychiatric patients vary greatly in their cognitive and social deficits and, therefore, require social-skills training tailored to their specific needs. Three training models that have been developed for use with psychiatric patients will be described below (Liberman et al. 1975): the basic model, the problem-solving model, and the attention-focusing model.

The Basic Model

The Basic Model has been in use the longest and shares many common features with the problem-solving and attention-focusing models. Training with this model can be conducted either with individual patients or in groups, but the latter will be described for the purposes of simplicity.

1. *Identify the interpersonal problems in each patient by assessing the following questions:* What emotion, need, or communication is lacking or not being appropriately expressed, and how often does this behavior occur? With whom does the patient desire to improve social contact? When does the problem occur? Where does the problem occur?

   A wide variety of techniques can be used to assess interpersonal problems, including simple observation, self-report measures, reports of significant others, and role-play performance. As in other behavior-therapy interventions, assessment is a process that occurs throughout social-skills training.

2. *Specify the goals of training.* New behaviors are taught that rectify deficits in performance or modulate excessive or overly intense emotional expressiveness. The patient with staff help chooses targeted behaviors that are related to achieving an attainable goal. Goals should be specific behaviors that are high in frequency, to provide more opportunity for practice and feedback. The relevant domains of goal-setting—behaviors and emotions, relationships and settings—which combine to set the stage for overcoming the problem and moving towards improved social and emotional functioning, are outlined in Table 6.1.

3. *Engage the patient in a role play of the problem situation using other members of the group to play relevant roles.* These scenes are usually events that have occurred in the recent past or are likely to occur in the near future. The first role play is a "dry run" done "naturally" by the patient, who is simply instructed to act as he or she would if he or she were in the actual situation. Following the dry run, which may be videotaped for immediate feedback, the patient's assets, deficits, and excesses in the role-play performance are noted. The patient is praised for appropriate behaviors and efforts, and positive feedback is solicited from other group members.

Table 6.1
Some Characteristics of Goal-Setting in Social-Skills Training

Targeted behaviors	*Interpersonal targets*
Asking for or giving information	Employers or employees
Initiating or terminating conversations	Family members
Maintaining conversations	Friends, acquaintances
Response topography (eye contact, voice	Hospital or board and care staff
volume, affect)	Sales persons, agency bureaucrats
Targeted emotions	Strangers
Affection, love	
Anger, annoyance, hostility	*Settings*
Assertiveness, dominance	Home, board and care
Frustration	Hospital, mental health center
Happiness, pleasure, delight	Job, school
Interest, empathy	Public place
Sadness, grief	

4. *In a series of role plays, use direct instructions, modeling* (behavioral demonstration by the therapist), *shaping* (reinforcing successive approximations), and *coaching* (verbal and nonverbal prompts given by a therapist to elicit specific behaviors in role play) *to gradually modify the patient's behaviors towards the goal.* Elements of the total gestalt are added one by one, such as eye contact, facial expression, vocal tone and loudness, posture, and speech content. After each role play good elements of the patient's performance are praised by the therapists and group members, and corrective feedback is given regarding deficits. A combination of modeling, shaping, and coaching is used to create further change in the behavioral rehearsal.

5. *Establish a program for generalization of the trained behavior to situations outside the training session by giving homework assignments to practice the skills in the natural environment and by giving positive feedback for successful transfer of skills.* Generalization of skills is improved when training is integrated into the patient's everyday world. Whenever possible, therapy should be taken out of the clinician's office and practiced in homes, wards, schools, stores, restaurants, and other environments where it is desirable to perform the target behaviors. Transfer of skills can also be facilitated by repeated practice and overlearning, teaching the patient to use self-evaluation and self-reinforcement, fading the structure and frequency of training, and ensuring that the natural environment is indeed socially responsive and reinforcing to the patient's skill performance. Friends, family members, nursing staff personnel, and peers can aid in this process by prompting and reinforcing new social behaviors until they are established.

The Problem-Solving Training Model

Many chronic psychiatric patients are deficient in basic problem-solving skills (Platt and Spivack 1972; Edelstein et al. 1980). Recently patients have been taught ways to better process information using a problem-solving procedure that prompts patients to identify short- and long-term goals, generate alternative behaviors, and evaluate the consequences of these behaviors (Foy, Wallace, and Liberman 1983). Information processing in interpersonal communication requires *receiving, processing,* and *sending* skills (Wallace et al. 1980). Receiving skills involve the accurate perception, interpretation, and comprehension of relevant situation parameters. Processing skills involve weighing and selecting response options and determining an implementation strategy. Sending skills are the verbal and nonverbal behaviors emitted in the interpersonal situation that are necessary steps toward attaining the specified goal.

As in the basic model, an interpersonal scene is role-played, and preferably videotaped. After each role play the therapist asks specific questions to assess the patient's receiving and processing skills. Examples of receiving questions are, What did the other person say? What was the other person feeling? What were the person's short-term goals? Examples of processing questions are, what alternative behavior could the person use in this situation? If the person were to do this alternative, what would the other person feel? Would the alternative help the patient achieve his long-term goal? After the patient has shown acceptable receiving skills, the processing and sending skills are assessed by reviewing his videotaped role play. Examples of nonverbal sending skills are eye contact, facial expression, posture, and voice volume. Some verbal sending skills include requesting behavior change, minimal verbal encouragers ("uh huh," "yeah"), and expressing positive or negative feelings directly.

Researchers at the Clinical Research Center for Schizophrenia and Psychiatric Rehabilitation at the Brentwood Psychiatric Division of the West Los Angeles VA Medical Center have developed a comprehensive social skills program for chronic psychiatric patients based on the problem-solving training model. This program is called the Social and Independent Living Skills Program, and includes training "modules" that are being developed in areas such as medication management, leisure and recreation, self-care and personal hygiene, food preparation, money management, and friendship and dating. Training is done in small groups of three to ten patients, meeting in one-and-a-half-hour sessions, one to three times weekly for a period of two to three months, depending on the patient's pretraining skills.

The Attention-Focusing Skills-Training Model

Some chronic patients with incoherence or severe attentional deficits fail to learn new behaviors using the basic or problem-solving skills-training models, and require training procedures that employ stimulus-control techniques to reduce the quantity of material taught on each trial. This model simplifies the learning of complex skills and has been found to be effective in teaching conversation skills to some seriously regressed, chronic psychiatric patients (Massel et al. 1984).

The procedure is characterized by discrete, multiple, relatively short training trials, and employs role-playing, corrective feedback, modeling, prompting, coaching, and reinforcement in a manner similar to that of the other training models. The attention-focusing model differs mainly in presenting the training components in a controlled and sequential way.

The therapist starts the procedure by making a statement to the patient. If the patient responds correctly to the statement, he is praised and sometimes given reinforcement in the form of food or drink. If the patient does not respond correctly, the therapist prompts him or her with increasingly more specific directives. The therapist presents the same statements until he gets several correct responses in succession, and then he goes on to new conversational behaviors.

Skills Training in Vocational Rehabilitation

The research we previously discussed which suggested that structured activities tend to reduce idiosyncratic and stereotypic behaviors (Rosen et al. 1981; Wong et al. 1985) leads us to believe that employment may have a beneficial effect on psychiatric symptoms. Other evidence that supports this belief includes an association between unemployment and more admissions to psychiatric hospitals (Brenner 1973), and correlations between unemployment and depression, suicide, and other symptoms (Hagen 1983). Although employment may have clinical advantages, most chronically mentally ill patients (as high as 80%) are unemployed in the United States (Goldstrom and Mandersheid 1982). This rate compares unfavorably with the high rates of employment for recovering psychiatric patients in nations such as the People's Republic of China (Walls, Walls, and Langsley 1975), Norway (Astrup, Fossum, and Holmboe 1962), and the Soviet Union (Wortis 1950). The low employment rate among mental patients in America reflects their difficulty in both obtaining and maintaining jobs. Approximately 20–30 percent of patients return to work within six months of their discharge from the hospital, but only 15 percent are still employed one year later (Anthony, Cohen, and Vitalo 1978).

Most recovering psychiatric patients find unemployment to be strongly aversive. In a survey of 500 chronic mental patients residing in Los Angeles board-and-care homes, Lehman (1983) found that lack of work was one of the greatest complaints related to poor quality of life. Even chronically impaired patients supported by Social Security pensions had not relinquished their aspirations for a job. Indeed, their dissatisfaction with unemployment and leisure time was significantly greater than that of a cross section of the normal population.

Since many patients who are capable of assuming full-time employment will not have jobs waiting for them when they leave the hospital, job placement is an important element in their rehabilitation and integration back into the community. How patients present themselves at job interviews is a critical determinant of whether they obtain work. Psychiatric patients often have special problems responding to questions about their personal circumstances and recent past. Several studies have demonstrated that psychiatric patients can benefit from training in interview skills (Kiel and Barbee 1973; Vernardos and Harris 1973; Furman et al. 1979; Kelly et al. 1979). Additional skills for obtaining employment include knowing how to solicit job leads and having the motivation and persistence to sustain a long and frustrating job search (Watts 1983). One effective program for overcoming the obstacles to employment has been the job-finding club, a program for recovering psychiatric patients who are stable enough to work full time.

Job-Finding Club

The job-finding club combines several successful techniques in a packaged module first developed by Azrin and Besalel (1980). Key elements of the module include (1) the use of an environment conducive to motivating patients in their job search; (2) the use of reinforcement strategies; (3) a breakdown of the tasks involved in finding a job; and (4) training in skills needed to find a job. In order to adapt this model to the needs of the psychiatrically disabled, it was necessary to increase the structure and motivation inherent in the program, including daily goal-setting activities, monetary rewards, and remedial training in job-seeking skills. The job-finding club for psychiatric patients was designed and evaluated at the Brentwood Division of the West Los Angeles VA Medical Center (Jacobs et al. 1984). Patients participated in the program full time (six hours per day) while they either lived in the hospital or in the community. The program is not time-limited; patients spend an average of twenty-four days in the club before locating employment. There are three distinct parts to the job club: training in job-seeking skills, the job search itself, and follow-up and job maintenance.

Training in Job-Seeking Skills

During the first week of the program patients participate in an intensive, six-hour-per-day workshop designed to assess and teach basic job-finding skills. The curriculum includes identifying sources of job leads, contacting job leads, writing job resumes, filling out employment applications, participating in job interviews, and learning how to use public transportation. Trainers use programmed materials, didactic instruction, role plays, and *in vivo* training exercises to teach these competencies. Whenever possible the program uses materials and situations that the client will face during the job search, such as filling out actual job applications and contacting sources for job leads. Patients' progress is closely monitored, and additional instruction is provided as necessary to meet individual needs.

Job Search

After completing the five-day workshop on skills required for job seeking, patients begin their job search. The program provides telephones, secretarial support, and a listing of current job leads. These leads are gleaned from newspaper want ads, friends and relatives, employment notices, civil service announcements, the yellow pages, and visits to state employment agencies. Each patient must begin his day by setting goals for his job search with his counselor. Together they develop expectations for the outcome of the daily activities, set a time for accomplishing tasks, and problem-solve potential obstacles that may be encountered. Patients keep a daily log of their job-seeking activities to account for their time in the program.

During the job-search phase, patients also learn to better manage daily problems, including the stress of looking for employment. Counselors provide direction and support as needed. They may assist the patient in finding housing and reliable transportation, in learning how to interact with others, and in adjusting to work hours. Patients remain in this phase until they secure a job or leave the program.

Follow-up and Job Maintenance

Job club graduates may attend a weekly aftercare session that teaches strategies to deal with problems that may threaten job security. Training follows a problem-solving model; solutions to an identified issue are specified, and then these solutions are role-played with feedback before the patient uses the approach in his work setting. Participants may identify such problems as learning how to get along with co-workers on the job, improving daily living conditions, and managing residual psychiatric symptoms. Graduates may also return to the program if they lose their jobs or wish to upgrade their positions.

Evaluation of the Job Club

The outcome of the first ninety-seven patients enrolled in the job club provides support for its effectiveness. The majority of these patients had hospital admission diagnoses of schizophrenia and a prior history of psychiatric hospitalization. The average patient had been unemployed for over a year and a half before his present hospitalization. The results of the job club assistance during the first eight months of operation are displayed in Table 6.2. Sixty-six percent of all the patients who entered the club either obtained employment or were enrolled in full-time job-training programs. Most jobs were secured in clerical and sales positions (34%), service occupations (25%), technical, managerial, or professional positions (11%), and machine trades (7%).

Six-month follow-up data were collected on the sixty-six patients who entered jobs or job-training programs from the job club. Of these 75 percent were still employed a half year after leaving the club. By comparison, out of the twenty-five patients who left the job club without successful placement, none had found a job six months later (Jacobs et al., 1984). Job outcomes have remained stable in the three years since the club's initiation. Out of a total referred patient group of approximately 300, 65 percent of the participants obtained jobs or entered full-time vocational education programs. Patients entering the club with high levels of symptoms had greater difficulties finding a job, as did older patients. Previous work history and education did not predict success in finding a job but did affect the type of employment secured. Thus, the job club is a viable program for training and preparing psychiatric patients in the skills necessary to finding employment in the competitive workplace.

Job Maintenance Training: A Case Study

The hallmark of successful rehabilitation programs for psychiatric patients is continuity of treatment. Services must be provided to patients according to their needs at different phases of their recovery, from inpatient

Table 6.2
Job Club Outcomes for Ninety-Seven Consecutively Referred Psychiatric Patients over Eight Months at a VA Medical Center

Outcome	No. of patients	Percentage
Employed	54	56
Enrolled in full-time job-training program	10	10
Returned to ward because of intrusive symptoms within first week	11	11
Voluntarily withdrew from program after first week	22	22

hospital care, to day treatment, vocational rehabilitation, and support programs for living and working within the community. A case study is presented to illustrate the implementation of social-skills training during psychosocial rehabilitation, and the importance of case management in handling problems that may arise.

Sam was a 28-year-old man who was physically abused as a child. At age 11 he was placed with foster parents and separated from his four siblings, who were placed in other foster homes. As a child he attended classes for the emotionally disturbed and in high school was treated with valium for a "nervous condition." Despite above-average academic performance, he dropped out of school in the tenth grade, worked at odd jobs until he was 18, and then joined the Marines. He remained in the Marines for three years. He did not see any military action and was honorably discharged with 25 percent medical disability for an injury he sustained. In the following four years, Sam held many jobs (driving, shipping, clerical work, heavy-equipment operator), some of which he lost because of PCP abuse, poor relations with co-workers, and injuries he received while on the job.

When Sam was 23 years old, after breaking up with his girlfriend and a bad PCP trip, he began to experience sleep disturbances, including night terrors and somnambulism. Symptoms included screaming while asleep, episodes of violence, and on two occasions smashing glass with his hands without even awakening. These symptoms persisted for two years prior to his admission as an inpatient to the Brentwood Division of the West Los Angeles VA Medical Center, for treatment of depression and night terrors. His DSM-III diagnoses included dysthymic disorder, sleep terror disorder, schizoid personality disorder, and intermittent explosive disorder.

During his eight-month hospitalization, Sam was treated with imipramine and experienced relief in depression and sleep terrors. Following his inpatient stay, Sam gradually began to live more independently. First, he lived for three months at a less structured living environment on the hospital grounds—the Intermediate Rehabilitation Unit—after which he moved into his own apartment in the community. Sam's participation in psychosocial programs also reflected his gradual growth of social competence and capacity to be self-sufficient. After four months in a general inpatient psychiatric unit, Sam was admitted to the Day Hospital, where he continued to show steady improvement over the next half year. Following Sam's treatment at the Day Hospital, his vocational skills were assessed, and because of his good mechanical ability he was enrolled in an office machine repair training program, requiring full-time participation for a year. Sam continued to receive antidepressant medication throughout all phases of his treatment. He graduated from the training program after thirteen months and immediately secured a job as a repairman in an office machine repair company in the community.

Working in a skilled, demanding job and living independently in the community were stressful life changes for Sam, and required special efforts for him to successfully adapt. Early in his job he complained to his caseworker that he thought that the customers whose machines he repaired gave him a hard time, and that he was being treated unfairly by the boss, whom he accused of giving him more work than the other workers. After working on the job for five months, the caseworker learned from Sam's boss that his job was in jeopardy. On several occasions Sam had lost his temper and been rude to customers or other people when repairing typewriters in the field. On one occasion, he had been reported by a customer for roughly jostling a typewriter. Sam's boss was concerned about the possible adverse effects of Sam's outbursts on his customer relations and business. The caseworker referred Sam to the Social and Independent Living Skills Program at Brentwood for job-maintenance-skills training.

Skills training was conducted using a variant of the basic skills model and employing a multiple baseline design to discriminate treatment effects (Mueser, Foy, and Carter 1986). First, on the basis of separate interviews with Sam and his boss, thirteen pilot scenes were constructed and role-played to assess Sam's specific performance deficits, in situations that involved interactions with supervisors, co-workers, customers, and security guards at offices in the field. Twelve scenes were selected for further role-playing. Over a three-week period Sam engaged in each role play three times. Throughout this baseline and the remainder of treatment, self-report measures were also obtained of Sam's job performance, rated both by Sam and his boss, who was unaware of the specific training interventions. Several behaviors targeted for change improved spontaneously in the baseline period (e.g., topical statements made to co-workers), while Sam and his boss reported no change in Sam's job performance during this interval. Those four scenes were deleted from further training, leaving a total of eight scenes for skill training.

The eight scenes used for training represented five different interpersonal situations, and included interactions with a friendly customer (two scenes), an unfriendly customer (two scenes), a security guard (two scenes), a justifiably critical supervisor (one scene), and an unjustifiably critical supervisor (one scene). Table 6.3 lists the targeted behaviors and identifies the behaviors targeted for each interpersonal situation. As can be seen from Table 6.3, only nonverbal behaviors (voice volume, eye contact, affect) were targeted for all the interpersonal situations.

Sam's skills were trained in sequential fashion with the usual combination of instructions, modeling, prompting, shaping, positive feedback, and corrective feedback. Several staff members were enlisted to play the interpersonal targets. Role plays were videotaped and later rated, but were not played back to Sam. A total of sixteen sessions (including the baseline

Table 6.3
Behaviors Targeted for Improvement in Given Interpersonal Situations for the Case of Sam

	Interpersonal situations				
Targeted behavior	Friendly customer	Unfriendly customer	Security guard	Justifiably critical supervisor	Unjustifiably critical supervisor
Voice volume	X	X	X	X	X
Eye contact	X	X	X	X	X
Affect (facial expression and voice tone)	X	X	X	X	X
Verbal responsiveness (reassurances, acknowledgers)	X	X			
Eliciting suggestions			X		
Requesting clarification				X	X
Appropriate self-assertion					X

sessions) were held over a four-month period, during which time all the targeted behaviors were trained to criterion levels as shown in Figure 6.1. Regular ratings by Sam's boss confirmed the impact of the acquired skills on his job performance, which were maintained at three months (Table 6.4). Most important, Sam's temper outbursts at customers ceased during training, and his job became more secure as his boss recognized him as a valuable and competent employee. An eight-month follow-up revealed that Sam was continuing to perform well on his job.

Sam's success shows how casework and the rapid mobilization of skills-oriented interventions can maintain and bolster rehabilitation gains. The social-skills technique we used with Sam has been employed in the past to treat outbursts of anger in adults similar to those exhibited here (Foy, Eisler, and Pinkston 1975) and to improve interpersonal skill deficits that were impeding satisfactory vocational performance by working alcoholics (Foy et al. 1979).

Skills Training in Behavioral Family Therapy

The family is a potentially powerful rehabilitative force in the patient's life (Evans, Bullard, and Solomon 1961). Modifying the family environment by reducing negative emotional communication and facilitating problem-solving will improve the patient's outcome by lowering the level of ambient stress. Recently, several treatments have evolved that attempt to modify the emotional climate of families containing a schizophrenic patient (Falloon, Boyd, and McGill 1984; Anderson, Reiss, and Hogarty 1986). The method discussed here is behavioral family management, which is based on behavioral-skills training (Falloon and Liberman 1983). Training occurs in five stages, with considerable recycling of each stage throughout therapy: (1) behavioral assessment; (2) education about schizophrenia and

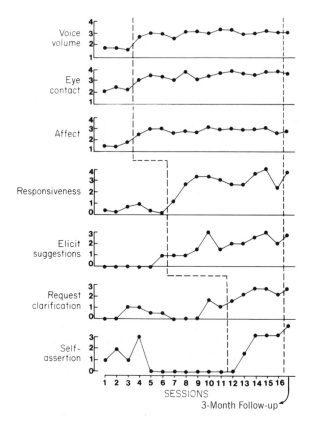

Figure 6.1
Skills acquisition over multiple baseline for Sam. For each skill, the dotted vertical line denotes the beginning of training. The first three behaviors are based on a 1–4 rating, with high scores indicating better performance. The last four behaviors are rated on a frequency count. Points are based on means for the role plays for each targeted behavior (see Table 6.3 for role-play list).

its care; (3) communication skills training; (4) problem-solving; and (5) special problems. The clinical efficacy of this model has been evaluated with a schizophrenic population (Falloon et al. 1985; Cardin, McGill, and Falloon 1985; Falloon and Pederson 1985), but the procedures can apply to other psychiatrically disabled populations, with modification required only in the educational component.

The behavioral assessment of a family system is interwoven with treatment, in a manner similar to individual behavior therapy. Assessment involves identifying the assets and deficits of individual members and of the family as a whole, and then determining the role that specific problem behaviors play in the functioning of the family. Information is obtained

Table 6.4
Job-Performance Rating by Sam's Boss during Baseline Period, at End of Treatment, and at One- and Three-Month Follow-ups

Job area	Baseline (mean of 3 ratings)	Post-treatment	1-month follow-up	3-month follow-up
Overall job performance	2.0	4	4	4
Response to criticism	1.3	3	4	3
Interactions with customers	2.0	4	3	4
Interactions with co-workers	2.0	4	4	4
Initiating conversations	1.0	4	4	4
Customer complaints (no. per week)	0.6	0	0	0

NOTE: Scores of 1 or 2 indicate unsatisfactory performance; scores of 3 and 4 are satisfactory performance.

through interviews, observing interactions in family sessions, and family performance on specific problem-solving tasks.

In the educational sessions, the caseworkers refute common misconceptions about the causes of schizophrenia, such as that families are responsible for causing schizophrenia, and that schizophrenia involves a "split personality." Families learn about the symptoms of schizophrenia; its diagnosis, prevalence, and course; and the biological theories of etiology. The relationship between stress and vulnerability in causing symptom exacerbations is described, and the role of neuroleptic medications in buffering biological vulnerability is emphasized. The effects of the patient's illness on each family member is elicited, and problems of management are discussed.

Training family members to listen empathetically, express positive feelings, make positive requests for behavior change, and express negative feelings constructively may help alleviate tensions in the family. The initial phase of communication training focuses on expressing positive feelings through prompting mutually rewarding behavior and empathic listening; such actions should create a warmer milieu where family members recognize and reinforce specific positive behavior in one another. Training emphasizes direct and brief verbal communication in which a specific behavior of one person is positively acknowledged or reinforced by another.

Once a family has developed satisfactory communication skills, they move on to problem-solving skills. These skills are taught as a sequence of steps for resolving problems in a manner that minimizes negative emotional undercurrents while searching for a solution. These steps are (1) defining the problem to everyone's satisfaction; (2) brainstorming a list of alternative solutions to the problem; (3) examining the advantages and disadvantages of each solution; (4) choosing the best solution or combination of solutions; (5) deciding how to implement a plan that incorporates the solutions; and (6) reviewing progress on implementation and reinforcing approximations toward goal achievement.

Problems experienced by patients in vocational rehabilitation, job attainment, and job maintenance are often addressed in family problemsolving sessions. One family spent several sessions talking about how to improve a schizophrenic patient's work rate in a sheltered workshop. Potential solutions generated by family members ranged from soliciting advice from co-workers or a supervisor and setting attainable daily goals, to making reinforcing self-statements following the completion of the job task. After several weeks of implementing, evaluating, and generating new solutions to this problem, the patient reported some increase in his work rate and a greater satisfaction with his performance. Another patient used problem-solving to obtain possible job leads from her family members.

When family members have acquired the problem-solving skills, they begin working on "special problems" that require a therapist's expertise. The therapist may suggest many behavioral techniques, such as contingency contracting for mutually desired behavior exchanges (Weathers and Liberman 1975), social-skills training for job interviewing, token economy programs for enhancing constructive daily activity, or cognitivebehavioral modification for depression or anxiety. Usually the entire family is involved in implementing these strategies and monitoring their effects.

When possible, behavioral family management is done at home so that newly acquired behaviors will be more likely to be generalized to the family's natural environment. The therapist also can observe the physical surroundings and family organization that are the backdrop for the therapy. Meeting in their home also conveys directly to the family the therapist's concern and involvement, reducing resistance to therapy (Liberman 1981). Such resistance may be particularly strong among families who feel they are to blame for the patient's illness (Appleton 1974; Terkelson 1983). In engaging such families, the therapist at the outset disclaims the notion that families cause schizophrenia and describes the stress-diathesis-coping model of schizophrenia (Zubin and Spring 1977; Liberman et al. 1980, Liberman, Falloon, and Wallace 1984).

As with most psychosocial treatment programs, the long-range clinical outcome of rehabilitation programs featuring social-skills training depends on the degree of support present in the post-treatment environment. It is most important that the patient live and work with people who reinforce his or her efforts toward more socially appropriate behavior. A comprehensive psychosocial program should modify individual coping skills, provide social supports, and reduce socioenvironmental stressors. Social-skills training enhances individual coping skills. Behavioral family management can strengthen social support, and communication and problem-solving skills training can reduce the ambient tension in family interactions. Our experience with these interventions has led us to conclude that continuity of treatment and the use of skills-based approaches directed at the patient and those in his or her environment are the critical elements for effective vocational and social rehabilitation.

References

Anderson, C. M.; Reiss, D. J.; and Hogarty, G. E. 1986. *Schizophrenia and the family.* New York: Guilford Press.

Anthony, W. A.; Cohen, M. R.; and Vitalo, R. 1978. The measurement of rehabilitation outcome. *Schizophrenia Bulletin, 4,* 365–83.

Appleton, W. S. 1974. Mistreatment of patients' families by psychiatrists. *American Journal of Psychiatry, 131,* 655–57.

Astrup, C.; Fossum, A.; and Holmboe, R. 1962. *Prognosis in functional psychoses.* Springfield, Ill.: Charles C Thomas.

Azrin, N. H., and Besalel, V. A. 1980. *Job club counselor's manual.* Baltimore: University Park Press.

Bachrach, L. L. 1980. Overview: Model programs for chronic mental patients. *American Journal of Psychiatry, 137,* 1023–31.

Banzett, L. K.; Liberman, R. P.; Moore, J. W.; and Marshall, B. D. 1984. Long-term follow-up of the effects of behavior therapy. *Hospital and Community Psychiatry, 35,* 277–79.

Bassuk, E. L., and Gerson, S. 1978. Deinstitutionalization and mental health services. *Scientific American, 238,* 46–53.

Beard, J. H.; Malamud, T. J.; and Rossman, E. 1978. Psychiatric rehabilitation and long-term rehospitalization rates: The findings of two research studies. *Schizophrenia Bulletin, 4,* 622–35.

Bellack, A. S.; Hersen, M.; and Himmelhoch, J. M. 1981. Social-skills training, pharmacotherapy, and psychotherapy for unipolar depression. *American Journal of Psychiatry, 138,* 1562–67.

———. 1983. A comparison of social-skills training, pharmacotherapy, and psychotherapy for depression. *Behavior Research and Therapy, 21,* 101–7.

Bellack, A. S.; Hersen, M.; and Turner, S. M. 1976. Generalization effects of social-skills training with chronic schizophrenics: An experimental analysis. *Behavior Research and Therapy, 14,* 391–98.

Bellack, A. S.; Turner, S. M.; Hersen, M.; and Luber, R. F. 1984. An examination of the efficacy of social-skills training for chronic schizophrenic patients. *Hospital and Community Psychiatry, 35,* 1023–28.

Brady, J. P. 1984a. Social-skills training for psychiatric patients, I: Concepts, methods, and clinical results. *American Journal of Psychiatry, 141,* 333–40.

———. 1984b. Social-skills trainings for psychiatric patients, II: Clinical outcome studies. *American Journal of Psychiatry, 141,* 491–98.

Brenner, M. H. 1973. *Mental illness and the economy.* Cambridge: Harvard University Press.

Brown, G. W.; Birley, J.L.T.; and Wing, J. K. 1972. Influence of family life on the course of schizophrenia disorders: A replication. *British Journal of Psychiatry, 121,* 241–58.

Cardin, V. A.; McGill, C. W.; and Falloon, I.R.H. 1985. Family versus individual management in the prevention of morbidity of schizophrenia: An economic analysis. In *Family management of schizophrenia,* ed. I.R.H. Falloon, pp. 115–23. Baltimore: Johns Hopkins University Press.

Casey, P. R.; Tyrer, P. J.; and Platt, S. T. 1985. The relationship between social functioning and psychiatric symptomatology in primary care. *Social Psychiatry, 20,* 5–9.

Edelstein, B. A.; Couture, E.; Cray, M.; Dickens, P.; and Lusebrink, N. 1980. Group training of problem-solving with psychiatric patients. In *Group therapy: An annual review,* ed. D. Upper and S. M. Ross, vol. 2, pp. 85–102. Champaign, Ill.: Research Press.

Englehardt, D. M., and Rosen, B. 1976. Implications of drug treatment for social rehabilitation of schizophrenic patients. *Schizophrenia Bulletin, 2,* 454–61.

Evans, A. S.; Bullard, D. M.; and Solomon, M. H. 1961. The family as a potential resource in the rehabilitation of the chronic schizophrenic patient: A study of 60 patients and their families. *American Journal of Psychiatry, 117,* 1075–83.

Falloon, I.R.H.; Boyd, J. L.; and McGill, C. W. 1984. *Family care of schizophrenia.* New York: Guilford Press.

Falloon, I.R.H.; Boyd, J. L.; McGill, C. W.; Ranzani, J.; Moss, H. B.; Gilderman, A. M.; and Simpson, G. M. 1985. Family management in the prevention of morbidity of schizophrenia: Clinical outcome of a two-year longitudinal study. *Archives of General Psychiatry, 42,* 887–96.

Falloon, I.R.H., and Liberman, R. P. 1983. Behavioral family interventions in the management of chronic schizophrenia. In *Family therapy in schizophrenia,* ed. W. R. McFarlane, pp. 117–40. New York: Guilford Press.

Falloon, I.R.H.; McGill, C. W.; Boyd, J. L.; and Pederson, J. 1985. Family management in the prevention of morbidity of schizophrenia: Social outcome of a two-year longitudinal study. *Psychological Medicine, 17,* 59–66.

Falloon, I.R.H., and Pederson, J. 1985. Family management in the prevention of morbidity of schizophrenia: The adjustment of the family: *British Journal of Psychiatry, 147,* 156–63.

Foy, D. W.; Eisler, R. M.; and Pinkston, S. 1975. Modeled assertion in a case of explosive rages. *Journal of Behavior Therapy and Experimental Psychiatry, 6,* 135–37.

Foy, D. W.; Massey, F. H.; Duer, J. D.; Ross, J. M.; and Wooten, L. S. 1979. Social-skills training to improve alcoholics' vocational interpersonal competency. *Journal of Counseling Psychology, 25,* 128–32.

Foy, D. W.; Wallace, C. J.; and Liberman, R. P. 1983. Advances in social-skills training for chronic mental patients. In *Advances in clinical behavior therapy,* ed. K. D. Craig and R. J. McMahon. New York: Brunner/Mazel.

Frederiksen, L. W.; Jenkins, J. O.; Foy, D. W.; and Eisler, R. M. 1976. Social-skills training to modify abusive verbal outbursts in adults. *Journal of Applied Behavior Analysis, 9,* 117–27.

Furman, W.; Geller, M.; Simon, S. J.; and Kelly, J. A. 1979. The use of a behavioral rehearsal procedure for teaching job interview skills to psychiatric patients. *Behavior Therapy, 10,* 157–67.

Glasscote, R. M.; Cumming, E.; Rutman, I. D.; Sussex, J. N.; and Glassman, S. M. 1971. *Rehabilitating the mentally ill in the community.* Washington, D.C.: American Psychiatric Association.

Goffman, E. 1961. *Asylums.* New York: Doubleday.

Goldsmith, J. B., and McFall, R. M. 1975. Development and evaluation of an interpersonal skill-training program for psychiatric inpatients. *Journal of Abnormal Psychology, 84,* 51–58.

Goldstein, A. P. 1973. *Structured learning therapy.* New York: Academic Press.

Goldstrom, I., and Manderscheid, R. 1982. The chronically mentally ill: A descriptive analysis from the uniform client data instrument. *Community Support Services Journal, 2,* 4–9.

Hagen, D. Q. 1983. The relationship between job loss and physical and mental illness. *Hospital and Community Psychiatry, 34,* 438–41.

Hersen, M., and Eisler, P. M. 1976. Social-skills training. In *Behavior modification: Principles, issues, and applications,* ed. W. E. Craighead, A. E. Kazdin, and M. J. Mahoney, pp. 361–75. Boston: Houghton Mifflin.

Hogarty, G. E.; Anderson, C. M.; Reiss, D. J.; Kornblith, S. J.; Greenwald, D. P.; Javna, C. D., and Madonia, M. J. 1986. Family psycho-education, social-skills training, and maintenance chemotherapy in the aftercare of schizophrenia; I: One year effects of a controlled study on relapse and expressed emotion. *Archives of General Psychiatry, 43*, 633–42.

Hooley, J. M.; Orley, J.; and Teasdale, J. D. 1986. Levels of expressed emotion and relapse in depressed patients. *British Journal of Psychiatry, 148*, 642–47.

Jacobs, H. E.; Kardashian, S.; Krienbring, R. K.; Ponder, R.; and Simpson, A. R. 1984. A skills-oriented model facilitating employment among psychiatrically disabled persons. *Rehabilitation Counseling Bulletin, 28*, 87–96.

Kelly, J. A.; Laughlin, C.; Claiborne, M.; and Patterson, J. 1979. A group procedure for teaching job-interviewing skills to formerly hospitalized psychiatric patients. *Behavior Therapy, 10*, 299–310.

Kelly, J. A.; Urey, J. R.; and Patterson, J. T. 1980. Improving hetero-social conversational skills of male psychiatric patients through a small-group-training procedure. *Behavior Therapy, 11*, 79–83.

Kiel, E. C., and Barbee, J. R. 1973. Training the disadvantaged job interviewee. *Vocational Guidance Quarterly, 22*, 50–56.

Lehman, A. 1983. The well-being of chronic mental patients. *Archives of General Psychiatry, 40*, 369–73.

Lehrer, P., and Lanoil, J. 1977. Natural reinforcement in a psychiatric rehabilitation program. *Schizophrenia Bulletin, 3*, 297–302.

Liberman, R. P. 1976. Behavior therapy for schizophrenia. In *Treatment of schizophrenia*, ed. L. J. West and D. Glinn, pp. 175–206. New York: Grune and Stratton.

———. 1981. Managing resistance to behavioral family therapy. In *Questions and answers in the practice of family therapy*, ed. A. S. Gurman, 1:186–94. New York: Brunner/Mazel.

———. 1983. Sociopolitics of behavioral programs in institutions and community agencies. *Analysis and Intervention in Developmental Disability, 3*, 131–59.

Liberman, R. P.; Falloon, I.R.H.; and Wallace, C. J. 1984. Drug-psychosocial interactions in the treatment of schizophrenia. In *The chronically mentally ill: Research and services*, ed. M. Mirabi, pp. 175–214. New York: Spectrum Publications.

Liberman, R. P.; King, L. W.; DeRisi, W. J.; and McCann, M. 1975. *Personal effectiveness: Guiding people to assert themselves and improve their social skills*. Champaign, Ill.: Research Press.

Liberman, R. P.; Marshall, B. D.; and Burkem, K. L. 1981. Drug and environmental interventions for aggressive psychiatric patients. In *Violent behavior: Social-learning approaches to prediction, management, and treatment*, ed. R. B. Stuart, pp. 227–64. New York: Brunner/Mazel.

Liberman, R. P.; Massel, H. K.; Mosk, M. D.; and Wong, S. E. 1985. Social-skills training for chronic mental patients. *Hospital and Community Psychiatry, 36*, 396–403.

Liberman, R. P.; Mueser, K. T.; and Wallace, C. J. 1986. Social-skills training for schizophrenics at risk for relapse. *American Journal of Psychiatry, 143*, 523–26.

Liberman, R. P.; Wallace, C. J.; Teigen, J.; and Davis, J. 1974. Behavioral interventions with psychotics. In *Innovative treatment methods in psychopathology*, ed. N. S. Calhoun, H. E. Adams, and E. M. Mitchess, pp. 323–412. New York: Wiley and Sons.

Liberman, R. P.; Wallace, C. J.; Vaughn, C. E.; Snyder, K. S.; and Rust, C. 1980. Social and family factors in the course of schizophrenia: Toward an interpersonal problem-solving therapy for schizophrenics and their families. In *The psychotherapy of schizophrenia*, ed. J. Strauss, M. Bowers, T. W. Downey, S. Fleck, S. Jackson, and I. Levine, pp. 21–54. New York: Plenum Press.

Linn, M. W.; Klett, C. J.; and Coffey, E. M. 1982. Relapse of psychiatric patients in foster care. *American Journal of Psychiatry, 139*, 778–83.

McKnight, D. L.; Nelson, R. O.; Hayes, S. C.; and Jarrett, R. B. 1984. Importance of treating individually assessed response classes in the amelioration of depression. *Behavior Therapy, 15,* 315–35.

Massel, H. K.; Bowen, L.; Mosk, M. D.; et al. 1984. A comparison of procedures for training conversational skills in chronic schizophrenics. Paper presented at the annual meeting of the Association for the Advancement of Behavior Therapy, Philadephia, November.

Mechanic, D. 1969. *Mental health and social policy.* Englewood Cliffs, N.J.: Prentice-Hall.

Meyerson, A. T. 1978. What are the barriers or obstacles to treatment and care of the chronically disabled mentally ill? In *The chronic mental patient,* ed. J. A. Talbott, pp. 129–36. Washington, D.C.: American Psychiatric Association.

Morrison, R. L., and Bellack, A. S. 1984. Social-skills training. In *Schizophrenia: Treatment, management, and rehabilitation,* ed. A. S. Bellack, pp. 247–80. New York: Grune and Stratton.

Mueser, K. T.; Foy, D. W.; and Carter, M. J. 1986. Social-skills training for job maintenance: A single case study. *Journal of Counseling Psychology, 33,* 360–62.

Paul, G. L., and Lentz, R. J. 1977. *Psychosocial treatment of the chronic mental patient.* Cambridge: Harvard University Press.

Paul, G. L.; Tobias, L. T.; and Holly, B. L. 1972. Maintenance psychotropic drugs in the presence of active treatment programs: A "triple-blind" withdrawal study in long-term mental patients. *Archives of General Psychiatry, 27,* 106–15.

Phillips, L., and Zigler, E. 1961. Social competence: The action-thought parameter and vicariousness in normal and pathological behavior. *Journal of Abnormal and Social Psychology, 63,* 137–46.

Platt, J. J., and Spivack, G. 1972. Problem-solving thinking of psychiatric patients. *Journal of Consulting and Clinical Psychology, 28,* 3–5.

Rosen, A. J.; Sussman, S.; Mueser, K. T.; Lyons, J. S.; and Davis, J. M. 1981. Behavioral assessment of psychiatric inpatients and normal controls across different environmental contexts. *Journal of Behavioral Assessment, 3,* 25–36.

Siegel, J. M., and Spivack, G. 1976. Problem-solving therapy: The description of a new program for chronic psychiatric patients. *Psychotherapy: Theory, Research, and Practice, 13,* 368–73.

Stein, L. I., and Test, M. A. 1980. Alternative to mental hospital treatment. *Archives of General Psychiatry, 37,* 392–97.

Sylph, J. A.; Ross, H. E.; and Kedward, H. B. 1978. Social disability in chronic psychiatric patients. *American Journal of Psychiatry, 134,* 1391–94.

Talbott, J. A. 1981. *The chronic mentally ill.* New York: Human Sciences Press.

Terkelson, K. G. 1983. Schizophrenia and the family, II: Adverse effects of family therapy. *Family Process, 22,* 191–200.

Test, M. A., and Stein, L. I. 1978. Training in community living. In *Alternatives to mental hospital treatment,* ed. L. I. Stein, and M. A. Test, pp. 57–74. New York: Plenum Press.

Vaughn, C. E., and Leff, J. P. 1976. The influence of family and social factors on the course of psychiatric illness: A comparison of schizophrenic and depressed neurotic patients. *British Journal of Psychiatry, 129,* 125–37.

Vaughn, C. E.; Snyder, K. S.; Jones, S.; Freeman, W. B.; and Falloon, I.R.H. 1984. Family factors in schizophrenic relapse. *Archives of General Psychiatry, 41,* 1169–77.

Vernardos, M. G., and Harris, M. B. 1973. Job-interview training with rehabilitation clients. *Journal of Applied Psychology, 58,* 365–67.

Wallace, C. J.; Nelson, C. J.; Liberman, R. P.; Aitchison, R. A.; Lukoff, D.; Elder, J. P.; and Ferris, C. 1980. A review and critique of social-skills training with schizophrenic patients. *Schizophrenia Bulletin, 6,* 42–63.

Walls, P. D.; Walls, L. H.; and Langsley, D. G. 1975. Psychiatric training and practice in the People's Republic of China. *American Journal of Psychiatry, 132,* 121–28.

Watts, F. N. 1983. Employment. In *Theory and practice of psychiatric rehabilitation,* ed. F. N. Watts and D. H. Bennett, pp. 215–40. New York: Wiley and Sons.

Weathers, L., and Liberman, R. P. 1975. The family contracting exercise. *Journal of Behavior Therapy and Experimental Psychiatry, 6,* 208–14.

Wing, J. K., and Brown, G. W. 1970. *Institutionalization and schizophrenia.* London: Cambridge University Press.

Wolpe, J. 1958. *Psychotherapy by reciprocal inhibition.* Stanford, Calif.: Stanford University Press.

Wolpe, J., and Lazarus, A. A. 1966. *Behavioral therapy techniques.* New York: Pergamon Press.

Wong, S. E.; Terranova, M. D.; Bowen, L.; Zarete, T.; Massel, H. K.; and Liberman, R. P. 1987. Providing independent recreational activities to reduce stereotypic vocalizations in chronic schizophrenics. *Journal of Applied Behavior Analysis, 20,* 77–81.

Wortis, J. 1950. *Soviet psychiatry.* Baltimore: Williams and Wilkins.

Zubin, J., and Spring, B. 1977. Vulnerability: A new view of schizophrenia. *Journal of Abnormal Psychology, 86,* 103–26.

7

A Family Approach to Rehabilitation

THOMAS W. JOHNSON

Most statistics reveal that more than half of those patients discharged from psychiatric hospitals return to live with their families. However, only recently have families been seen as collaborators in the rehabilitation process. Johnson outlines the problems faced by families as well as ways in which they can be helpful in improving vocational functioning. Emphasizing the contributions of the expressed emotion research and the importance of timing in the phases of recovery, he describes the psychoeducational model and the structural/strategic approach. Finally, he synthesizes his own approach combining the family approaches and vocational theory and applies it to two very different case examples.

In the wake of deinstitutionalization, there has been a shift in the site of chronic care from the hospital to the community, and often to the family homes of many persons with prolonged mental illness. Hospital staff are less involved than ever in vocational and psychosocial rehabilitation as inpatient lengths of stay decrease. At the same time, community-support programs for discharged patients struggle to provide assistance in the face of dwindling federal funds for psychosocial services. More and more of the responsibility for helping the chronically mentally ill is thus being shared by families as hospital and community resources become less available. However, family members often seek help from kin before turning to other social support systems (Uzoka 1979). Hatfield (1983) contends that this is typically the case with the chronically mentally ill, thereby making families the principal caregivers.

Recent demographic studies of the chronically mentally ill also support the notion that community care is often taking place at home. William McFarlane (1983a), of New York State Psychiatric Institute, reports that in fiscal year 1980/81, 51 percent of all patients discharged from New York State hospitals returned to live with their families. With patients whose lengths of stay were less than three months, 80 percent were discharged to their families. McFarlane also notes a steady decrease in the number of patients released to alternative residential programs since 1977. As these studies indicate, many families are very much involved in their ill relatives' lives and are dealing with the many daily stresses created by chronic mental illness.

What Do Families Face?

Life with a relative who is in an acute or chronic phase of a severe psychiatric disorder is often frightening and uncertain. Primary positive symptomatology, such as auditory hallucinations, uncontrolled outbursts of anger, undue suspicion, incoherent speech, and abrupt mood swings, are difficult to understand and cope with at home. Many family members report living in fear of what each day will bring. Agnes Hatfield (1979) studied the difficulties facing families by questioning members of a family organization, the Schizophrenia Association of Greater Washington. Respondents, most of whom were parents, reported feeling tense and on guard much of the time. Marriages were described as seriously troubled, and parents worried that the patient's siblings were neglected. Extrafamilial socializing dwindled to the point where many families were isolated. Respondents also indicated that serious signs of emotional and physical strain surfaced at times in all family members. However, what appeared to trouble families the most were concerns about the patient's general functioning. Families particularly worried about the patient's poor grooming, aimlessness, vocational failure, and impairments in concentration. Functional deficits, as well as the negative symptoms of the illness, seemed to tax families in a profound way. Severely impaired vocational development seemed especially difficult for families to tolerate. Many times a son or daughter with bright promise and high aspirations is capable of much less than had been expected. Parents watch in pain as their once talented child establishes a lifelong career as a public assistance recipient. As one respondent in Hatfield's study remarked of a daughter diagnosed as schizophrenic, "I ache for her wasted life" (p. 339).

Families confronted with the problems of severe mental illness frequently appeal to professionals for answers to questions about stabilization and rehabilitation. The answers require not only a good clinical understanding of mental illness, but also knowledge of the family's influence on the course of prolonged psychiatric disorders.

A team of British researchers provided some interesting data relevant to these questions. Brown, Birley, and Wing (1972) studied the effects of a family's emotional climate on the recovery of patients diagnosed as schizophrenic. They developed the concept of expressed emotion (EE), which is a measurement of certain specific aspects of a family's emotional life. EE levels were calculated by trained raters who counted verbal and nonverbal expressions of criticism, hostility, and overinvolvement with the patient during interviews with 101 families of hospitalized patients diagnosed as schizophrenic. Interviews were conducted during an inpatient stay and nine months after discharge. They found that families with high levels of EE had patient relapse rates of 58 percent in the first nine months postdischarge, as compared to 16 percent relapse rates in patients from low EE households. Patients from high EE households who had high levels of "face-to-face contact" (greater than 35 hours/week) with high EE relatives had relapse rates of 68% while on medication and 90 percent when not on medication. Moreover, other factors, such as severity of previous disturbance, were discovered to be influential only as a function of EE level.

Anderson, Hogarty, and Reiss (1980) linked the results of the British study to current biopsychological studies. They cited research that contends that persons diagnosed as schizophrenic struggle with a deficit in their ability to control the intensity and processing of stimuli. The highly stimulating and arousing environment of a high EE family could activate this deficit and lead to symptoms and relapse. It is also easy to see how living with a chronically mentally ill person might precipitate high levels of criticism and overinvolvement, given the strains of coping with the illness. Thus, the family unwittingly sabotages stabilization and continues to contribute to the recovery-decompensation cycle.

In 1976 another British team, Vaughn and Leff, replicated the study done by Brown, Birley, and Wing (Vaughn and Leff 1976). They studied the relationship between high EE and relapse in thirty-seven families of hospitalized schizophrenic patients and in thirty families of hospitalized depressed neurotic patients. This team also found a significant association between relapse and high EE for the schizophrenic group and for the depressed group. In the schizophrenic group 50 percent of patients from high EE families and 12 percent of patients from low EE families relapsed. In the depressed group 67 percent relapsed from the high EE groups and 22 percent from the low EE groups. Vaughn and Leff also indicated that the depressed sample was more significantly affected by criticism and was, in fact, more apt to relapse at lower levels of criticism than the schizophrenic sample. In 1982 Vaughn and his associates replicated the study in the United States. Following the same procedures as in the British studies with an American schizophrenic group of fifty-four, they reported a similar association of high EE and relapse (Vaughn et al. 1982). The results indicated that 56 percent of patients with a high EE relative and 17 percent of patients without a high EE relative relapsed within the nine months' follow-up period. Some differences were noted between the British and American samples. There were fewer low EE families in the American sample, and the ratings of hostility were significantly more frequent in the American sample.

One finding of the British research on EE directly relates to vocational rehabilitation. Leff and Vaughn (as cited in Leff, Kuipers, and Berkowitz 1983) claimed that 70 percent of the critical comments were about the patient's negative symptoms and functioning. Families found it difficult to tolerate their ill relative's remaining idle most of the day and doing little either to help with tasks around the house or to find a job. Leff and Vaughn reported that this concern accounted for many more of the critical comments than even florid psychotic symptoms such as delusional thinking or incoherent speech.

The standpoint of families must be appreciated in order to make sense of their reactivity. As Grunebaum (1984) noted, the pressures of familial responsibility and loyalty usually propel families to "do something" right away when confronted by a severely dysfunctional relative. For example, most parents cannot dispassionately sit by and watch their child become perplexed and dazed when faced with even the simplest of tasks, or watch him fail repeatedly at attempts to work outside the home. They typically feel compelled to assist by prodding and instructing. Unfortunately, that pressure is not always helpful and can contribute to high levels of EE.

Hatfield (1979) and Anderson, Hogarty, and Reiss (1980) suggested that much of the emotional reactivity of families is a function of lack of information. Because living with a mentally ill person is unpredictable and confusing, it is not a surprise that families feel anxious and pressured. The two authors suggested that education about the illness relieved these feelings by providing a sense of predictability and normalcy. With regard to restoration of patient functioning, families also need information about appropriate expectations. Boyd, McGill, and Falloon (1981) and Hatfield (1979) noted that relatives of the chronically mentally ill are often operating in the dark when they undertake the improvement of patient functioning at home. Misguided plans to get a family member back on his feet can often backfire when they are forged in the absence of accurate theoretical knowledge or professional help. For example, families need to know that too much pressure can trigger relapse (Brown, Birley, and Wing 1972), while Anderson, Hogarty, and Reiss (1980) emphasized that too little pressure can support negative symptoms and poor levels of functioning. Families need help to strike the right balance.

Anderson, Hogarty, and Reiss (1980) recommended providing families with the most current data on phenomenology, etiology, onset, treatment, course, outcome, and prognosis in language that is easily comprehensible to the layman. They also advocated presenting concrete and practical advice about managing the patient's symptoms at home. This is often what families request, and the input can also help to decrease high levels of anxiety and irritability (Hatfield 1979).

The timing of appropriate family responses and interventions is crucial, since chronic mental illnesses have identifiable phases (Strauss et al. 1985).

Educating the family about these phases is important to help the family understand the usual course of the illness and modify their expectations accordingly. Through this learning process, relatives obtain a longitudinal perspective on the patient's illness and see that abilities and vulnerabilities may vary as a function of phase.

Strauss and co-workers (1985) explained that psychiatric disorders move along a nonlinear course with three typical phases: moratoriums, change points, and ceilings. Following an acute episode, patients frequently shift into a moratorium phase, in which little movement occurs and only few behavioral changes are noted. However, some latent changes do take place. Strauss and colleagues maintained that patients quietly and subtly work on "reconstituting skills" during this period (Strauss et al. 1985, p. 292), but this would not be apparent to the observer. The second phase, which the authors referred to as change points, describes brief bursts of significant movement in level of functioning or level of symptom severity. The direction of change can either be towards exacerbation or improvement, depending on the patient's history of dealing with stress and his or her strengths and supports. The third phase, ceilings, represents what seems to be a leveling off at the highest level of functioning attained over a given time interval. The authors noted that patients rarely move past their ceilings without decompensation and exacerbation of symptoms. Although patients can venture beyond these ceiling points, they find these transitions extremely stressful and need extensive support. Related to these phases is another important longitudinal principle that is important for families to take into account in timing their interventions. Strauss and associates contended that patient vulnerability decreases over time after the acute episode.

These authors also noted parallel phases in the environmental response to the patient. The first phase, convalescence, comprises the first two to four months after discharge from the hospital, during which time family, friends, and clinicians make few demands and provide a good deal of assistance and support to the patient. When the convalescent period ends, there is what the authors call the backlash period. During this phase, significant others and clinicians begin to apply pressure to the patient and often expect more than they had before the decompensation. There are probably other environmental phases which correspond to the patient's course. For example, families may have moratoriums, change points, and ceilings of their own. Further longitudinal study of families is warranted in order to understand this more fully.

Problems often develop when the patient and the family are in different phases (Strauss et al. 1985). For example, during a backlash period, a family often pressures the patient who is in the moratorium phase to work at a taxing job. This may trigger decompensation. The patient may not have had time to marshal the resources necessary for this dramatic a shift.

Moreover, a patient's moratorium phase may extend for much longer than a family expects. The family needs help to know and respect the patient's phases of recovery.

In addition to information regarding the process of recovery, families need a supportive alliance with professionals. As Hatfield (1979) pointed out, the relationship between the professional community and families has historically been fraught with suspicion and hostility. She suggested that theoretical biases and professional training that attribute etiological responsibility to family relationships underpin a critical stance towards families. Understandably, families respond to this position with guilt, hostility, and uncooperativeness. Terkelsen (1983) described how this professional posture undermines work with families: "My attitude most certainly perpetuated guilt—by not actively countering it and sometimes by covertly fostering it. In the presence of continuing guilt, the parents were certainly unable to look at their situation with curiosity. And without curiosity they were unable to learn new and presumably more benevolent ways of living with the patient" (p. 193). It is conceivable that when professionals assume such a position with families, they may stimulate guilt and anxiety, and thereby increase the level of tension at home, raise the level of EE, and undermine the patient's recovery. As McFarlane (1983a) stated, "Blaming the family is explicitly countertherapeutic, even if such blame is unexpressed" (p. 10).

There is a long tradition of theory and research which posits that serious mental illnesses like schizophrenia and the major affective disorders are causally linked to disturbed family relationships. However, Terkelsen (1983) and others contended that this premise is empirically unfounded, since methodological flaws in the studies do not permit making valid conclusions about etiology. Moreover, he indicated that these studies do not provide data which supports a family etiology model over and above a "biogenic" one, or a "responsive" model which contends that disturbed family interactions are the result of living with an ill relative. Terkelsen even suggested that when professionals employ a family etiology model in their work, they may create iatrogenic disturbances in family patterns. This means that families may relate in peculiar ways with one another while being observed by professionals because of the fear that they will be seen as the cause of their relative's problems. Hatfield (1979) recommended that professionals suspend "blaming" perspectives and develop supportive and collaborative relationships with families that make use of their "deep commitment and first-hand knowledge" (p. 340).

What Can Families Do?

In the late 1970s, a number of practitioners turned to approaches that focused directly on helping families to rehabilitate the patient. One example is the psychoeducational approach that achieved prominence with the work of Anderson, Hogarty, and Reiss (1980). These practitioners proceed from the perspective that illnesses like schizophrenia are biopsychological phenomena that wax and wane in response to environmental stress. Their theoretical foundation includes the work of the British EE researchers. The interventions they recommend revolve around educating families about the illness, reducing family stress, and helping families motivate and improve the functioning level of the patient. Adherents to this approach have increased through the United States: Hogarty, Anderson, and Reiss at the University of Pittsburgh; Goldstein and Doane at the University of California at Los Angeles; Falloon and Boyd at the University of Southern California (Rohrbaugh 1983).

Another approach is represented by Jay Haley and Chloe Madanes, who also provide family treatment that is aimed at improving the level of functioning of an ill relative. However, their theoretical premise is very different from the psychoeducational approach. They believe that the behaviors seen in the chronically mentally ill are by-products of a disturbed power hierarchy in a family and that putting the parents in charge of getting a disturbed son or daughter back to work or to school should be the central aim of treatment (Madanes 1983).

Both the psychoeducational approach and what Ryglewicz (1984) referred to as the "structural/strategic" approach of Haley (1980) and Madanes (1983) address what families are requesting from professionals. Families are asking for pragmatic, concrete, and specific, behaviorally oriented advice about how to help a relative stabilize and function again. This is the foundation of treatment in these two approaches. It would be helpful, then, to look more closely at what goes on in the psychoeducational model—particularly Anderson's model, since she specifically addresses vocational and prevocational rehabilitation—and in the structural/strategic approach.

Anderson was one of the first American psychoeducational practitioners to publish a detailed description of this type of work with schizophrenic patients and to report results (1980). As of 1983, thirty-three families have been involved in her experimental program. These are all high EE families, and the overall relapse rate of the experimental group is only 16 percent (1983).

The basic theoretical assumption underlying Anderson's work is that patients who have been diagnosed schizophrenic have a "core psychological deficit" which results in difficulty in controlling the processing of stimuli. Therefore, very stressful and/or stimulating environments often lead to symptoms and relapse. She cited the research of the British EE theoreticians to substantiate this point. She argued that "deintensifying the family environment" will reduce relapse rates. However, she also noted that understimulating, laissez-faire environments will also contribute to the maintenance of negative symptoms. The answer involves a program in which "a variety of supportive and education techniques are used to lower the emotional temperature of the family while maintaining sufficient pressure on patients to avoid the pitfalls of negative symptoms" (Anderson, Hogarty, and Reiss 1980, p. 492).

The thrust of Anderson's approach is twofold. First, she attempts to decrease the level of expressed emotion in families through education about the illness, provision of support, amplification of social networks, and establishment of clear boundaries and rules within the patients' families. Secondly, she helps the family to mobilize their ill relative to increase social and vocational functioning in a slow and measured fashion.

How specifically does Anderson propose to accomplish these goals? She has developed a four-phase program that begins when a patient enters the hospital. During the first phase, *Connection with the Family*, the primary aim is for the clinician to engage the family during the crisis of the ill relative's relapse. The clinician makes contact with the family soon after the patient's admission and meets with them to discuss their reactions to the crisis, their questions about the illness, and the problems with which they need help. The goal of these meetings is to lower the emotional temperature in the home through providing information about the illness and support. By the end of the phase, feelings of confusion, helplessness, and anxiety should be reduced. At this point, a predischarge meeting is held with the patient to discuss the household structure and rules which will help to keep the patient out of the hospital.

Education about the illness continues in Phase II, *The Survival Skills Workshop*. This part of the program is a day-long workshop for four to five families who have just entered the program. During the workshop, lectures and question-answer sessions are offered around the following themes: information about the nature and the course of the illness; information about management at home; facilitating communication with the patient; and the importance of decreasing family isolation. Anderson reports that it is common for profound decreases in EE level to occur after one of these workshops because of the relief from isolation, the increased understanding of the illness, and the revision of expectations of the patient.

Phase III, *Reentry and Application of Survival Skills Themes*, occurs after the workshop. At this point symptoms are no longer acute, and the patient is home from the hospital. The tasks of this phase are preventing relapse and increasing the patient's social and vocational functioning. Rehabilitation is the main focus of this period. However, the clinician must first help the family sustain a lowered emotional temperature. In order to do this, the clinician holds biweekly family sessions dealing with appropriate expectations for patient functioning; reasonable family structure, rules, and boundaries; and effective ways of coping with symptomatic behavior. In addition, families need ongoing support to accept the slowness with which improvement in social and vocational functioning occurs. For example, families need help from the clinician to tolerate the fact that the patient may spend a great deal of time in bed right after discharge from the hospital. Family members must also be encouraged to give each other space and to pursue interests and relationships outside the home in order to reduce stress and overinvolvement.

Once the patient has an extended period of symptom stabilization, the work of the reentry phase focuses on improvement of functioning. In the first step, the family assigns small, uncomplicated household tasks to the patient. These assignments may be done initially with another family member and then slowly done independently. Evaluation and discussion of the task-assignment process occupies most of the time of sessions with the clinician at this point. Assignment gradually becomes more complex and demanding as functioning slowly improves. When and if appropriate, tasks can be moved from the home to the work world. The most important principle underlying this phase is gradual movement and attention to only one change at a time in order to avoid the excessive stress that leads to relapse. When the patient is functioning at an optimal level, the fourth phase, *Continued Treatment or Disengagement,* occurs. At this point families are given the option of more traditional family treatment to work on any unresolved systemic issues, or of gradual disengagement from the project. In terms of the latter option, Anderson recommends "maintenance sessions" which taper off over a year or longer.

Anderson's approach is fairly consistent with Strauss's vision of the phases of chronic mental illness. Although she does not earmark specific phases of patient recovery, she recognizes that patients go through periods of more or less vulnerability to relapse and increased or decreased ability to make changes in functioning. Her suggestion that families move slowly in their expectations of the patient during the initial period after decompensation is congruent with Strauss's recommendations for responding to a patient in a moratorium phase. Moreover, she proposes that patients need consistent and noncritical support from family when making changes because of the vulnerability to relapse at these times. This closely corresponds with Strauss's recommendations during change points. Finally, Anderson recognizes that different patients have different functional ceilings and that, families must therefore expect different treatment outcomes. Strauss used this notion of variable ceilings as well.

Although Anderson's psychoeducational model shares a great deal with Strauss's work and also with the body of stress/diathesis research, her model represents a major departure from many established family system approaches, as exemplified by the structural/strategic approach represented by Haley (1980) and Madanes (1983). Rather than focusing on the biopsychological nature of illnesses such as schizophrenia, Haley and Madanes focus on problematic power hierarchies in families that maintain what they refer to as "mad" behavior such as schizophrenia or anorexia nervosa or heroin addiction. The power-hierarchy disturbance that is typically seen in families of "mad" young people is one in which the young adult has become more powerful than the parent. His or her illness and the resulting mad behavior immobilizes the parents and prevents the family system from moving through that phase of the family life cycle when children are launched out of the home. Cross-generational alliances between the patient and a parent as well as marital discord reinforce this process. In order to circumvent this dysfunctional pattern, the clinician must ally with the parents and put them in charge as a team of executives over the young person's behavior. They must also help the family begin to expect and reinforce normal behavior from the patient. Madanes specifically stated that when "the young person loses power over the parents, he will begin to behave normally" (1983, p. 223). She also contended that "as long as a patient is alive, s/he should not be thought of as chronic, hopeless, or incurable" (p. 224). Abandoning an illness perspective allows the parent to expect the child to function in various capacities. A central goal of this type of treatment can thus be to improve vocational functioning.

Unlike those using the psychoeducational approach, Haley and Madanes do not educate the family about the illness and work on reducing immediate expectations. They encourage the family to expect normal behavior as soon as possible. Moreover, they believe that illness-focused education "disempowers" families. However, like Anderson, they help the families to develop tasks for the patient that are functionally targeted.

The first step of a clinician working within this framework is to meet with the family and patient before the patient's discharge from the hospital to discuss rules for behavior at home and expectations of patient functioning. The clinician's primary objective is to have the parents work as a team charged with the task of restoring the patient's normal functioning. The clinician works to keep the parents in charge despite the patient's efforts to subvert the new power hierarchy. By the end of the first interview, the parents should be able to establish clear rules, with consequences for violations, and clear expectations about patient responsibilities. During the first few sessions, deadlines are set for the patient to begin looking for work, registering for school, or entering a job-training program. Consequences are developed for noncompliance with these deadlines. For example, one family was advised to lock a resistant son out of the house on the day he was to look for a job. In addition to making demands and setting limits, the family is asked to be supportive during changes in functioning level. A father might be asked to give his son a lesson on how to dress and behave during a job interview. Despite all of this focus on the patient, the clinician's eye is on how the parents are functioning as a team and how they are handling their child's attempts to undermine the shifts in the power hierarchy.

Haley and Madanes contend that most of the clinician's work in the middle stages of treatment is in maintaining the modified power hierarchy so that the patient can figuratively "leave home." The final stages entail supporting the patient's involvement in work and in social relations, and planning for independence from the parents. When these goals are met, sessions are reduced, and the treatment is discontinued.

There are significant differences between Haley and Madanes' "structural/strategic" approach and Anderson's psychoeducational program. However, they are both rehabilitation-oriented, and they also both address the families' requests for practical advice about how they can help the patient.

In examining the results of outcome studies of relapse, the psychoeducational approach is the most effective in preventing rehospitalization. As Rohrbaugh (1983) reported, Anderson's group, Falloon's group, and Goldstein's group all show significantly lower relapse rates for patients participating in psychoeducational family programs. However, although there is a control group, this research is new, and samples are small. Haley's sample is not only small but is uncontrolled. Haley (1980) followed fourteen patients over a three-year period, and 29 percent had relapsed after an average of fourteen family therapy sessions.

An approach used by the author to help families improve an ill relative's functioning is one which combines Anderson's and Haley's approach with vocational theory (Super 1963; Ciardiello and Bingham 1982). An outline of these strategies follows, along with two case illustrations.

The clinician first helps the family to stabilize the patient by setting up clear boundaries, rules, and expectations within the home. Medication compliance is negotiated, and heightened levels of criticism, hostility, and overinvolvement with the patient are defused through education, consistent alliance-building and support for the family, and pragmatic problem-solving. In the case of an ill son or daughter living with parents, every effort is made to help the parents become a mutually supportive team and to help them function effectively as the household "executives." In the case of a single parent or a spouse, a supportive member of the family's kinship or friendship network is found to make up a supportive team. Families are also encouraged to develop extrafamilial connections in order to decrease their isolation.

Once stabilization occurs, the next goal is to increase the patient's motivation, self-appraisal, and self-esteem through a task-assignment program. Tasks start out as simple household duties and gradually increase to more demanding assignments. The family negotiates the tasks with the patient and assesses the results during sessions with the clinician.

Clear, simple feedback, support, and positive reinforcement is an important part of the family's interactions with the patient and the clinician.

As the patient moves into more complex task assignments that involve
more interaction with others outside the family, the clinician begins to discuss the patient's entry into a psychosocial rehabilitation program, job
training, or some kind of employment. The family is encouraged to provide a great deal of support at this time and to ensure that only one step at
a time is taken. The family can also be useful in helping the patient sort out
what he has learned through the task program and to integrate this with
what is known about jobs and employment opportunities.

Once the patient has entered the work world in some fashion and has
stabilized in that setting, sessions are gradually decreased. However, a
family may decide to continue treatment to work on other family issues. In
previous sessions, family issues have been addressed only if they impacted
on patient functioning. During concluding stages families have the opportunity to explore and resolve these other issues that may have emerged
earlier.

I have explained this integrated approach in the context of a single family working with a clinician. However, this approach can also be applied
within a multiple family group. Very often this format is cost-effective in
an institutional setting, as four to five families can be treated simultaneously. McFarlane (1983b) provides a helpful description of this approach and its benefits.

Two case examples illustrate more specifically how an integrated approach can be carried out with patients who are functioning at very different levels.

Case # 1

Angela was a 28-year-old single Italian female who had always lived with
her parents. She was the youngest of five children. All of her siblings lived
on their own. She had been severely ill since her first break at 17, but because of her family's insistence that they take care of her, she had never
been hospitalized.

Angela had been maintained on medications for ten years. Her diagnosis was chronic undifferentiated schizophrenia and her symptoms included unremitting auditory hallucinations of the voice of God, ideas of
reference in which she picked up sexual messages from the radio, and total
refusal to relate to anyone but her parents. Outside of her home, Angela
was mute. There were many severe negative symptoms. Angela was spend-
ing each day either sleeping or watching TV. When pressed by her parents
to help out at home, she became agitated and enraged, and screamed that
she was too confused to do anything because electrodes had been im-
planted in her spinal cord.

When her parents presented themselves for help, they revealed that Angela had never worked and had always adamantly refused to attend a local psychosocial rehabilitation program. The level of hostility, criticism, and overinvolvement in the family was quite high. The father was tremendously anxious and overresponsible, and either demanded or implored Angela to help around the house. Very often he gave up and criticized his daughter for her timidity and laziness. The mother felt entirely overwhelmed and was passive and distant after years of being unable to help her daughter.

The first treatment issue was to decrease the volatile emotional temperature in the family. Both Angela and her parents were given information about the symptoms, underlying biopsychological processes and course of the illness, the biogenic model of etiology, and the ways families can help. Everything that the parents had done formerly was framed positively as devoted concern and compassion in order to reduce guilt. The mother and father were encouraged to rely on each other for support as the importance of parental teamwork was emphasized. They were also urged to draw on the supportive resources of the extended family to ward off burnout. As the father's anxiety and frustration began to diminish with a clearer understanding of the illness and with an increased involvement by the mother in dealing with Angela, the level of tension, criticism, and hostility in the family decreased.

At this point, the family was helped to begin to expect small steps on Angela's part in becoming involved in household chores. After negotiation about this during family sessions, Angela was asked to put out the garbage daily. In slow incremental steps, she was asked to dry dishes, then wash and dry the dishes, and then make her bed. The family calmly and carefully instructed her on all the steps involved in these tasks. Family sessions included trouble-shooting when Angela became resistant and providing support and positive reinforcement to all members. The parents particularly needed support to accept the slowness with which such small changes progressed.

Feeling more confident, Angela then began to express a tentative interest in learning how to cook. The mother worked slowly and carefully with her around the routines and tasks of preparing a meal. They worked together, and Angela began very slowly to assume more and more independent responsibility for meal preparation. At present she cooks family dinners every night.

All the family members have noted that Angela's concentration, memory, planning skills, and attention have slowly improved. At present, she has a tentative interest in a career in food service. However, she is still very much impaired socially and vocationally. She is considering entering the local psychosocial rehabilitation program for more intensive rehabilitation.

Although Angela has made considerable progress, the work has often been slow and sporadic and has taken many years of biweekly family sessions.

Case # 2

Bill was a 22-year-old single Irish male who lived with his mother and two of his brothers. His father had died eight years before after a lengthy illness. Bill was the youngest of four sons, and his two brothers lived at home sporadically because of their difficulties in separating from the family. Bill had his first psychotic episode just before graduation from high school. He had been hospitalized three times since then for severe paranoid episodes in which he became agitated, explosive, and convinced that he and his family were being poisoned by a local food-processing plant. Hospitalizations typically occurred at state facilities because of the family's poor financial resources. His diagnostic presentation was withdrawn, anxious, and overly compliant. With regard to his functioning level, he had never worked for more than six months at a time.

The family presented itself for help after Bill's last discharge from the hospital. All the family members seemed calm and pleasant, although they also appeared to be unusually quiet. At times, the mother became overly protective and anxious with regard to Bill, but this dissipated easily with reassurance. The family was referred to a multiple family group run by the author. Within the group, they learned about Bill's diagnosis and about the symptoms, nature, and course of the illness. They also learned that they were perhaps being too laissez-faire in their approach to Bill's functioning. The mother was directed to request that Bill complete some small, uncomplicated household chores while she was at work. The group supported her and helped the family to gauge the successfulness of Bill's activity in the sessions. Bill and his mother received a great deal of positive reinforcement and support from other group members. After a period of increasingly demanding chore responsibilities at home, Bill found a job doing some light work at a stable near his home. Although the group was delighted in Bill's accomplishment, they also cautioned Bill and his mother about making gradual progress.

After a year of this work Bill started to explore career choices. He talked about his skills and deficits and decided that he wanted a job that would involve doing something with his hands but that would not involve a great deal of social interaction. Other parents in the group talked about their work experiences and how they decided upon their careers. Bill then decided to apply for a job as a mechanic's assistant. A father in the group who was employed as a mechanic had been particularly helpful to Bill in making this decision.

The multiple family group was effective with this family in a number of ways. The group provided a supportive network to Bill and his mother, who was an overwhelmed single parent. They also strongly urged the mother to mobilize Bill to function more effectively. The group provided a good re-source for Bill's vocational self-appraisal and provided information about the work world. This was extremely helpful to Bill and his mother in their struggle with a severe psychiatric disorder and rehabilitation.

As these two cases illustrate, the stabilization and vocational rehabilita-tion of the chronically mentally ill is not a simple task. However, the fam-ilies in each of these cases were able to make an important difference in the course of a relative's illness and as well as in his or her vocational devel-opment.

Conclusion

Families have increasingly become a significant resource in the lives of the chronically mentally ill. As numerous studies have indicated, they can play a primary role in stabilization and rehabilitation. In particular, families can make a dramatic impact upon vocational development. However, they need specific information, guidance, and support to be effective. The work of the psychoeducational practitioners, the "structural/strategic" thera-pists, and those utilizing combined approaches provides a guide for fam-ilies and for professionals. Further study of outcome and related modifica-tions of models is needed in order to help families continue their important role.

References

Anderson, C. M.; Hogarty, G. E.; and Reiss, D. J. 1980. Family treatment of adult schizo-phrenic patients: A psychoeducational approach. *Schizophrenia Bulletin, 6,* 490–505.

Anderson, C. M. 1983. A psychoeducational program for families of patients with schizo-phrenia. In *Family therapy in schizophrenia,* ed. W. R. McFarlane, pp. 99–116. New York: Guilford Press.

Boyd, J. L.; McGill, C. W.; and Falloon, I.R.H. 1981. Family participation in the community rehabilitation of schizophrenics. *Hospital and Community Psychiatry, 32,* 629–32.

Brown, G. W.; Birley, J. T.; and Wing, J. K. 1972. Influence of family life on the course of schizophrenic disorders: A replication. *British Journal of Psychiatry, 121,* 241–58.

Ciardiello, J. A., and Bingham, W. C. 1982. The career maturity of schizophrenic clients. *Rehabilitation Counseling Bulletin, 26,* 3–9.

Grunebaum, H. 1984. Comments on Terkelsen's "Schizophrenia and the family, II: Adverse effects on family therapy." *Family Process, 23,* 421–27.

Haley, J. 1980. *Leaving home.* New York: McGraw Hill.

Hatfield, A. B. 1979. The family as partner in the treatment of mental illness. *Hospital and Community Psychiatry, 30,* 338–40.

———. 1983. What families want of family therapists. In *Family therapy in schizophrenia,* ed.

W. R. McFarlane, pp. 41–65. New York: Guilford Press.

Leff, J. P.; Kuipers, L.; and Berkowitz, R. 1983. Intervention in families of schizophrenics and its effect on relapse rate. In *Family therapy in schizophrenia*, ed. W. R. McFarlane, pp. 173–77. New York: Guilford Press.

McFarlane, W. R. 1983a. Introduction to *Family therapy in schizophrenia*, ed. W. R. McFarlane, pp. 1–13. New York: Guilford Press.

———. 1983b. Multiple family therapy in schizophrenia. In *Family therapy in schizophrenia*, ed. W. R. McFarlane, pp. 141–72. New York: Guilford Press.

Madanes, C. 1983. Strategic therapy of schizophrenia. In *Family therapy in schizophrenia*, ed. W. R. McFarlane, pp. 209–25. New York: Guilford Press.

Rohrbaugh, M. 1983. Family therapy and schizophrenia research: Swimming against the mainstream. *The Family Therapy Networker, 7,* 28–31.

Ryglewicz, H. 1984. An agenda for family intervention: Issues, models, and practice. In *Advances in treating the young adult chronic patient*, ed. B. Pepper and H. Ryglewicz, pp. 81–90. San Francisco: Jossey-Bass.

Strauss, J. S.; Hafez, H.; Lieberman, P.; and Harding, C. M. 1985. The course of psychiatric disorder, III: Longitudinal principles. *American Journal of Psychiatry, 142,* 289–96.

Super, D. E. 1963. Self-concepts in vocational development. In *Career development: Self-concept theory*, ed. D. E. Super. New York: CEEB.

Terkelsen, K. G. 1983. Schizophrenia and the family, II: Adverse effects of family therapy. *Family Process, 22,* 191–200.

Uzoka, A. F. 1979. The myth of the nuclear family: Historical background and clinical implications. *American Psychologist, 34,* 1095–1106.

Vaughn, C. E., and Leff, J. P. 1976. The influence of family and social factors on the course of psychiatric illness: A comparison of schizophrenic and depressed neurotic patients. *British Journal of Psychiatry, 129,* 125–37.

Vaughn, C. E.; Snyder, K. S.; Freeman, W.; Jones, S.; Falloon, I.R.H.; and Liberman, R. P. 1982. Family factors in schizophrenic relapse: A replication. *Schizophrenia Bulletin, 8,* 425–26.

8

The Psychodynamics of Work

RICHARD L. MUNICH and TSILIA GLINBERG

Although Freud cited success in work and love as the desired outcome of psychoanalysis, there has been very little written which explicitly addresses the capacity to work from a psychodynamic perspective. Munich and Glinberg's chapter is an important contribution to understanding the intrapsychic factors which can inhibit vocational functioning. Included are developmental, drive, ego, object relations, and self-psychological points of view. In addition, the authors consider the special problems of women and work.

> One can live magnificently in this world, if one knows how to work and how to love; to work for the person one loves and to love one's work.
> —Leo Tolstoy

Because skill acquisition and work adaptation rarely take place in a social or psychological vacuum, psychodynamic factors are relevant to different extents in every case of work dysfunction. In some cases, these psychodynamic factors are primary, so that even the most effective program for vocational rehabilitation will have difficulty without considering them. In other cases, psychological issues are secondary to years of failure and dysfunction in a way that a successful program gradually ameliorates. Generally, however, the vocational rehabilitation of chronically disturbed patients will be enhanced to the degree that it addresses and is informed by a psychodynamic understanding of the client's work deficits or inhibitions. Since there are some patients with minimal psychological disturbance who have severe vocational deficits and some severely disturbed patients who manage to sustain work, it is not easy to generalize about this subject. Therefore, this chapter focuses on psychodynamic considerations of work and its inhibition, irrespective of the client's level of disturbance or chronicity.

Work is both a psychological and sociological function. According to Jaques (1960) it "is a fundamental activity in a person's testing and strengthening of his sanity." Resulting from the dual need of the human organism for instinctual gratification and self-preservation, it evolves from the infant's earliest activities necessary to achieve these ends. While it extends through the childhood experiences of play and learning, both of which are modified and enhanced by social constraints, successful work adaptation is the culmination of several psychodynamic trends integrated in complex ways.

Several factors complicate explication of the psychodynamics of work and its inhibition. To begin with, there is a lack of consensus about what elements contribute to the capacity to work: self-preservation and adherance to the reality principle, a sublimation of unconscious sexual and aggressive fantasies (i.e., a substitute pleasure), or a reaction formation inherent in instincts which produces the repetition of certain behavior and experience irrespective of the striving for pleasure. Some authors have gone so far as to posit work as a basic instinct, comparable to the pleasure principle and demanding equal gratification. The second factor one must consider is the multiplicity of dynamic points of view concerning the problem: developmental, drive theory, ego psychology, object relations theory, and self psychology. Finally, an explication of dynamics depends on the level of personality organization of the individual involved: neurotic, borderline, or psychotic.

Work inhibition denotes many different things and manifests itself in a variety of ways. On a pragmatic and descriptive continuum, it might extend from being unable to work at any job to being unable to complete a doctoral dissertation. On a more theoretical or developmental continuum, work inhibition might extend from a severe school phobia to job failure as a consequence of a midlife crisis. Various examples of patients with work inhibition highlight just a few of the several aspects of this dilemma. A 38-year-old man came for consultation because each time he came up for promotion, he felt compelled to change companies. By virtue of these changes, he had, in fact, attained a level of considerable responsibility in his present position. His present anxiety derived from the suspicion that the same chain of events was about to occur. Late in the interview the patient told a story about going to urinate during halftime of a football game. The closer he came to the front of the line, the more anxious he became. When it became his turn, he had to leave. Another patient, a 22-year-old compensated schizophrenic woman left the hospital to take a bus trip for a job interview. Several hours later she was returned to hospital floridly psychotic, having been found wandering in a neighborhood at the end of the bus line. Many hours with the patient were needed to discover that, in addition to her anxieties about leaving the hospital unaccompanied, she had not known exactly at which bus stop to get off. Most important, she did not know to ask the bus driver and was incapable of asking any of her fellow passengers for assistance.

In contrast to these inhibitions is the well-documented phenomenon that during some crises disturbed patients are able to organize and perform at high levels. A typical example of this concerned the three-week strike of hospital maintenance, housekeeping, and dietary personnel. With modest encouragement, the staff mobilized the severely disturbed patients to provide replacement for these services at an acceptable level with a minimum number of incidents. When the strike was over, patients returned to their usual low level of functioning. Similarly, it is well known that individuals with severe neurotic symptoms can regularly function in positions of great responsibility and authority. Thus, the context in which work happens is critically important. Although several studies have failed to demonstrate significant relationships between psychiatric symptomatology and vocational functioning (Ciardiello and Turner 1980; Ciardiello, Klein, and Sobkowski 1981), it is intuitively obvious that some symptoms are debilitating. Certain phobias, severe depression, and psychoticism with bizarre delusions and command hallucinations are examples of symptoms that interfere with and inhibit work adaptation.

A useful way to organize and think about many of these issues and the ways in which work and its inhibition have been described is to divide the points of view into writings which focus either on intrapsychic conflict or on ego defects. While both processes could lead to the same observable problem or inhibition, it is our hypothesis that most difficulties in work adaptation, especially with more disturbed individuals, result from a complicated admixture of both, and, therefore, that treatment and rehabilitation approaches which do not address both the patient's conflict and deficit will have a far more difficult task.

Intrapsychic Conflict

Although Freud indicated that the capacity to love and work were essential ingredients of the healthy personality, both he and subsequent psychoanalytic authors generally neglected problems associated with work. Freud first mentions the "incapacity for work" in 1892 in "A Case of Hypnotic Treatment," but elaborates neither its etiology nor its course. In Freud's account of a patient with an obsessional neurosis, self reproaches for neglectful behavior at the time of his father's death led to a serious incapacity in the Rat Man's ability to work. Freud related this work disturbance to unconscious ambivalence toward the patient's father (1909); and he posited similar dynamics—that is, a conflict between two internal and mutually exclusive impulses (in this case, love and aggression)—in "A Seventeenth-Century Demonological Neurosis" (1923).

Finally, in 1926 in "Inhibitions, Symptoms, and Anxiety," Freud wrote:

In inhibition to work—a thing which we so often have to deal with as an isolated symptom in our therapeutic work—the subject feels a decrease in his pleasure in it or becomes less able to do it well; or he has certain reactions to it, like fatigue, giddiness or sickness, if he is obliged to go on with it. If he is a hysteric, he will have to give up his work owing to the appearance of organic and functional paralysis which make it impossible for him to carry it on. If he is an obsessional neurotic, he will be perpetually being distracted from his work or losing time over it through the introduction of delays and repetitions. (P. 89)

Using the new concepts of the structural theory, Freud wrote that "inhibition is the expression of restriction of ego function," and elaborated a problem in each mental structure that might contribute to that restriction. The first, from the id, occurred as a result of pressure from forbidden instinctual strivings; strivings which, for example, led to the eroticization of various ego functions. The second occurs when, in an effort to avoid conflict, the punitive superego will not allow success and gain. Both of these formulations might be employed to explain the example of the man who became anxious at the prospect of promotion. Finally, Freud suggested that the ego itself might sustain a "generalized inhibition" resulting from a diminution in its' energy secondary to severe physical illness, life stress, or loss and its attendant mourning.

Writing specifically about "occupational inhibition," Fenichel (1945) elaborated Freud's notion by stating that occupational inhibition did not constitute a psychological unit. "It occurs whenever a person's occupation required the performance of actions that have become inhibited. Thus all types of inhibitions may form the basis of occupational inhibitions" (p. 183). He listed four specific ways in which actions could become inhibited: conflicts around dependence and independence and around ambition (preoedipal); conflicts around authority, all struggles between rebellion and work (oedipal); work which is reactive to any instinctual demand (the compulsive worker); and finally, neurotic disturbances of attention and concentration. Confirmation of and variation in all but the last of these pathways have been provided by Halperin (1964), Oberndorf (1951), Savitt (1959), and Munich (1986), among others.

Erik Erikson's (1950) epigenetic scheme synthesizes developmental, drive, ego, and social psychological theories. The third stage in this scheme, initiative versus guilt, coincides with the resolution of the oedipal phase of psychosexual development, identification with the parent of the same sex, and internalization of society's mores in the form of conscience. The child is thus able to add to his or her autonomy "the quality of undertaking, planning and 'attacking' a task" (p. 255). Initiative inevitably leads to competition and rivalry, not only for primacy with the parent of the opposite sex, but also in the internal work of fantasy as well as the external one of physical reality. As the stage indicates, the risk of initiative is guilt. There is the guilt of forbidden wishes; there is the guilt associated with assuming more than the developing organism can manage; and there is the guilt that comes with success. A most important and potentially inhibiting consequence of the developmental chores of this stage, especially in the struggles with guilt, is the growth of a conscience, or superego, that not only appropriately regulates impulses but also overpowers them with hateful and moralistic tendencies.

If, however, there is a mutual and synergistic relation between the pressure to initiative and the constraints of guilt, then the growing individual is prepared to negotiate the next, fourth stage—industry versus inferiority. The successful strivings for initiative lead naturally to the work of production. "To bring a productive situation to completion is an aim which gradually supersedes the whims and wishes of play" (Erikson 1950, p. 259). School, systematic instruction, and the fundamentals of technology are, of course, the orders of the day. Here is also where self-confidence and self-esteem emerge as critical issues. Many authors, such as Horney (1947) and Jaques (1960), have listed confidence as a critical feature in the capacity to work, while low self-esteem has been correlated with poor vocational rehabilitation outcome and unemployment in psychiatric patients (Watts and Po-Kwan 1976; Griffiths 1974). Unsuccessful struggles with the agenda of this phase of development undermine the growing sense of confidence and lead to a sense of inadequacy and feelings of inferiority. The child may be pulled back to the family and its oedipal struggles and have to struggle again with those early identifications. This struggle impedes his or her already fragmentary efforts to acquire and employ instrumental means "beside and with others." Here is where the sociocultural aspects of work and its inhibition have their roots.

Ego Defects

According to various writers, especially Hartmann (1950), the ego is at the center of the personality, integrating and mediating between the inner demands of the id and superego and outer demands from the environment. The ego is responsible for reality testing, the capacity to regress, judgment, impulse control, thought processes, defensive functioning, stimulus barrier, synthetic functioning, objects relations, and a whole host of so-called autonomous functions. These autonomous functions include attention, concentration, memory, learning, perception, motor functioning, language skills, habit patterns, and intention. An ego impaired in these responsibilities or functions makes adaptation more difficult, and especially so in the individual's efforts to cope with the demands of vocational functioning.

So far, the psychodynamic point of view we have focused on has involved conflict between and within psychic structures. While the ego is involved in most of these conflicts, there is another point of view that focuses on problems within the ego itself. Freud (1911) first alluded to a defect in the ego when he attempted to delineate the mechanism of paranoia. Although he later (1926) modified this notion that in psychosis the ego was incapable of cathecting objects or the external world, the debate between a conflict and defect model to explain certain forms of psychopathology has remained a lively one.

The point of view one takes in this controversy has substantial relevance for an understanding of the etiology of dysfunctional or maladaptive aspects of work performance. That is, is functional incapacity the result of conflicts within the ego between competing drives, drive derivatives, self or object representations or identifications; or is it the result of some inherent defect in the structure of the ego itself? The idea of an inherent defect in the ego is reminiscent of and relevant for Freud's concept of "generalized inhibition" and Fenichel's use of "disturbances of attention and concentration" mentioned earlier. Aspects of ego failure may be used to account for the example of the decompensation of the patient on the bus.

Although not at all what Freud had in mind, Hendrick's concept of the work principle (1943) is a good starting point for this idea: "work is not primarily motivated by sexual need or associated aggressions, but by the need for efficient use of the muscular and intellectual tool, regardless of what secondary needs—self-preservative, aggressive or sexual—a work performance may also satisfy." (p. 311). Giving work the same status in psychological life as the pleasure principle, in which the individual strives to maximize pleasure and minimize pain, Hendrick believed that there were certain basic ego functions gratified by work. He referred to these functions as the "executant functions" of the ego. Drawing from French, Waelder, Nunberg and Hartmann, Hendrick included the highly integrated perceptual, cognitive, and muscular manifestations of the central nervous system. Although their development is affected by object relations, frustrations, and identifications, this theory suggests that the executant functions are "responses to an instinct differing in its goal, purpose, and pleasure mechanism from the libido" (p. 314). This is the "instinct to master" and is regarded, like any other instinct in psychoanalytic terms, as the biological source of tensions impelling to specific patterns of action. Differing from sexual, sadistic, and aggressive instincts, the aim of the instinct to master that Hendrick postulates is to control or alter a piece of the environment and to perform one's work efficiently.

A most important consequence of this theory is the idea that failures in the gratification of the instinct to master are not simply the result of the usual processes of conflict, repression, and anxiety. The instinct to master might also be interfered with by defects inherent in the ego apparatus itself. Although Hendrick is referring here to problems with defects in partial autonomous functions like ocular fixation, sucking, and phonation, it is implicit that he also means defects which result from underlying problems in the ego's "physical" structure (anatomical, biochemical, or physiologic) or in its more behaviorally oriented development (modeling, conditioning, learning).

Writing on the development of children, Thomas and Chess (1980) echo Hendrick's questions about the exclusively motivational framework for perception, language, and cognition. They conclude that "highly significant phenomena, such as exploratory behavior, curiosity, and pleasure in problem-solving, cannot really be explained by instinct and drive reduction theory" (p. 45). Drawing from Eisenberg, Papousek, and Piaget, these authors not only posit task mastery and social competence as linked concepts, but also see the infant as either biologically equipped or flawed for the pursuit of these two basic adaptive goals.

Severe emotional illnesses, especially schizophrenia and other psychotic illnesses, are viewed as the consequence of ego dysfunction. Again, this dysfunction might have constitutional as well as developmental origins. In a recent study of ego deficits and vocational rehabilitation of schizophrenic patients, Ciardiello, Klein, and Sobkowski (1984) showed that the two ego functions that differentiated between those schizophrenic patients with work experience and those without it were a higher level of autonomous functioning and a greater capacity to regress in the service of the ego. The latter especially included greater flexibility in meeting the demands of a job and in offering "creative alternative strategies" in dealing with the individual's disabilities themselves. This flexibility leads naturally to a discussion of the synthetic function of the ego.

The Synthetic Function of the Ego

Except for performance of the most primitive of tasks, adaptation and task mastery require the ego to synthesize various contradictory elements within itself. The synthetic function of the ego, first formulated by Nunberg (1931), "acts" to perceive, assess, and coordinate demands coming from the drives, the superego, external reality, and established ego institutions such as the autonomous functions. The concept of the synthetic function was elaborated by Schilder (1951), who included even more complex phenomena in the concept: building perceptions from sensations and connecting and integrating them with already available memories, combining groups of perceptions with object representations to form concepts, and integrating concepts with such other aspects within the personality as needs, affects, opinions, and convictions. Thus, synthetic processes in the ego are responsible for abstract and consequential thinking and the ability to form new concepts. Insofar as task mastery involves these elements, the synthetic function also has an essential relation to the capacity for work.

In linking concepts of identity and its diffusion with the synthetic function, Prelinger (1958) notes various interferences with an effectual synthetic process. At times, for example, when the ego is struggling against powerful impulses, the synthetic function may act inappropriately, as in the formation of pathological rationalizations, delusions, or ideas of reference. As we have suggested earlier, these "primitive synthetic efforts" run counter to reality testing and may lead to an inhibition of function.

Two other ego functions which have an inhibitory effect on the synthetic function are differentiation and defense. Whereas differentiation may be in the service of growth, it also may, according to Prelinger, "lead to fragmentation of experience, to concreteness, and to dependence on haphazard stimuli . . . or to exclusive domination by whatever psychological process is operative at any moment" (p. 226). Similarly, synthetic functioning may be compromised whenever the ego must defend against representations of impulses, especially insofar as defenses act to deconstruct connections between these representations and the corresponding representation of their objects.

We have focused on the ego's synthetic function and dysfunction because of its central role in the capacity for work. Furthermore, in no more critical location than in the synthetic function do the two themes of conflict and deficit come together. The evolution of the synthetic function is inevitably connected with the last phases of adolescence, when the consolidation of an integrated or ego identity takes places. As Erikson (1956) summarizes it, ego identity is "a configuration gradually integrating constitutional givens, idiosyncratic libidinal needs, favored capacities, significant identifications, effective defenses, successful sublimation, and consistent roles" (p. 71). Earlier, Erikson (1950) termed this stage in development as one of identity versus role confusion. In this phase, the maturing adolescent is not only concerned with the rejection and selection of identity fragments but also with "the question of how to connect the roles and skills cultivated earlier with the occupational prototypes of the day" (p. 26). Commenting on the sense of competence that goes with identity and a sense of self, White (1966) notes the ease and confidence that is critical for the person in performing significant acts or in taking on significant roles. Role confusion and identity diffusion often manifest themselves in the inability to settle on a career or occupational identity. This inability may account for many of the obstacles inherent in work inhibition.

Object Relations Theory and Self Psychology

The concepts of the synthetic function and ego identity lead to a consideration of the place of more contemporary psychodynamic frameworks in work and its inhibition. Although object relations theory is naturally more concerned with interpersonal relationships and social competence than with adaptation and task mastery, the effect of pathological internalized object relations on the capacity to work can be profound.

Since there is almost no work which exists in a vacuum, virtually every work situation itself mobilizes these internalized relations. At the most superficial levels, an individual may have many adaptive skills, but when he or she is in the workplace, interactions with fellow workers and/or employers lead to restrictions in the use of those skills. At the same time, the social context might provide a matrix in which pathologic object relations are temporarily "normalized" and skills enhanced, as in the earlier example of the high functioning of disturbed hospitalized patients during the strike. Irrespective of the context and at a deeper level, internalized object relations affect self-esteem in ways that have already connected with decreased work functioning.

According to Kernberg (1983), unconscious intrapsychic conflicts are more than those between impulse and defense or between psychic structures: "These conflicts are between two opposing units or sets of internalized objects relations. Each of these units consist of a self and an object representation under the impact of a drive derivative (clinically, an affect disposition). Both impulse and defense find expression through an affectively imbued internalized object relation" (p. 247–48).

When discussing earlier psychodynamic points of view, we alluded to the notion of identification with parents and parental roles. Following Kris (1955) and returning briefly to the language of ego psychology, one might add here the idea that sublimation and/or neutralization of aggression resulting from the process of identification enhances the capacity to do work. Whereas Kris and other psychoanalytic theorists felt that the assimilation of qualities and characteristics came from abandoned object relations, this complicated process by which the developing child emulates and incorporates aspects of each parent while constructing an identity is modified in an important way by object relations theory. In object relations theory the child also internalizes the relationship between the developing self and the parental object. Modified by drives, thus are the self and object representations established.

Kernberg uses as an example of the results of this process an excessively passive man who may function with the following two units or sets of internalized object relations in conflict with or split off from one another: one unit consists of a self representation which easily submits to a powerful and protective parental or object representation; the other unit, more repressed and against which the former defends, is an angry and rebellious self-representation that takes into account a sadistic and castrating parental representation. Hence, every time this man is faced with a demand from an authority figure, affects and representations from these sets are mobilized, and the conflict is stimulated. It is not difficult to imagine the difficulties in self-esteem, acquiescence, and achievement that accrue to such a person. If we add to this equation a father with a defective occupational identity or troubled work history of his own, then the conditions for work inhibition prevail. Incidentally, a parent's troubled work history might include not only failure but also success achieved at great cost. It is not uncommon to see profound work inhibitions in severely disturbed patients one of whose parents has accomplishments at a very high level. In this context, it is worth noting the possibility that both the mode and product of work can assume the elements of an object representation in the developing unconscious. Insofar as libidinal and aggressive drives fuel the identifications inherent in self and object representations, so would Hendrick's "work instinct" play a similar role. A young child, for example, might include as part of his or her representations the picture of its father working—the style, pace, intensity, and investment. For some children, the view of father working (or stories about it) may be the only way to construct a picture of him. A precursor for this would be the way in which the mother or the father has played with the child. Similarly, an adult might so value the product of his or her work that it becomes a way of compensating for deficiencies in otherwise defective self and object units.

Object relations theory has a position in the conflict-deficit controversy. If we think of the conflict between different sets of self and object representations as one way to account for difficulties in development, then the idea of a defective (split-off fragmented and/or grandiose) self, proposed by Kohut (1971, 1977) and the self-psychologists, is its opposite. This latter version of the self, available to the empathic perception of the therapist and the introspective perception of the patient, is conceived of as a holistic structure which expresses "the organization, competence and environmental fit of the personality as a whole" (Hoit 1984). For self-psychologists "unresolved grandiose fantasies from infancy contain the energic aspects of the personality and are split off or repressed. This leaves the central reality-self depleted of energy . . . and therefore incapable of competent functioning. . . . Kohut has also described the failure of organization of the personality and the persistant splitting of the self as due to a failure of internalization on the part of basic tension-regulating ego structure" (p. 230).

Writing about disturbances in the work ego, Hoit comments on how the experience of identity diffusion can be masked by defensive rationalization, so that the development of grandiosity covers underlying feelings of helplessness. He continues: "It is especially necessary to recognize when one is dealing with a situation in which the ego has been overwhelmed, is functioning with a deficit, or is exhausted" (p. 238). Many late adolescents who are unable to work academically present three possible psychological and treatment scenarios. First, exploration will reveal that the sense of self has remained cohesive, and the work inhibition is amenable to classical analytic technique. Second, the sense of self is only relatively cohesive, with many signs of fragmentation and a struggle to find a suitable object to complete the sense of self. Here the therapist must help the patient identify his or her "narcissistic-need structure," that is, to recognize all elements of the struggle for objects. And finally, work stoppage can be the most obvious sign that a fragmentation of the self is threatening to become permanent. This type of fragmentation is the situation that leads the developing adolescent to addiction, perverse sexuality, paranoia, or psychosis and requires support, psychotropic drugs, or hospitalization.

This most severe form of fragmentation and defective self returns us, once again, to Freud's idea of a generalized inhibition and its role in the more profound disturbances of work, the work ego, and occupational identity. It is clear that there are many pathways to work inhibition, both through primary processes of adaptation and secondarily in the establishment of self and object representations and relationships. These pathways touch, intersect, and diverge many times during normal development and may be a result of intrapsychic conflict, ego deficit, or various combinations of both.

Object Relations and Self Psychology in Adult Development and Work Inhibition

Whereas the processes that lead to successful and maladaptive work patterns are more noticeable in late adolescence and early adulthood, it is generally agreed that development and its interferences continue through adult life. Writing about disturbances in adult work and creativity, especially during the critical midlife transition, Jaques (1965) adds the awareness of death to the features that play a role in our complicated story. Jaques focuses on changes in the mode and content of work of the developing adult (35–45 years). Essentially, the mode of work changes from a product that is spontaneous and unsculpted to one which is more worked over and sculpted. In the content of work, there is a shift to more and more tragic and philosophic detail. The familiar features of the change are described:

Late adolescent and early adult idealism and optimism, accompanied by split-off and projected hate, are given up and supplanted by a more contemplative pessimism. There is a shift from radical desire and impatience to a more reflective and tolerant conservatism. Beliefs in the inherent goodness of man are placed by a recognition and acceptance of the fact that inherent goodness is accompanied by hate and destructive forces within, which contribute to man's own misery and tragedy. (Pp. 504–5).

Jaques shows that a successful resolution of the midlife crisis requires the individual to explicitly recognize, acknowledge, and integrate two fundamental features of human life—"the inevitableness of eventual death, and the existence of hate and destructive impulses inside each person" (p. 505). In summary, he believes that "the successful outcome of mature creative work lies thus in constructive resignation both to the imperfections of men and to shortcomings in one's own work" (p. 505). According to Jaques, this resignation is accomplished by working through the reemergence of the infantile depressive position, a position that had been repressed when the original self or object representation was formed.

Colarusso and Nemiroff (1981) use the premises of self-psychology to account for disturbances in the development of adult work habits and creativity. They hypothesize that while early identifications help build psychic structure, "later identifications such as the mentor relationship add specificity to the adult personality, in this instance, through the establishment of a work identity" (p. 98). This process involves an initial fusion with the mentor, internalization of aspects of this mentor through partial identifications, and then a separation which leads to further individuation. There are many pitfalls in this process, especially insofar as each step might catalyze a "reemergence of aspects of infantile narcissism." Specifically, the mentor might be used to supply narcissistic needs, complete a sense of self or bolster self-esteem rather than simply become a new object with which to identify. When in this process previously disguised fragmentation is uncovered and grandiose tendencies are mobilized, then "stagnation, regression and self-limitation" may ensue. Drawing upon Kohut, these authors state that this regression

refers to the archaic, inflated self-configurations and archaic, overestimated representations of others which have not been integrated into the personality. The result is an impoverishment of the adult personality and its mature functions because of the deprivation of energies which are invested in the ancient structures and a hampering of adult realistic activities because of the breakthrough and intrusion of archaic representations and claims. (P. 99)

Colarusso and Nemiroff have developed the following table to outline the development of work adaptation in adult life. The table also highlights the well-known fact that work adaptation may be altered throughout the course of development.

Late teens and twenties
  Ability to make a choice, to identify work skills

Growth of capacity for sustained work
Pleasure, interest in work
Success and failure

Thirties
Solidification of work identity
Continued development of skills
Level of achievement
Balancing of work and family, work and play, etc.

Forties and fifties
Continued development of skills and achievement
Acceptance of failure to reach certain goals
Choice of new or second career—effect of development, realistic or not
Working for society, for others
Use of power and position

Sixties and seventies
Continued involvement in meaningful work and play
Ability to transfer power to the young
Attitudes toward retirement

(P. 206)

Special Problems of Women

As working people, women are as vulnerable to work inhibitions as men. However, because of their traditionally domestic sphere of activity, women's particular work inhibitions require special consideration. Even outside the home, for example, women are still expected to provide nurturant functions, much of the substantive work in such occupational roles as secretary, nurse, teacher, paralegal, waitress, and flight attendant.

One special set of conflicts that emerge in these supportive roles outside the home relates to the tensions between loyalties to home and work. Guilt about being outside the home during the day inevitably mobilizes questions of maternal competence. These questions may lead to the impairment of work productivity and satisfaction. This conflict between work and home often intensifies when a woman wants or receives promotion, accrues more responsibility or needs to spend more time acquiring a prerequisite degree. Naturally, these strains are heightened in the case where parental identifications stress and reinforce the traditional roles, as in the following vignette:

A woman physician decided over the subtle objections of her parents and the explicit objection of her husband to obtain an advanced degree in a related field. Following an invitation to teach a course from one of her professors and while on Christmas vacation with her husband, she reported a disturbing dream. In the dream she had just finished showering. Standing naked in the bedroom of their house, she heard her mother calling from downstairs that she must hurry as the police were coming. The physician knew that she was being accused of murdering a child, and there was circumstantial evidence implicating her. As soon as she heard her mother's voice, she started hiding a box containing the evidence and began dressing frantically.

In exploring this dream, the patient was able to connect her wish to further education with the murder of the baby both her mother and her husband wished her to have.

Another set of conflicts unique to women occur with those who have moved out of their traditional gender identities altogether and ventured into the "male" world of science, technology, administration, and politics. The executive woman or the female boss does not simply turn into a man in a skirt. She has the task of more fully integrating various feminine and masculine identifications and becoming more flexible in shifting identities, languages, and powers. The more complicated the task, the more potential conflicts in achieving it.

Most writers on feminine psychology suggest that women may be less able to deal with the loneliness and frustration of the executive position (Krueger 1984). In addition, the conflict of gender identity reactivated by the executive woman in all of her staff is played out by the female boss's not obtaining the conscious and unconscious support and admiration from her female staff that male bosses usually get (Applegarth 1976). Instead, all concerned are reminded of various aspects of the oedipal conflict, such as competition with and betrayal of her mother, sisters, female children, for father, husband, and brother.

Additionally, in obtaining her executive post the woman has surpassed her male colleagues. Since few men tolerate this situation well, they may consciously or unconsciously hate and avoid her and sabotage her work. These particular dynamics point to an inherent paradox: what she needs more of by virtue of being a woman she will get less of because she is a woman in a traditionally male role. The workplace by and large is not ready to accommodate fully to the executive woman; so she tends to accommodate to the system—at the price, however, of limited productivity, restriction of creative endeavors, and stunted upward mobility. One outcome of this particular inhibition is that the promotion of executive women often tends to stop at the level of middle management: associate director, associate professor, junior partner, rather than chief executive officer.

According to Karen Horney (1934) and Helene Deutsch (1944), women tend to be more insecure and require a greater degree of positive interaction with their immediate external environment to maintain their self-esteem. Although this is a traditional and conservative point of view, perhaps more so in women than men, downward fluctuations of self-esteem seem to play a key role in the ability to work productively.

In addition to the conflicting identifications women have to overcome, there are various external obstacles and pressures against succeeding in their work. They need to overcome traditional gender stereotypes in the population at large. A woman carpenter or plumber would have to work a lot harder to get clients than a man in the same trade simply because people are not accustomed to seeing women in these trades. Women, like minorities, have to prove themselves more outstanding to succeed in a job traditionally held by men. These internal and external pressures to rework gender identities require that men and women collaborate more closely at home as well as at work. Often, however, the attempt to alter traditional work roles leads to strain, marital disruption, or divorce.

Conclusion

This summary of psychodynamic issues in work and its inhibition includes developmental, drive, ego psychological, object relations, and self-psychological points of view. It has organized these from the point of view of intrapsychic conflict, constitutional and ego deficits, and the tension between them. Although psychodynamics is interested in the vicissitudes of work, the issues involved obviously go way beyond the individual and his or her psychological status. Furthermore, conceptualizations of the severe disturbances in adaptation that characterize the population this book is designed to serve are less well formulated than conceptualizations for those who can be addressed from a purely psychodynamic point of view.

It is therefore the recommendation of these authors that a psychodynamic approach to the rehabilitation of patients with severe and prolonged mental illness be adjunctive rather than central. This recommendation in no way diminishes the importance of a psychological understanding of an individual with these disturbances, in spite of its complexity and the difficulty in quantifying it.

References

Applegarth, A. 1976. Some observations of work inhibitions in women. *American Journal of Psychoanalysis*, 24, 251–68.
Berger, M. 1979. On work inhibition. Paper read at the Chicago Insitute for Psychoanalysis, April 29.
Ciardiello, J. A.; Klein, M. E.; and Sobkowski, S. 1981. Final report of the vocational rehabilitation project—Part I (SREG 116). Trenton, N.J.: Department of Education, Division of Vocational Education and Career Preparation.
———. 1984. Ego functioning and the Vocational rehabilitation of schizophrenic clients. In *The broad scope of ego function assessment.* ed. L. Bellak and L. Goldsmith. New York: Wiley and Sons.

Ciardiello, J. A., and Turner, F. D. 1980. Final report of the vocational assessment project (SREG 808). Trenton, N.J.: Department of Education, Division of Vocational Education and Career Preparation.

Colarusso, C., and Nemiroff, R. 1981. *Adult Development.* New York: Plenum Press.

Deutsch, H. 1944. *Psychology of women,* Vol. 1. New York: Bantam Books.

Erikson, E. 1950. *Childhood and society.* New York: Norton.

———. 1956. The problem of ego identity. *Journal of the American Psychoanalytic Association, 4,* 56–121.

Fenichel, O. 1945. *The psychoanalytic theory of neurosis.* New York: Norton.

Freud, S. 1892. A case of hypnotic treatment. *Standard Edition,* 1:118.

———. 1909. Notes upon a case of obsessional neurosis. *Standard Edition,* 10:151–318.

———. 1911. Psychoanalytic notes on an autobiographical account of a case of paranoia (dementia pardoides). *Standard Edition,* 12:9–79.

———. 1923. A seventeenth-century demonological neurosis. *Standard Edition,* 19:69–108.

———. 1926. Inhibitions, symptoms, and anxiety. *Standard Edition,* 20:77–174.

Griffiths, R. D. 1974. Rehabilitation of chronic psychotic patients: an assessment of their psychological handicap, an evaluation of the effectiveness of rehabilitation, and observations of the factors which predict outcome. *Psychological Medicine, 4,* 316–25.

Halperin, H. 1964. Work inhibition in children. *Psychoanalytic Review, 51,* 173.

Hartmann, H. 1964. Comments on the psychoanalytic theory of the ego (1950). In *Essays on ego psychology,* ed. H. Hartmann. New York: International Universities Press.

Hendrick, I. 1943. Work and the pleasure principle. *Psychoanalytic Quarterly, 12,* 311–29.

Hoit, M. 1984. Collapse of the work-ego in adolescence. In *Late adolescence: Psychoanalytic studies,* ed. D. Brockman. New York: International Universities Press.

Horney, K. 1934. The overevaluation of love. *Psychoanalytic Quarterly, 3,* 605–38.

———. 1947. Inhibitions in work. *American Journal of Psychoanalysis, 7,* 18–25.

Jaques, E. 1960. Disturbances in the capacity to work. *International Journal of Psychoanalysis, 41,* 357–67.

———. 1965. Death and the midlife crisis. *International Journal of Psychoanalysis, 46,* 502–14.

Kernberg, O. 1983. Object relations theory and character analysis. *Journal of the American Psychoanalytic Association, 31,* 247–71.

Kohut, H. 1971. *The analysis of the self.* New York: International Universities Press.

———. 1977. *The restoration of self.* New York: International Universities Press.

Kris, E. 1955. Neutralization and sublimation: Observations in young children. *Psychoanalytic Study of the Child, 10,* 30–46.

Krueger, D. W. 1984. *Success and the fear of success in women.* New York: Free Press.

Lantos, B. 1952. Metapsychological considerations on the concept of work. *International Journal of Psychoanalysis, 33,* 439–43.

Munich, R. L. 1986. Transitory symptom formation in the analysis of an obsessional character. *Psychoanalytic Study of the Child, 41,* 515–34.

Nunberg, H. 1931. The synthetic function of the ego. *International Journal of Psychoanalysis, 12,* 123–40.

Oberndorf, C. P. 1951. Psychopathology of work. *Bulletin of the Menninger Clinic, 15,* 77–84.

Prelinger, E. 1958. Identity Diffusion and the synthetic function. In *Psychosocial problems of college men,* ed. B. N. Wedge. New Haven: Yale University Press.

Savitt, R. 1959. The analysis of an occupational inhibition. *Journal of Hillel Hospital, 8,* 131–37.

Schilder, P. 1951. Studies concerning the psychology and symptomatology of general paresis. In *Organization and pathology of thought,* ed. D. Rappaport, pp. 519–80. New York: Columbia University Press.

Thomas, A., and Chess, S. 1980. *The dynamics of psychological development.* New York: Brunner/Mazel.

Watts, F. N., and Po-Kwan, Y. 1976. The structure of attitudes in psychiatric rehabilitation. *Journal of Occupational Psychology, 49,* 39–44.

White, R. W. 1966. *Lives in progress.* New York: Holt, Rinehart, and Winston.

9

A Vocational Psychology Perspective on Rehabilitation

WILLIAM C. BINGHAM

Vocational theory was based on "normal" human development, and its application to the chronically mentally ill has been sporadic. Bingham describes the historical development of vocational theory, gives two important formulations in detail, and applies them to working with persons with prolonged psychiatric disorders. He explains that Holland's structural theory can be useful in matching client attributes with environmental demands and that Super's theory is important in understanding and addressing problems in the course of vocational development. He emphasizes the importance of self-direction, especially as it relates to motivation to work.

There is little evidence that major theories of vocational psychology (Thomas and Berven 1984) have had any systematic impact on rehabilitation practice, particularly on efforts to rehabilitate people with prolonged mental illness (Shaw 1976). The present chapter is intended to review some of the relevant history and current thinking in vocational psychology and make suggestions about how these ideas might be applied in the treatment of chronically mentally ill clients.

The Development of Vocational Theory

Vocational psychology is the study of human behavior in relation to work. By and large, vocational psychologists are counseling psychologists (the earliest of whom combined training in clinical psychology and vocational guidance to create counseling psychology) who focus their professional and scholarly attention on vocational behavior. Theories which attempt to explain vocational behavior are of two types: structural and developmental.

Structural theories are so named because they represent efforts to examine, on the one hand, the structure of human attributes, and on the other, the structure of the environments in which people must function, and then to seek a match between the two. Early efforts in vocational psychology (see Miller 1964; Stephens 1970) were characterized by what has often been called trait-factor theory. These efforts were primarily empirical and focused on gathering evidence about human performance. Since trait-factor theories are more descriptive than predictive, they are not theories in the strict sense. However, they are important precursors of structural theory.

Trait-factor studies of how people perform were pursued actively in the period immediately following World War I. Various human characteristics—intelligence, special aptitudes, vocational interests, personality and temperament, attitudes, proficiency, and so on—were studied with a view to understanding how they are associated with performance in various environments. Vocational psychologists were particularly interested in gaining an understanding of the functioning of personal attributes in the workplace. At the same time, organizations such as the Minnesota Employment Stabilization Research Institute were engaged in the analysis of work environments. These efforts produced an extensive collection of psychological assessment instruments (see Super and Crites 1962) and detailed data about job requirements and working conditions (Shartle 1946).

Vocational counselors put the information to use, typically, in a three-step process: (1) they administered tests, accumulating scores on the attributes considered important, thus developing psychometric profiles of clients; (2) they helped clients to understand the meaning of the profile and the demands of various occupations and work settings; and (3) they helped clients to integrate both bodies of knowledge in making an occupational choice that would provide opportunities to implement important personal attributes. This process was seen as enabling clients to find their way into job environments compatible with their unique combination of attributes and to make satisfying adjustments to work. The core assumption was that, at a single point in time, an individual could be matched with a suitable employment situation.

A limiting aspect of the trait-factor approach was that occupational choice tended to be treated as if it were an isolated event in the lives of workers, ordinarily occurring in coincidence with the completion of formal education. Within a decade or so after the end of World War II, both evidence and professional opinion signaled a basic change from this point of view to one more concerned with human development. The influence of clinical psychology on guidance practice highlighted the inadvisability of treating vocational behavior in isolation (Matthewson 1949; Tyler 1961); occupational choice was demonstrated to be a process extending over several years (Ginzberg et al. 1951); application of notions about developmental tasks to vocational behavior linked the occupational-choice process irrevocably to earlier development (Havighurst 1953); and knowledge of differences in career patterns suggested that the process extends well into adulthood (Miller and Form 1951).

The emergence of this kind of thinking redirected the attention given to vocational behavior. Study of the structural characteristics of people and environments diminished while investigation of the processes experienced by each became a common focus. Developmental psychologists (Jersild 1957) began to address vocational behavior; processes in the economy at large (Darcy 1974) and in employment environments (Neff 1974) were examined in relation to worker behavior; subjective experience such as motivation to work (Herzberg, Mausner, and Snyderman 1959; Vroom 1964) and values and satisfaction in job behavior (Katzell 1964) were examined more closely. In particular, developmental formulations were adopted by vocational psychologists. Choice of occupation as implementation of self-concepts was posited (Super 1951); decision-making was described as a process rather than an event (Tiedeman and O'Hara 1963); exploration of self and occupations (Jordaan 1963) was incorporated into thinking about vocational maturation, as was readiness for vocational planning (Gribbons and Lohnes 1965). These "new" formulations have been combined into conceptualizations of vocational behavior as a dynamic process extending over the life span, and scholarly attention has focused on ways in which individuals progress through life, moving in and out of various work-related roles and preparing for and managing the transitions encountered at each choice point. Occupational choice has come to be conceived as an event which may occur many times during life but which always occurs as a function of the constitutional endowments and the accumulated psychological and social experience of the individual interacting with the cultural, economic, political, and other forces which impinge on people and institutions.

Two Important Theoretical Formulations

Although structural and developmental views in vocational psychology are different, they are neither mutually exclusive nor incompatible. Each makes an important contribution to a general understanding of vocational behavior. The developmental view provides a life-span perspective on the place of work in human experience, and the structural permits comparison between personal attributes and job requirements.

As is generally true in counseling psychology, the primary study in vocational psychology has been concerned with behavior in normally developing individuals. Although specific formulations do differ, for the most part vocational psychologists value ideas stating that individuals have both the capacity and the desire to become knowledgeable about themselves, that there is an innate tendency to grow toward full implementation of potential, and that the most productive motivations are intrinsic. Reflecting such beliefs, many vocational psychologists strive to foster three conditions related to clients' thinking about themselves as workers:

self-understanding, self-direction, and the fullest possible use of individual strengths. Objectives built on such a posture express confidence in clients' abilities to set their own goals, make their own decisions, and otherwise direct the course of their own lives.

Much of the knowledge gained through this orientation to the study of vocational behavior is relevant to understanding how mentally ill people think about, qualify for, accommodate to, and profit from work. As a backdrop for considering an application of vocational theory to rehabilitation, two of the most widely used theories are outlined below. Super's theory illustrates the developmental type, and Holland's the structural.

Super's Theory of Career Development

Super offered the first elaborated statement of a developmental vocational theory, conducted a twenty-year longitudinal study to test it, and has continued to expand and refine it. Three aspects of his formulation illustrate the emergence of his approach and its progression into a systematic statement of vocational psychology: the organization of vocational development into *life stages*; the formation, translation, and implementation of *self concepts*; and the *synthesis* of these ideas along with others relating to role behavior and the quality of life into a comprehensive view of career behavior.

Drawing on Buehler's work in developmental psychology, Super (1957) divided the life span into five stages differentiated in terms of developmental tasks, attitudes, vocational expectations, and characteristc behaviors. He posited that progress through the tasks of each stage is facilitated by exploratory behavior aimed at developing progressively fuller understanding of the self and of environmental demands and opportunities. Relative progress through each stage offers indications of vocational maturity.

For normally developing individuals, the *growth* stage extends approximately through age 14. During this stage young people identify with adult workers they know, develop attitudes about work through family and neighborhood activities, "practice" implementing their traits in work roles through fantasy, gain work experience by performing chores in the home, and explore emerging expectations of what it must be like to work by adopting adult worker roles in their play. Through such experiences, young people learn the meaning of work, acquire an orientation to work, and begin to formulate significant work values. Toward the end of the period actual employment gives many of these individuals opportunities to test their emerging perceptions of themselves as workers.

During the *exploration* state (ages 15–25), vocational interests become clear, aptitudes mature, skills are acquired and tested through schoolwork and part-time employment, and compromises are made between aspirations and opportunitites. Individuals crystallize and then specify occupational preferences, and attempt to implement them by entering employment or continuing their education beyond secondary school. Early employment and/or advanced education proves satisfying or disappointing, self-perceptions and expectations are modified accordingly, additional compromises may be made or different routes to implementation attempted. Success, or the lack of it, in these efforts may foreshadow patterns of vocational behavior that tend to be predictive of future vocational adjustment.

In the *establishment* stage (ages 25–45), careers tend to stabilize or stagnate. Stabilizers find a niche for themselves in an organization, advance into more demanding and responsible positions, gain recognition, and find satisfaction. Stagnators may or may not enjoy regular employment, but are less likely than stabilizers to see themselves as well situated at work. Although work is frequently not very satisfying for stagnators, they may find that activities outside of work provide some level of recognition and satisfaction. With increasing age, motivations change, energy diminishes, and career advancement becomes less important; effort is directed instead to capitalizing on what has already been accomplished. In this *maintenance* stage (ages 45–65), consolidation of status and planning for and anticipating retirement consume progressively larger proportions of the individual's attention, and modifications of self-perceptions and expectations are similarly directed. In our culture, the *disengagement* stage (earlier called decline) is usually marked by abrupt and formal withdrawal from paid employment.

Super (1963) identified three distinguishable phases in self-concept development. The *formation* of self-concepts begins early in life when perceptions of self and environmental circumstances permit individuals to distinguish themselves from others. By assuming various roles and trying out new behaviors, persons refine these perceptions: some are retained and internalized when they are found compatible; others are abandoned because they are not. *Translation* of self-concepts into occupational terms proceeds through one or more of three processes which may occur separately or simultaneously: identification is a generalized effort to be like someone, usually an admired adult; experience, resulting from planned or accidental events, permits discovery of important interests or talents; and observation enables individuals to learn that their attributes may have occupational relevance. *Implementation* of self-concepts is accomplished by action—entering employment or continuing with education or training needed to qualify for employment.

As indicated above, progress through the developmental tasks of each life stage is facilitated by productive exploratory behavior. Exploratory behavior is a complex process through which individuals learn about themselves and their environments. In its simplest form, it involves behaviors such as inspection, manipulation, and attentive observation (Jordaan 1963). In order to explore profitably, individuals must engage in these behaviors with reasonable accuracy. While these simple activities are fundamental in exploratory behavior, the deeper concern of vocational psychology is behavior that is directly reflected in the mastery of vocational developmental tasks. Obviously, an individual who encounters difficulty with the simple behaviors will encounter greater difficulty with the conceptual and symbolic thinking involved in the more advanced developmental tasks.

As is evident in the discussion of life stages and self-concept development, individuals play a variety of roles during various life stages. The content and quality of their functioning in each work role affects all of the other life roles that they occupy. It was for the purpose of putting the interactions among these roles into useful perspective that Super (1984) first proposed the concept of careers as a constellation of roles, graphically represented as a Life-Career Rainbow. Each arc of the rainbow represents one of nine roles: child, student, worker, spouse, homemaker, parent, citizen, leisurite, and pensioner. Each is colored or shaded to show the amount of time devoted to the role (lifespace) and the affect invested in it (commitment).

Early in the life of an individual, the only colored arc would be the one depicting the child role because that one occupies 100 percent of the life-space. As additional roles are assumed, the coloring or shading is adjusted in corresponding arcs to reflect the proportion of life-space devoted to each role, and the intensity varied to show the relative commitment to each.

Though the importance that people attribute to work (and to other roles they occupy) has long been of interest, the construct has been elusive, one which is difficult to translate into concrete and practical terms, resists measurement, and has generally been treated impressionistically rather than systematically. A recent formulation of "importance" (Super 1980) seems to be worthy of consideration in understanding clients' motivations to work. Importance is seen as having three basic components: knowledge (cognitive), participation (behavioral), and commitment (affective). Examining these components permits a more precise analysis of importance than treating the broader concept. It is possible, for example, for an individual to have a great deal of emotional investment in a role—that is, be committed to it—without having much knowledge about role requirements or taking any action in relation to it. Similarly, one may be quite knowledgeable about a role (an occupation, for example) without any commitment to it.

Holland's Theory of Careers

Probably the most widely implemented structural theory in vocational psychology is John Holland's (1973) theory of careers. Four key assumptions underlie his formulation: (1) most persons can be characterized as one of six personality types; (2) environments can be characterized in parallel terms; (3) people seek out environments which permit them to exercise their personal attributes, fill compatible roles, and work on agreeable problems; and (4) behavior is determined by the interaction between personality and environment.

Through the course of typical development, interactions among personal and cultural factors lead people through a process of acquiring preferences, interests, and competencies which dispose them to think and act in particular ways. Each of these ways of responding can be characterized by one of the personality types. Since environments tend to be dominated by one personality type, they can be characterized in similar terms. Because people seek out compatible environments, it is possible to use a personality profile to predict which type of environment is most likely to be attractive. Knowing something about the similarity between an individual and an environment permits prediction of important outcomes, such as adjustment, success, and satisfaction.

Holland sees human development as a process in which individuals, each with a unique combination of heredity and experience, progress through a sequence of events leading to progressively more differentiated competencies. With age, values crystallize and fashion characteristic behavior patterns which are exhibited in personality: perceptions of the world, self-concepts, coping styles, achievement, differential reactions to rewards and stress, occupational preferences, and so forth.

Six personality types emerge in our culture. *Realistic* people have mechanical and athletic abilities and lack human relations skills. They value concrete, tangible attributes and prefer manipulation of objects and machines to educational activities. They prefer outdoor occupations which involve physical activity and use of tools and equipment. People of the *investigative* type develop preferences for systematic observation and creative examination of natural and cultural phenomena so they can understand and control them. They avoid social and repetitive activities, see themselves as scholarly, and prefer occupations which require formal education and demand little leadership ability. Many of them work in academic settings and laboratories. *Artistic* people prefer ambiguous, free, unsystematized creative manipulation of materials and avoid ordered activities. They like to solve problems requiring expressive, intuitive, introspective, and imaginative abilities and prefer occupations in art, music, drama, and writing. People of the *social* type prefer activities involving interactions with other people for the purposes of informing, training, enlightening, or curing them. They value endeavors aimed at solving social and ethical problems. Preferred occupations include teacher, food service manager, bartender, and manicurist. *Enterprising* people prefer to manipulate others for the attainment of organizational goals or economic gain. They are strong in interpersonal and persuasive competencies, have leadership but not scientific skills, are aggressive, self-confident, and sociable in seeking political and economic aims, and prefer jobs in sales, management, and law. *Conventional* people work for organizational or economic goals through ordered manipulation of data. They avoid exploratory and ambiguous activities, are deficient in artistic skills and proficient in clerical and computational skills. They prefer bookkeeping, clerical, and accounting occupations.

Each model environment attracts its associated personality type and stimulates people in that environment to perform their characteristic activities, encourages them to exercise and improve their characteristic competencies, reinforces their characteristic self-perceptions, and rewards their displays of characteristic values.

Holland's formulation can be arranged conveniently into a hexagonal representation, with each personality type (or model environment) situated at one point of the hexagon in the order listed above (usually designated by the initial of each type—RIASEC). In this arrangement, the psychological resemblances among types have been demonstrated to be inversely proportional to the distances among them: correlations are consistently higher between adjacent types (ranging from .34 to .68) than between types opposite each other in the hexagon (ranging from .11 to .21), with others falling in between.

Obviously, a six-category scheme is not sufficient to describe all personality types, and classifying a person as a single type is too simplistic to reflect the complexity of personality. By comparing a person's similarity to each model type it is possible to rank those similarities to obtain a personality pattern. The Vocational Preference Inventory (Holland 1978), a standardized interest measure, and the Self-Directed Search (Holland 1977b), a self-assessment instrument, are especially suited to this purpose. The Strong-Campbell Interest Inventory (Strong and Campbell 1974), the most widely used vocational interest measure, also arranges scores according to Holland's personality types. Ordering a person's resemblances to each of the six models actually provides for 720 different personality patterns. Using the three highest resemblances is customary. For example, an individual may be ranked SEA indicating greatest resemblance to the social, enterprising, and artistic models, in that order. Holland has linked many such three-letter codes directly to occupations listed in the *Dictionary of Occupational Titles* through the use of a device he calls the Occupations Finder (Holland 1977a).

The Self-Directed Search measures attributes such as fantasies and competencies as well as interests, but, as the name indicates, they are self-assessments; no reference is made to external norms. It is self-scored, as well as self-administered, so it has the additional advantage of involving the client actively in the assessment process. As part of the scoring process, clients convert their scores into appropriate RIASEC codes. Relative freedom from threat, in combination with reflection about self and the opportunity to relate that reflection directly to occupations, permits clients to become more meaningfully involved in their own assessment than is generally the case. With suitable supervision or individual administration, clients with prolonged psychiatric disorders can often be given appropriate ego support to make self-assessment possible (Ciardiello and Turner 1980).

Applying Vocational Theory to Persons with Prolonged Psychiatric Disorders

In discussing the use of career development theory in vocational counseling with disabled clients, Super (1957) suggested that the strategies employed will differ with respect to whether a disability constitutes a barrier or a hurdle. A hurdle requires some kind of adaptation, perhaps modification of self-perceptions, but is something that can be overcome. In the best of circumstances, it serves as a challenge that may stimulate creative efforts to find a useful accommodation between the client and an employment situation. A barrier suggests that accommodation is not possible. It may require a radical change in career direction, demanding a new beginning, retraining, and entry into a new job at the lowest level. In the worst of circumstances, it may mean that aspirations for employment need to be abandoned altogether.

Whether a disability functions as a barrier or hurdle may be a matter of objective reality or a matter of client perceptions. The same disability may serve as a barrier to employment in some occupations, a hurdle in others. Because people with prolonged mental illness may perceive their own disability as a barrier to all employment, it is important that rehabilitation workers make accurate distinctions between the two conditions in individual cases. By doing so, they can be equipped to support client efforts to seek accommodation where it is possible, and can avoid false encouragement where accommodation is not likely to occur. Although the power of staff expectations has been demonstrated primarily in classroom settings (cf. Rosenthal and Jacobson 1968), the possibility that the effect is the same in other settings should lead rehabilitation workers to be aware that whether *they* believe a client's disability to be a barrier or a hurdle may very well influence the client's self-perceptions and job-related behavior.

The basic orientation of vocational psychology departs dramatically from the medical model of rehabilitation. In the traditional medical model, the client undergoes a series of tests and interviews and, then, a staff member, a vocational evaluator, interprets the results, makes a vocational diagnosis, and writes a vocational prescription (Shaw 1976). This type of intervention does not treat vocational behavior as developmental; seems to disregard assumptions about self-direction, intrinsic motivation, and self-conception; and ignores the interactions among behaviors in various life roles. Quite differently, in the vocational psychology orientation, assessment would attend initially to the mastery of developmental tasks, then focus on self-evaluation with a view to estimating its impact on functioning in all roles. A structured assessment would be introduced after these dimensions of client performance had been carefully evaluated in order to further self-assessment and self-understanding. The type of formal, externally focussed assessment implied in the traditional model outlined above would be undertaken, if at all, only after the client was seen as able to use it constructively. In effect, developmental formulations are applied first in determining a client's present functioning, and as a basis for furthering client self-understanding. Later in the intervention process, structural formulations can be used to help clients understand relationships between their present psychological status and employment prospects.

Addressing developmental needs first is important because most people with prolonged mental illness probably have not developed beyond the growth or the exploration stage. The most effective intervention strategies are seen as those which address, as directly as possible, the precise reason that individual clients appear to be in the early stages of vocational development. For instance they may never have had the opportunity to work; they may have worked but have found it an unpleasant experience leading to feelings of failure and unworthiness; or they may have worked satisfactorily but are currently suffering from a setback associated with the episodic nature of severe mental illness.

Coping with the demands of vocational development requires a fairly high level of integration of self with environment. The conceptual linkages which knit perceptions of self and environment into a cohesive expression of self-understanding interacting with a sense of reality can be fashioned only through effective ego functioning (Ciardiello and Bingham 1982). Thus, the major vocational developmental tasks of the growth and exploration stages—acquiring an orientation to work, comprehending the meaning of work, trying out work roles, crystallizing and specifying occupational preferences, and setting vocational goals—depend in large measure on successful ego functioning. For all individuals, vocational development can present very difficult challenges; for persons with severe ego deficits these challenges can seem insurmountable and, in many cases, may be associated with developmental arrest. Under these circumstances, effective treatment must necessarily be built upon accurate understanding of each individual client's present functioning with respect to essential developmental tasks. Building on ego strengths which already exist is a productive method of remediating deficits and thereby facilitating vocational maturation (Ciardiello, Klein, and Sobkowski 1984).

Chronically mentally ill clients often give the impression that work is not important in their lives. Such a perception is understandable because the disruptions caused by poor functioning are almost certain to be felt more keenly at work than in other roles. At work, an individual's performance is usually observed carefully and evaluated regularly, so that, compared to other roles, poor performance is more visible and has more immediate consequences. For those with prolonged mental illness, then, work can pose a risk because it may focus attention on individual inadequacies. Thus, avoiding work provides more security than engaging in it. For many chronically mentally ill individuals, other life roles are safer places to implement their self-concepts.

Besides this perceived risk of failure, there are other aspects of prolonged mental illness which hamper clients' ability to assume the worker role. Impaired functioning is likely to increase dependency on family and friends and on various caregivers and social agencies. Hospitalization often fosters nearly total dependency, with the effect that clients come to expect that they will be taken care of by someone else. For many of them, this patient role becomes very comfortable and takes on special importance. Some well-conceptualized rehabilitation programs have attempted to minimize this tendency to capitalize on being a patient by emphasizing the functional demands of other life roles. For instance, as a member of a rehabilitation community, a client is expected to assume certain responsibilities and is systematically assisted in meeting those expectations. Such program strategies also strive to improve client performance in social, leisure, and prevocational roles and devote effort to helping clients deal with the interactions among these various roles.

As clients make progress in comprehending and dealing with their own developmental needs, they are likely to become more ready and more motivated to consider some of the other aspects of occupational choice. As this readiness becomes apparent, it is appropriate to shift to the use of structural theory and introduce more formal and systematic assesment. Holland's formulation is particularly useful in examining the interactions between personality components and requirements of the work environment. In initiating assessment of this kind, the Self-Directed Search is especially useful because it involves the client directly in the process. In turn, this helps to assure client participation in subsequent steps and underscores the need for client self-direction and intrinsic motives. The more fully a client experiences this involvement, the more likely it is that a good "match" will be found between worker and work. Even the best of matches, however, is not permanently stable. For the severely mentally ill, the stability of a match may be quite tenuous because of the episodic nature of the illness and the catastrophic effects of stress. What seems to be a reasonable match at one point may later become stressful enough to result in work disruption or hospitalization. Applied at appropriate points in the rehabilitation process, Holland's paradigm offers a valuable framework for finding a reasonable match between personality and the work environment. Thus, it serves as a useful structure for activities designed to facilitate clients' understanding of the importance of worker roles and, in turn, for enhancing their motivation to work.

Conclusion

Both Super's developmental formulation and Holland's structural one offer valuable theoretical perspectives which can be applied in treating the difficulties experienced by the chronically mentally ill in their efforts to work. The developmental view permits the rehabilitation worker and client alike to maintain their focus on the course of vocational development; the structural orientation can be interposed at suitable points in the process to focus on the fit between client attributes and environmental demands.

References

Ciardiello, J. A., and Bingham, W. C. 1982. Career maturity of schizophrenic clients. *Rehabilitation Counseling Bulletin, 26,* 3–9.

Ciardiello, J. A.; Klein, M. E.; and Sobkowski, S. 1984. Ego functioning and the vocational rehabilitation of schizophrenic clients. In *The broad scope of ego function assessment,* ed. L. Bellak and L. Goldsmith. New York: Wiley and Sons.

Ciardiello, J. A., and Turner, F. D. 1980. *Final report of the Vocational Assessment Project.* Trenton, N.J.: Department of Education, Division of Vocational Education and Career Planning.

Darcy, R. L. 1974. The nature of economic enterprise. In *Vocational guidance and human development,* ed. E. L. Herr, pp. 109–29. Boston: Houghton Mifflin.

Ginzberg, E.; Ginsburg, S.; Axelrad, S.; and Herma, J. L. 1951. *Occupational choice.* New York: Columbia University Press.

Gribbons, W. D., and Lohnes, P. R. 1965. Predicting five years of development in adolescents from readiness for vocational planning scales. *Journal of Educational Psychology, 56,* 244–53.

Havighurst, R. J. 1953. *Human development and education.* New York: Longmans, Green.

Herzberg, F.; Mausner, B.; and Snyderman, B. 1959. *The motivation to work.* New York: Wiley and Sons.

Holland, J. L. 1973. *Making vocational choices: A theory of careers.* Englewood Cliffs, N.J.: Prentice-Hall.

———. 1977a. *The occupations finder.* Palo Alto, Calif.: Consulting Psychologists Press.

———. 1977b. *The self-directed search.* Palo Alto, Calif.: Consulting Psychologists Press.

———. 1978. *Vocational preference inventory.* Palo Alto, Calif.: Consulting Psychologists Press.

Jersild, A. T. 1957. *The psychology of adolescence.* New York: Macmillan.

Jordaan, J. P. 1963. Exploratory behavior: The formation of self and occupational concepts. In *Career development: Self-concept theory,* ed. D. E. Super, R. Starishevsky, N. Matlin, and J. P. Jordaan, pp. 42–78. New York: College Entrance Examination Board.

Katzell, R. A. 1964. Personal values, job satisfaction, and job behavior. In *Man in a world at work,* ed. H. Borow, pp. 341–63. Boston: Houghton Mifflin.

Mattewson, R. H. 1949. *Guidance policy and practice.* 1st ed. New York: Harper.

Miller, C. H. 1964. Vocational guidance in the perspective of cultural change. In *Man in a world at work*, ed. H. Borrow, pp. 3–23. Boston: Houghton Mifflin.

Miller, D. C., and Form, W. H. 1951. *Industrial sociology*. New York: Harper.

Neff, W. S. 1974. The world of work. In *Vocational guidance and human development*, ed. E. L. Herr, pp. 156–79. Boston: Houghton Mifflin.

Rosenthal, R., and Jacobson, L. 1968. *Pygmalion in the classroom: Teacher expectations and pupils' intellectual development*. New York: Holt, Rinehart, and Winston.

Shartle, C. L. 1946. *Occupational information*. Englewood Cliffs, N.J.: Prentice-Hall.

Shaw, K. J. 1976. Career development: Client responsibility in vocational planning. *Journal of Rehabilitation, 42*, 30–39.

Stephens, W. R. 1970. *Social reform and the origins of vocational guidance*. Washington, D.C.: National Vocational Guidance Association.

Strong, E. K., Jr., and Campbell, D. P. 1974. *Strong-Campbell interest inventory*. Stanford, Calif.: Stanford University Press.

Super, D. E. 1951. Vocational adjustment: Implementing a self-concept. *Occupations, 30*, 88–92.

———. 1957. *The psychology of careers*. New York: Harper.

———. 1963. Self-concepts in vocational development. In *Career development: Self-concept theory*, ed. D. E. Super, R. Starishevsky, N. Matlin, and J. P. Jordaan, pp. 1–16. New York: College Entrance Examination Board.

———. 1980. A life-span, life-space approach to career development. *Journal of Vocational Behavior, 16*, 282–98.

———. 1984. Perspectives on the meaning and value of work. In *Designing careers: Counseling to enhance education, work, and leisure*, ed. N. C. Gysbers, pp. 27–53. San Francisco: Jossey-Bass.

Super, D. E., and Crites, J. O. 1962 *Appraising vocational fitness*. New York: Harper and Row.

Thomas, K. R., and Berven, N. L. 1984. Providing career counseling for individuals with handicapping conditions. In *Designing careers: Counseling to enhance education, work, and leisure*, ed. N. C. Gysbers, pp. 403–32. San Francisco: Jossey-Bass.

Tiedeman, D. V., and O'Hara, R. P. 1963. *Career development: Choice and adjustment*. New York: College Entrance Examination Board.

Tyler, L. E. 1961. *The work of the counselor*. 2d ed. New York: Appleton-Century-Crofts.

Vroom, V. H. 1964. *Work and motivation*. New York: Wiley and Sons.

10

Transitional Employment and Psychosocial Rehabilitation

THOMAS J. MALAMUD and DENNIS J. McCRORY

The psychosocial rehabilitation program developed at Fountain House, New York City, has had a long-standing influence on the development of many similar clubhouse programs throughout the United States. Malamud and McCrory give a detailed account of transitional employment as it is practiced at Fountain House. They describe the philosophical assumptions underlying the model, as well as the ways in which its various elements interface with a general psychosocial model. Results of an evaluation of transitional employment are used to suggest new directions for research and program development.

There has been increased interest in the vocational rehabilitation of the mentally ill in recent years owing to deinstitutionalization. Work, it has been established, is of vital importance for the reintegration of the "chronically mentally ill" in the community.

Vocational rehabilitation is a process that enables transitions to higher levels of productivity for people disabled by medical and/or psychiatric conditions. In practice, it is often a series of transitions. The number of steps, the course and duration of the process, and the long-term outcomes vary greatly from individual to individual.

Sadly, for persons with severe psychiatric impairments, vocational rehabilitation services are often not available in a timely fashion. Sometimes, such impaired individuals and their families, therapists, and rehabilitation counselors cannot imagine their holding down a full-time job. They are assumed to be "too sick." At other times, it is held that they simply need a period of time for convalescence or treatment to regain their mental health, and they resist referral to programs that serve obviously handicapped psychiatric clients. They are "not sick enough" that is, until long periods of unemployment or repeated failures to (re)enter the work force, regressions, and rehospitalizations increase their residual disabilities, erode their hope, and again make them appear "too sick." Lastly, there are times when services or a sequence of services that would meet their needs are not offered in local communities.

Thus, there has developed a stereotype, which has become a self-fulfilling prophecy, that the chronically mentally ill cannot be gainfully employed and instead should declare themselves "permanently and totally disabled" and apply for Social Security benefits. The risk of loss of these benefits then becomes a disincentive to the further pursuit of work. The person who may have valued work, may have developed occupational skills, and may indeed have "rehabilitation potential" has now become a chronic mental patient, with little likelihood of employment.

This state of affairs was well described by Gruenberg (1967) as the social breakdown syndrome. Not only does the person have to contend with the symptoms and impairments of his illness, but he has also lost hold of his life structure and must live with a changed set of expectations of himself, reinforced by the concern of the significant others in his life. He has lost the sense of "can do" which White (1963) has termed *effectance:* "energies . . . which seem to perform the service of maintaining and expanding an effective interaction with the environment." He has also lost his sense of belonging in the community as a productive member of society, a wage earner, a breadwinner, a taxpayer.

In a review of the relevant vocational rehabilitation literature, Anthony, Cohen, and Vitalo (1978) reported low employment rates, from 10 to 30 percent, following patient discharge and at the end of a one-year follow-up. By contrast, it is clear that there is a higher percentage for other, non-psychiatrically disabled groups (Skelley 1980).

We believe that this process of dishabilitation is neither inevitable nor irreversible, and in this chapter we develop another point of view: when offered opportunity, support, and sufficient time, many persons with prolonged mental illness can successfully engage in a vocational rehabilitation process.

One salient factor in the review by Anthony and colleagues is the length of follow-up periods for collecting data. Most of the studies had a six- to twelve-month follow-up period, and there are indications that there is a positive correlation between client attendance at a particular training program and employment outcome. For instance, a longitudinal study was done in Vermont of 269 patients with chronic mental illness who became involved in a psychosocial and vocational rehabilitation program (Harding et al. 1983, 1987). Subjects were hospitalized for six continuous years on the average and were "ill" for sixteen years. They were discharged from the hospital into the community in the mid-1950s, and after twenty to twenty-five years, results showed that 50 percent of those employable (not retired), were working productively, many on farms. Seventy-three percent of the sample showed little or no evidence of symptomatology, and 82 percent were self-sufficient, requiring little or no help with basic living routines.

Sheltered workshops in general and other inpatient programs such as work therapy have been charged with creating dependency and not facilitating the movement towards competitive employment (Barber, Berry, and Micek 1969; Carpenter and Black 1986). Further, although the literature involving work stations in industry is very limited, such research has concluded that work stations are more effective than workshops in increasing self-esteem, competence, and vocational skills (Conte 1983b; Rapp 1979).

The transitional employment (TE) model is an alternative method for placing psychiatrically disabled persons in competitive industrial employment. The TE model is a narrower form within the work stations (Conte 1983a) and differs from the latter in that it has a short period of placement, while work stations involve a long-term job setting.

Rutman and Armstrong (1985) identified and evaluated 114 provider agencies in the United States of which 95 agencies were currently providing transitional employment programs, while 19 other agenices were not. Results showed that the average number of days on TE was significantly related to employment outcome. Partial correlations were used to control for past work history. It was estimated that about 35 percent of the persons studied were employed six months after transitional employment; of these, 19 percent were working full-time and 16 percent part-time in competitive employment.

Thus, over the past thirty years, there has developed a variety of approaches that can be conceptualized as a continuum of work experiences: hospital work programs, volunteer employment, short-term sheltered employment, extended sheltered employment, prevocational program in day treatment and day training centers, transitional employment, supported work, and on-the-job training.

This chapter focuses on one of these approaches, transitional employment (TE). The clubhouse model as practiced in Fountain House will be described. The general development and practice of TE will also be presented. Results of a recently completed long-term retrospective study of TE will be presented to support its efficacy. Implications for practice will be drawn, and directions for further program development and research will be suggested.

Transitional Employment in the Community Context: The Fountain House Model

From an ecological perspective, human needs and problems can be seen as generated by transactions between people and their environments, calling for practices which will focus on both releasing the adaptive capacities of individuals and improving their environments. A rehabilitative method must engage people's strengths and the forces pushing toward growth as well as influence organizational structures, social systems, and physical settings so they will be more responsive to individual needs. This perspective, and the method used to implement it, compose the "life model."

In the life model, as described by Germain and Gitterman (1980), individuals' needs and predicaments are located at the interface of person and environment. Professional interventions are directed to creating healthy processes at that interface. In the relationship between the individual and work, where each brings the influences of interacting life-space forces, goals are set to strengthen adaptive capacity and increase environmental responsiveness.

The clubhouse model of prevocational rehabilitation and TE facilitates such transactions between prolonged mentally ill persons and their environments. Skills for community adjustment are facilitated by engaging individuals in real work both in the clubhouse and on the job site. This is an ecological-systems approach where the entire process of planning is rooted in the real needs of the member population (Auerswald 1968).

Fountain House, a nonprofit psychiatric rehabilitation center, was established in 1948 for the express purpose of facilitating the social and vocational rehabilitation of men and women, called "members" (rather than patients or clients), following hospitalization in public and private mental institutions. Fountain House occupies a homelike clubhouse located just a few blocks from Times Square in New York City, and is attended each day by 375 individuals who participate in its comprehensive rehabilitative programs.

These programs are organized around the concept of the "clubhouse model." It is an environment in which an individual's presence is clearly needed and celebrated, where there is emphasis on mutual help and self-help. There are opportunities to engage in a wide range of restorative activities concerned with the operation and management of the clubhouse program. Staff and members work side by side. The clubhouse is open seven days a week throughout the year. The daytime hours are utilized to prepare members for independent employment through a prevocational program directed toward those activities required to keep the clubhouse operational. These activities include preparing a noontime meal, a wide variety of clerical functions, cleaning and maintenance work in the clubhouse, receiving and touring visitors, putting out a daily newspaper, running an in-house TV station, computer programming, and fundraising.

Fountain House also provides housing alternatives for 170 members either in fully supervised community residences, partially supervised apartment settings, or independently shared satellite apartments. During the evenings and on weekends and holidays, social and recreational activities are available.

A fourth program area is the employment alternative known as transitional employment (TE). As part of the day program, transitional employment is a vocational service that was initiated in 1958 (Beard 1982) and provides any member the opportunity to work in commerce and industry.

Fundamental to creating TE placements is the clubhouse's need to fill such placements. The practice has always been to create work opportunities first, rather than preparing members first and then locating placements later, in the belief that work must be important for the experience to be rehabilitative. Each day 110 members go to work on TE, and an estimated 450 members will have a TE experience over the course of a year. A large number of severely disabled individuals are provided a real work experience, and Fountain House communicates to its men and women the actual need for them to work at these placements.

The operating dynamic at Fountain House, therefore, is a continual encouragement for members to try TE. Crucial to the integrity of this dynamic are the provisions of ongoing supports and easy reentry back to Fountain House. Since membership may be life-long, members realize that neither job success nor job failure leads to rejection by the clubhouse. This policy permits members to try placements without the fear of success or the burden of failure. Members may start TE within a month of agency intake or may take weeks, months, or even years to reach the point of trying TE.

Movement on and off placement is freer, because members will return to the day program for further services prior to returning to TE once again. Many times "success" is the simple act of trying a placement, the "surviving" of one day on placement. Ease of access in and out of Fountain House and TE also allows for success to be defined as increasing time on TE and decreasing time in the day program between placements. Of course, success can also be defined as movement on to independent employment, school, or other rehabilitation programs. This broader definition of success and consequent easy reentry to Fountain House allows for more liberal standards with reference to symptomatology. Staff members do not view job readiness as necessarily related or equivalent to absence of symptoms.

Transitional Employment Programs Based on The Fountain House Model

By the end of 1985, a total of 135 community-based rehabilitation facilities in thirty-five states, the District of Columbia, and two foreign countries were providing TE programs. In partnership with the business community, these programs facilitate the work adjustment of the vocationally disabled, financially dependent psychiatric patient. Based on the Fountain House model of TE, each of these 135 programs had in common certain basic characteristics. All placements for the severely disabled mentally ill are located in normal places of business, ranging from large, nationally recognized corporations to small local firms employing only a few individuals.

TE placements are essentially entry-level employment requiring minimal training or job skills. All employers provide the prevailing wage rate for each job position, ranging from the minimum wage to over $6.00 an hour, with a few positions paying up to $8.00 an hour. Almost all jobs are worked on a half-time basis so that one full-time job can serve two members at a time. This allows the member to be at the clubhouse half of each day. Many programs provide weekly or bi-weekly dinner meetings for TE members to get together.

Most TE positions are on an individual basis. The member works in the presence of other employees. Some placements, however, are performed on a group basis where six to ten members work together, relating primarily with each other. All placements are temporary or "transitional," providing employment for as little as three months to as long as a year.

TE is a guaranteed opportunity to work on temporary, entry-level jobs in normal places of business and to continue employment through a series of TE placements or to use the job as a step toward eventual full-time, independent employment. Placements are maintained only if the individual meets the work requirements of the employer. Employers do not adjust or lower work standards. Job failures are viewed as experiences which the vocationally disabled member, in most instances, must undergo to eventually achieve a successful work adjustment. In the work experiences of nondisabled individuals, failure or withdrawal from entry-level employment often occurs. TE employers emphasize that job turnover rates are not typically greater for the mentally ill on TE than the rates for the nondisabled employee.

New placements are first performed by a staff worker for a few hours to assess the requirements of the job. The staff is therefore able to evaluate the work environment and its compatibility to the needs of the disabled individual, as well as the degree of acceptance by other employees on the work site. Because of this familiarity with the work environment, staff have immediate access to the work site when starting new members. Whenever vocational difficulties or crises occur, staff can make a prompt assessment of a member's performance. In the training phase, staff are able to provide on-the-job guidance to the member.

Placements are assigned by the employer to the rehabilitation facility. The selection process by which placements are filled rests with staff and the individual member it serves. The employer pays wages without any subsidy. This collaboration between the business community and the rehabilitation facility is not a charitable act by the employer. It is an agreement of mutual benefit to employer and member.

TE programs provide an opportunity to enrich and expand the evaluation of vocational potential. Assessment in a normal work environment has advantages over evaluations in sheltered environments or those based on personal interviews and psychological assessment.

In short, TE programs successfully remove or circumvent barriers common to employment for psychiatrically disabled individuals. These barriers include a history of psychiatric disorders, an inability to pass a job interview, the absence of a work history, motivational deficits, and many others.

In each of the 135 community-based rehabilitation facilities throughout the nation that provide TE programs, the vocationally disabled member has the easily accessible opportunity to go to work part-time in an entry-level job in a normal place of business. This is an integral part of the vocational adjustment process.

These work opportunities show the member that mental illness is not the sole or even primary explanation of vocational disability. Rather, mental illness is a personal experience which typically has prevented the member from entering the real world of work and developing the capacity to perform work productively and meet job requirements.

An Evaluation of the TE Program

Having described the context and the components of TE, we now present an evaluation of the program. This retrospective evaluation was completed in 1985 (Malamud 1985). The basic design followed was a single-group time-series quasi-experimental design as described by Huck, Cormier, and Bounds (1974). The design included observations at agency intake, at study intake, and at a number of points following placement on TE.

Observations measured the amounts and kinds of rehabilitation services or other community services each subject received. The instrument developed to record these observations is called Categories of Community Adjustment, or COCA (for a description see Malamud 1985). Thus, changes in program experiences constituted the independent variable, and the dependent variables were measures of functional capacity observed at various intervals.

TE is an opportunity available to all Fountain House members, and as such, all participants have met the general agency eligibility criteria: (1) they are age 16 or older; (2) their primary presenting problem is not alcoholism, drug abuse, severe developmental disability, or acting-out behavior; and (3) they are able to participate in Fountain House unattended. Data were collected on all members who secured a TE placement during the forty-two-month period from July 1, 1980, through December 31, 1983. An examination of twenty-one demographic, social, clinical, and vocational variables gathered at intake showed that the TE sample of 527 individuals were representative of the Fountain House population. Thus, findings from this study may be generalized to similar groups of severely disabled psychiatric patients.

Identification of Patterns of Adjustment

Subjects in the sample underwent a large number of changes in their levels of community adjustment, averaging better than one change every three months. While the frequency of these changes may not differ for those severely disabled individuals in the community who do not have access to programs like Fountain House, it is expected that for such nonmembers the character of such changes might be substantially different. Instead of being isolated and withdrawn from the community and undergoing psychiatric rehospitalization, a situation typical of nonmembers, the great majority for the Fountain House sample were moving in and out of the day program, TE, and independent employment.

The day program was the most frequently used experience. Over 40% percent of all movement was into day program, over 80 percent of all members had some day program experience during the follow-up, and 28 percent of the sample were in the day program at the end of the follow-up.

We found that 174 subjects, or a third of the sample, had a least one independent employment experience following a TE placement, and that about 15 percent of the total time during our study was spent on full-time jobs. Further, we found that independent employment rates increased as time in the program increased. Thus, by the forty-second month, nearly 36 percent of those completing 42 months of follow-up time were independently employed, a rate higher than typically reported in the literature. An additional 7 percent were employed on TE at the forty-second month, so that a 43 percent employment rate had been achieved. If the few people who were lost to follow-up at the forty-second month were dropped and the remaining rates prorated, then the independent employment rate would be 40 percent and the TE rate would be 9 percent, so that just under 50 percent of the known sample were employed at the end of 42 months.

During the time of the study, for all 527 subjects a total of 140,975 days were spent on TE, an average length of 8¾ months. Of greater interest, the sample spent a total of 69,927 days independently employed for an average length of just under 4½ months. As the average length of time in the study is 29½ months, the more than 13 months spent employed represents about 45 percent of the total study time available.

Psychiatric hospitalizations occurred relatively infrequently during the study, and no more than 3.4 percent of the sample were hospitalized at any one time. With respect to duration, a total of 13,790 days were spent in the hospital during the study, or an average for the whole sample of 26 days during the 42-month period.

Identification and Definition of Subgroups

From the analysis of data certain subgroupings emerged. One of these consisted of 148 subjects who were in a psychiatric hospital at some point during the study. For those 148, the average time spent in the hospital was 93 days, or three months. Three-fifths were hospitalized once, and half were in the hospital for less than 30 days.

Compared with intake data, time in hospital was reduced. It appears that length of hospitalization during the study was less for those subjects on a TE or day program. Over 70 percent of the hospitalizations which followed a TE placement and nearly 60 percent of those following a period in the day program were less than 30 days in duration. In comparison, 70 percent of rehospitalizations following involvement in some other rehabilitation program and two-thirds of those following a period withdrawn in the community not involved in any rehabilitative activity were longer than 30 days in length. The differences between length of hospitalization and preceding adjustment experience was found to be statistically significant (chi square = 16.08, df = 4, $p < .01$). Background characteristics did not distinguish between those hospitalized and those not hospitalized during the study.

A second group consists of those securing independent employment. Length of time on full-time jobs for those employed averaged 400 days, or just over 13 months. Nearly three-fifths of those employed had jobs of over 3 months in length, while one-quarter of the jobs were from one year to 38 months. With so much time independently employed, many members who had been receiving either SSI or SSDI have had their entitlements affected, including removal from the rolls, reduction in benefits, or extension of time as the 9-month trial work period had been surpassed.

The data document that the process of rehabilitation can be a long one. Results indicated that the length of time from agency intake to the securing of full-time gainful employment could take five years or longer. Groups which had been in the study the longest were composed of subjects with more time in Fountain House prior to study intake. These groups and those subjects had the highest rates of independent employment (66% for those 104 members with over two years following Fountain House intake and 42 months of study follow-up time), as well as the highest proportion of study time spent on full-time jobs. This leads to the conclusion that the rest of the study sample might achieve equally high employment rates once sufficient time has been allowed for them to be in the day program and TE.

Over a third of all instances of independent employment were immediately preceded by TE, and the length of time spent on TE is positively and significantly correlated to the obtaining of full-time gainful employment ($t = 2.154$, $df = 525$, $p < .025$). We conclude, therefore, that the length of time required for securing a full-time job might be shortened substantially by providing more opportunities for TE placements. Analysis of background characteristics did not significantly differentiate the 174 individuals who had an independent placement from the 353 others who did not obtain full-time employment during the study.

Implications for Practice and Future Trends

In his chapter in *The Chronic Mental Patient,* Peterson (1978), a member currently on staff at Fountain House, personally witnessed the value of transitional employment for both himself and his fellow members. These members can be eloquent about their experiences (Schmidt, Nessel, and Malamud 1969, pp. 95–102):

I began working less and less until . . . I just stopped completely for 2½ years. It was just a matter of not being able to function any more. Employment is very important. People don't realize this but as long as you are busy this is a great thing for the mind. It keeps your mind off a lot of other things that are really of no value . . . The more time that you have to think, why of course, you can just retrogress, which isn't very good.

It makes you forget a little bit of your emotional problems and your nerves and your worries. It gets you with people who are well instead of sitting here talking all day—"Oh, I've been sick for 10 years, I've been sick for 20 years." This is discouraging. When you're working, you're with healthy people . . . You're interested in what they're saying. You're trying to keep up with them in clothes and your appearance. Since I have been working, I'm setting my hair, showering, ironing, washing, cleaning the apartment. I'm functioning so much better . . . because I feel that I'm doing something.

It gets your life going. It gives you responsibility and also makes you feel different, makes you feel that you can face the outside world. And also makes you feel that you are important. Important to your people, important to your friends, because you are earning money. You're making your own penny, your own dollar bill . . . And when you walk into the store, you feel, well, I can buy this and I can buy that, because it's your money, and it's a wonderful feeling. And I'm glad to be working.

When I first went to work there, I didn't know anything about the . . . business. I started part-time . . . I helped set up the routine and I helped serve the customers. The bosses are pleasant to work for and the people are pleasant to associate with. I think people do benefit from its being in existence. It gives them a feeling of usefulness and it helps them to feel that they are accomplishing something, and it increases their own general knowledge. It's an honest day's labor for an honest day's pay. Helps you sleep nights.

This TE study has gone beyond such intuitive and anecdotal evidence of the effectiveness of TE as practiced at Fountain House. Our goal in sharing these experiences is threefold: to help correct the stereotype that persons with prolonged mental illness cannot work; to broadcast one rehabilitation model that had been clearly defined, replicated, and studied; and to stimulate the development of similar programs and studies.

While Fountain House believes that the clubhouse model supports TE, it recognizes that TE can be offered in conjunction with sheltered workshops and day treatment programs, and actually gives these basic programs more of a transitional nature. TE is also offered as an independent program although some programs identified as TE resemble the supported work model, whose goal is to "roll over" the transitional position into full-time permanent employment. All such programs need to define their activities and study their effectiveness over a prolonged periods of time. Through this precision and inquiry the contributions of differing models will be discovered, so that their differential usefulness will emerge. Currently, for example, Fountain House is conducting a national evaluation of the levels of vocational and residential adjustment in a sample of 1,800 individuals connected with twenty-five clubhouse programs.

Conclusion

Given opportunity, support, and time, a substantial number of persons with severe psychiatric disabilities can benefit from a vocational rehabilitation process.

This finding is very much in keeping with the results of the twenty-year retrospective study, cited earlier, of patients discharged from Vermont State Hospital in the middle 1950s. Indeed, an emerging finding is that the diagnosis of major mental illness is more compatible with healthy vocational and social functioning than traditional wisdom had believed, provided that support, opportunity, and time are available. As Peterson (1978) stated, "There are places where the chronic patient becomes less chronic, and I hope we can prove what can be accomplished, so that there will be fewer people in the mental health field who seem to feel hopeless about the chronic patient. We need people to believe in us and what we can accomplish . . . Most important is to stop looking at us as chronic."

For ten years, Fountain House has offered a national training program for those wishing to start their own clubhouse and TE programs. By the end of 1985, over 630 colleagues from 340 agencies throughout the United States and eleven foreign countries have attended this training program, with the result that some 180 new clubhouse programs have emerged.

There are now 135 TE programs nationwide, giving 1,756 individuals the opportunity to return to work, earning, in collective annualized wages, $6,992,387—a small, but substantial beginning. The hope is to encourage further local expressions of this approach. Regional training centers at appropriate clubhouse programs are planned to help in this process. Such training centers have already been established at Beach House, Virginia Beach, Virginia; Independence Center, St. Louis, Missouri; and Rainbow House, Rome, New York.

Given the chance, members have been able to make efforts to direct their energies to real-life challenges, not just to cope with the vicissitudes of their mental illness. They have been able to organize themselves to meet the demands of real jobs that have given them the real and immediate rewards of money, status, and enhanced self-esteem. The need for and recognized value of their work has given them more reason to struggle with their conflicts and symptomatology and demonstrate a mastery of themselves that has helped to change their "patient" roles into "worker" roles. This has, of course, represented hard work for them and those who have supported them. All were not successful in their first efforts; their were regressions and rehospitalizations, albeit remarkably few. Not everybody reached a level of sustained competitive employment. Many needed to work at the process for what seemed like a very long time.

It is also clear that the success of members in their ability to commit themselves has depended not just on their individual efforts supported by their supervisors, but also on the support of their peers, families, clinicians, and employers. Particularly noteworthy is the support of fellow members, whether by reaching out, by informal sharing, or at member meetings and TE dinners.

There are certainly questions that require further study. The study reported here spanned nearly four years. What trends will appear over a longer follow-up period? Can employment rates be expected to continue increasing? Members had opportunities to (re)join the work force initially on entry levels. What difference would it make to have a more active placement program? What sorts of skill development and career advancement will occur after members begin to work competitively? What substantive changes will occur in the entitlements such individuals have been receiving? Low hospitalization rates were found during the study. What are the implications for long-term prognosis for psychiatric illness with participation in a Fountain House type program? TE is available to all clubhouse members. What are the criteria for persons with prolonged mental illness who can benefit from TE but may not be clubhouse members? These and other questions deserve further inquiry and will be certainly followed up with interest by Fountain House and, it is to be hoped, by other rehabilitation programs as well.

References

Anthony, W. A.; Cohen, M. R.; and Vitalo, R. 1978. The measurement of rehabilitation outcome. *Schizophrenia Bulletin, 4*, 365–83.
Anthony, W., and Jansen, M. 1984. Predicting the vocational capacity of the chronically

mentally ill: Research and policy implications. *American Psychologist, 39,* 537–44.

Auerswald, E. H. 1968. Interdisciplinary vs. ecological approach. *Family Process, 7,* 205.

Barber, M.; Berry, K.; and Micek, L. 1969. Relationship of work therapy to psychiatric length of stay and readmission. *Journal of Consulting and Clinical Psychology, 33,* 735–38.

Beard, J. H. 1982. Industry and the vocational rehabilitation of the disabled mental patient. Paper presented to the annual meeting of the President's Committee on Employment of the Handicapped, Washington, D.C.

Carpenter, M., and Black, B. 1986. Review of research and evaluation. In *Work as therapy and rehabilitation for the mentally ill,* ed. B. Black. New York: Altro Health and Rehabilitation Services.

Conte, L. 1983a. Sheltered employment and disabled citizens: An analysis of the work stations in the industry model. *Dissertation Abstracts International, 43,* 2976A.

———. (1983b) Sheltered employment services and programs. *Rehabilitation Research Review,* Monograph no. 11. National Rehabilitation Information Center, Washington, D.C.

Germain, C., and Gitterman, A. 1980. *The life model of social work practice.* New York: Columbia University Press.

Gruenberg, E. 1967. The social breakdown syndrome: Some origins. *American Journal of Psychiatry, 123,* 1481–89.

Harding, C.; Brooks, G.; Ashikaga, T.; and Strauss, J. 1983. Overview: The long-term course of chronic patients. Paper presented at the annual meeting of the American Psychiatric Association, New York.

———. 1987. The Vermont longitudinal study of persons with severe mental illness, I:Methodology, study sample, and overall current status. *American Journal of Psychiatry, 144,* 718–26.

Huck, S.; Cormier, W.; and Bounds, W. G. 1974. *Reading statistics and research.* New York: Harper and Row.

Malamud, T. J. 1985. Evaluation of a clubhouse model: Community-based psychiatric rehabilitation. New York: Fountain House. Mimeographed.

Peterson, K. J. 1979. Assessment in the life model: A historical perspective. *Social Casework* (Family Service Association of America), 60, 590.

Peterson, R. 1978. What are the needs of chronic mental patients? In *The chronic mental patient,* ed. J. A. Talbott. Washington, D.C.: American Psychiatric Association.

Rapp, R. E. 1979. A normalization approach to the vocational training of mentally retarded adults. Ph.D. diss., University of Arizona, 1979. *Dissertation Abstracts International, 40,* 1410A.

Rutman, I., and Armstrong, K. 1985. A comprehensive evaluation of transitional employment programs in the rehabilitation of chronically mentally disabled clients. A Mary E. Switzer Research Fellowship Project, 1983–84.

Schmidt, J. R.; Nessel, J. J.; and Malamud, T. J. 1969. An evaluation of rehabilitation services and the role of industry in the community adjustment of psychiatric patients following hospitalization. Final report, RD1281-p, Rehabilitation Services Administration, Washington, D.C.

Skelley, T. 1980. National developments in rehabilitation: A rehabilitation services administration perspective. *Rehabilitation Counseling Bulletin, 24,* 22–33.

White, R. W. 1963. *Ego reality in psychoanalytic theory.* New York: International Universities Press.

III

THE PROCESS

There are several aspects of the vocational rehabilitation process which are common to all the approaches described in the previous section. Vocational assessment, medication management, ego functioning, the rehabilitation relationship, and program evaluation are central elements in the vocational rehabilitation process and, therefore, are the special topics of this section.

In Chapter 11 Bolton outlines a useful assessment strategy and describes how assessment data can be used in vocational planning. In the following chapter Kane describes some of the aspects of medication management as they relate to different members of the treatment team and vocational rehabilitation. Ego functioning is described in relation to symptomatology and social and vocational functioning by Ciardiello, Klein, and Sobkowski in Chapter 13. These authors also discuss the practical application of an ego function approach in the vocational rehabilitation process. Chapters 14 and 15 stress different aspects of the rehabilitation relationship. McCrory illustrates the building of a rehabilitation alliance and the rehabilitation cycle with several case examples. In his chapter, Ryan stresses the need for a personal relationship in which to address the "why" of rehabilitation.

11

Vocational Assessment of Persons with Psychiatric Disorders

BRIAN BOLTON

Bolton uses the rehabilitation literature as an empirical basis for an assessment model which focuses on assessing work personality, and the vocational abilities, interests and temperamental traits which make up occupational capability. In addition to situational assessments, instruments recommended include the Work Personality Profile, the General Aptitude Test Battery, the U.S. Employment Service Interest Inventory, and Form E of the Sixteen Personality Factor Questionnaire. Relevant validity evidence is summarized and suggestions are made for the use of assessment data in vocational planning.

The fundamental premise of this chapter is that successful vocational adjustment is determined, in part, by the appropriate use of vocational assessment. Successful vocational adjustment refers to satisfactory job performance in one of three employment settings: sheltered workshops, supported or supervised work in the community, and the competitive labor market. Although any diagnostic procedure—for example, psychiatric interview, neurological examination, mental status evaluation, or social casework report—may generate information for understanding the individual case, this chapter focuses on procedures that have demonstrated validity (using appropriate vocational criteria) for psychiatrically impaired clients, or, where appropriate, for the general population.

The earliest discussions of vocational assessment techniques for psychiatrically impaired clients were by Gellman (1957) and Patterson (1962). Gellman advocated using the evaluative workshop as the primary tool for analyzing vocational assets and liabilities of former psychiatric patients. The central questions addressed in Gellman's approach are whether the client is capable of assuming the role of worker, and if not, what deficits must be remediated to make the client employable. Gellman did not recommend exclusive reliance on the workshop evaluation, however, but rather, viewed it as the core component of a comprehensive vocational appraisal. Although Patterson proposed a somewhat broader and more balanced approach to vocational evaluation of psychiatrically impaired clients, he emphasized the same critical elements as Gellman. Specifically, Patterson eschewed clinical diagnosis and symptom evaluation and suggested instead that vocational assessment focus on occupationally relevant behavior. He recommended the use of the evaluative workshop, as well as psychological tests and inventories that measure aptitudes and abilities, temperamental characteristics, and vocational interests.

The insights of Gellman and Patterson have been confirmed by research conducted in the past twenty years. In fact, their tentative formulations are now regarded as basic principles in psychiatric rehabilitation. This chapter elaborates and extends the initial proposals by Gellman and Patterson, incorporating recent research and assessment technology, and developing a general approach to the vocational appraisal of psychiatrically impaired clients. It is oriented to the practical needs of rehabilitation professionals who work with psychiatrically disabled persons to enhance their vocational potential with the ultimate objective of maximizing their productive functioning in the community.

An Assessment Model

Vocational assessment of psychiatrically impaired persons will be most useful if it derives from a theoretically based and empirically supported assessment model. The framework outlined in this section draws upon two sources: (1) formulations of the work personality that have been published in the rehabilitation literature since 1950, and (2) empirical evidence concerning the nature of the psychometric variables relevant to successful vocational adjustment. The model presented here is a synthesis of concepts from Dawis (1986), Gellman (1953), Hershenson (1981), Neff (1985), and Roessler and Bolton (1983).

Two fundamental components of occupationally relevant capabilities may be delineated. The first category is the set of habits, attitudes, values, and behaviors that are essential for adequate functioning in the work environment. These include such behaviors as punctuality, task orientation, and appropriate interactions with peers and supervisors. The capabilities that enable the individual to respond satisfactorily to the demands of work are referred to by most writers as the *work personality*. This entity develops during late childhood and early adolescence through school experience and initial work activities such as assigned chores at home, work in the neighborhood, and part-time jobs held during vacations and after school hours. Because the work personality is learned, handicapped or disadvantaged persons may be denied the requisite opportunities. But the overwhelming evidence indicates that the rudiments of the work personality can be acquired at any age—in other words, maturation is not a limiting factor.

The second category of occupationally relevant capabilities is composed of general abilities, vocational interests, and enduring personality characteristics which determine the direction and limits of human performance. These abilities, interests, and temperamental traits are highly stable for most persons throughout adulthood. Psychological traits develop from the interaction of the individual's innate biological potential and environmental stimulation, but once neurological maturation is relatively complete in late adolescence, further modification of trait structures is unlikely.

Formulations of the work personality by Gellman (1953) and Neff (1985) recognize these two broad categories of work capabilities, but both authors emphasize habits, attitudes, and behaviors because these characteristics are amenable to planned interventions, especially that of the vocational adjustment workshop. In contrast, Dawis (1986) focuses on two classes of occupationally relevant traits—general abilities and work values. Hershenson (1981) and Roessler and Bolton (1983) examine both traditional work-personality elements and stable vocational traits. This chapter gives equal weight to the two classes of occupational capabilities.

All theorists recognize the individual component of the work-adjustment equation and the equally important job environment. Neff (1985, ch. 7) carefully specified the nature of the demands made upon the individual by the general work environment, while Dawis (1986) and his colleagues formulated a model of work adjustment for use by vocational counselors that involves the measurement of specific job environments, that is, the aptitudes required for success and the reinforcers present. But all writers recognize the importance of the general work environment in shaping the work personality. Procedures outlined in this chapter are premised on the distinction between (a) general behavioral requirements imposed by all work settings (i.e., habits, attitudes, and behaviors), and (b) specific capabilities needed for success in various job families (i.e., requisite vocational traits).

This division leads to entirely different approaches to vocational appraisal. The assessment of an individual's ability to meet the general demands of work—the individual's work personality—is most appropriately conducted in a situation that is as similar as possible to an actual work setting. The standard procedure is the vocational evaluation workshop, in which the individual is observed over a period of two weeks or more, with judgments and ratings completed by professional staff at regular intervals. By contrast, the appraisal of general abilities, vocational interests, and enduring personality traits is carried out with standardized psychometric instruments. These tests of maximum and typical performance generate normative scores and estimates of performance that provide a basis for occupational counseling.

Especially relevant to vocational assessment of psychiatrically impaired persons is the separation or differentiation of the work personality from the total personality of the individual. Neff (1985) described the semiautonomous nature of the work personality; consistent with this view, Gellman (1953) emphasized that vocational adjustment is *not* a direct function of psychosocial or interpersonal adjustment. Of course, neither theorist is suggesting that work maladaption and personality disturbance are unrelated spheres of functioning. While psychiatric and other clinically oriented evaluations may provide data relevant to the diagnosis of work-personality problems, clinical appraisal cannot substitute for a thorough evaluation of vocational potential.

Psychometric Foundation

Assessment techniques in this chapter are recommended because they have demonstrated validity in relationship to vocational performance criteria. Relevant to the validity of vocational assessment are these two general conclusions documented by Anthony: (1) Ratings of work-adjustment skills and interpersonal skills based on professional observations in a workshop setting are good predictors of future employment for psychiatrically disabled persons; and (2) psychiatric diagnosis and symptomatology are poor predictors of future employment for psychiatrically disabled persons (Anthony 1982; Anthony and Jansen 1984; Cohen and Anthony 1984).

The first conclusion, which is based on a dozen independent studies of psychiatrically impaired persons, establishes unequivocally the predictive validity of the situational approach to assessment of basic work capabilities advocated in this chapter. The second conclusion confirms Neff's characterization of the work personality as a semiautonomous structure, and it is consistent with his observation that persons with fairly severe mental disorders often make a reasonably good adjustment to work.

A third major conclusion reached by Anthony—that psychometric tests are poor predictors of "future work performance"—appears to be based on inappropriate criterion measures. Like the studies that led to the first two conclusions above, the criterion of "vocational functioning" in the typical study of predictive validity of psychometric tests with psychiatric clients was essentially employment versus unemployment. This is an insensitive criterion measure for most occupationally relevant psychometric tests. General ability tests were designed to predict differential performance on the job (i.e., productivity), while interest and personality inventories are used to identify the type of work (i.e., the job family) for which an individual is best suited. Because there are few if any validity studies of psychometric tests with psychiatrically impaired persons that address appropriate criteria, it is necessary (and reasonable) to rely on investigations using the general population.

In a series of studies reported in the late 1970s and early 1980s using a procedure called validity generalization, John Hunter and his colleagues concluded that occupational aptitude tests are uniformly valid predictors of job performance for almost all of the 12,000 jobs in the U.S. economy (see Hunter and Hunter 1984). The only job characteristic that appears to require consideration in determining the relative importance of multiple aptitudes is the cognitive complexity of job requirements. Using a simple weighted combination of cognitive ability and psychomotor ability it is possible to predict job performance for almost all job families with validity coefficients of .50 or greater. (It should be noted that the coefficients are estimates of true validity, i.e., they are corrected for criterion unreliability and restriction of range when appropriate.) In an additional analysis, Hunter and Hunter (1984) determined that for entry-level jobs, an appropriate ability composite (with mean validity of .53) is a more accurate predictor of job performance than any alternative procedure, whether job tryout (.44), biographical inventory (.37), reference check (.26), experience (.18), interview (.14), or training and experience ratings (.13).

The conclusions reached by Hunter and his colleagues are based on several thousand independently conducted validity studies, including 515 standardized studies using the General Aptitude Test Battery (GATB). Hence, it would be difficult to argue that general occupational ability tests that measure cognitive ability and psychomotor ability are not valid predictors of job performance for one subgroup of the population, psychiatrically impaired persons, unless it could be demonstrated that the test scores do not accurately reflect the abilities of such persons. More generally, predictive validity studies of job performance assume that psychometric tests measure *stable* characteristics of examinees if the validity results are applicable in vocational diagnosis and planning with clients.

An investigation by Showler and Droege (1969) in which adults were retested with parallel forms of the GATB at seven intervals ranging from one day to three years demonstrated the stability of occupational aptitudes. The retest correlations for the one-day interval (parallel-form reliabilities) averaged .87 for the nine GATB aptitudes. The mean retest correlations (stability coefficients) for the nine aptitudes at intervals of six weeks, one year, and three years were .85, .81, and .81, respectively. If these stability coefficients are corrected for attenuation (unreliability), they approach 1.00, indicating that general abilities are highly stable characteristics of adults.

Evidence for the validity and stability of vocational interests dates from early investigations by E. K. Strong and is summarized in numerous sources, including Campbell (1971), Hansen (1984), and Tyler (1965).

One of the best-documented findings in psychological testing is that inventoried interests—that is, an individual's pattern of preferences (likes and dislikes) for various vocational activities—are highly stable aspects of adult personality. In his pioneering studies, Strong found median stability coefficients for individuals' interest profiles in the .80s for intervals of up to seventeen years and in the .70s for intervals from eighteen to twenty-two years. Subsequent investigations have confirmed and solidified his findings, but have stressed that while vocational interests are highly stable over time for most adults, there are dramatic shifts for some individuals.

Research literature amply demonstrates the substantial predictive validity of vocational-interest inventories. People are typically found to be employed in occupations that correspond to vocational areas or occupational scales on which they previously scored higher. It is important, however, to emphasize that interest scores are not predictive of successful performance in an occupation. Vocational interests are relatively independent of the abilities that determine occupational success. This conclusion explains why interest inventories are not predictive of the dichotomous criterion of employment versus unemployment.

Evidence supporting the longitudinal stability of measured personality traits is almost as impressive as that for vocational interests. The best summaries of relevant investigations are by Costa and McCrae (1985) and by Schuerger, Tait, and Tavernelli (1982). It should be emphasized that the conclusions in this section pertain to *normal* personality traits such as sociability, friendliness, dominance, conscientiousness, and sensitivity, and not to pathological syndromes such as schizophrenia, grandiosity, depression, and paranoia. The latter characteristics are known to fluctuate substantially over time.

Longitudinal data collected for a sample of adult men by Costa and McCrae (1985) illustrate the stability of self-reported personality traits. The ten scales of the Guilford Zimmerman Temperament Survey (GZTS) had stability coefficients at six years of .71 to .83 and at twelve years of .59 to .87. When the latter stability coefficients were corrected for unreliability, the estimated true stabilities for the twelve-year interval ranged from .80 to 1.00, with a median of .91. Perhaps the strongest evidence for stability of normal personality constructs are the twenty-year retest coefficients, ranging from .61 to .70 (uncorrected) for the two major second-order personality factors, neuroticism (or trait anxiety) and extraversion, using the GZTS at first administration and two different personality questionnaires twenty years later.

The empirical relationships between individual personality make-up and various aspects of vocational functioning are well-documented in the research literature. The most consistent evidence comes from investigations of Holland's (1984) theory of six occupational personality types (realistic, investigative, artistic, social, enterprising, and conventional). Numerous studies have identified relationships between various standard personality inventories and expressed vocational preference, college major, vocational training curriculum, or interest inventories that measure Holland's six occupational themes (see Holland 1984, pp. 63–68). The strongest test comes from studying the relationship between personality and employment.

The most recent validity study addressing this topic analyzed the Sixteen Personality Factor Questionnaire (16 PF) profiles for sixty-nine occupational groups that were each allocated to one of Holland's six occupational categories (Bolton 1985b). Three discriminant functions, labeled independence, extroversion, and anxiety, enabled correct classification of 75 percent of the occupational groups to the appropriate Holland category. Furthermore, the modal personality profiles for the six types based on standard 16 PF scale descriptions were highly consistent with Holland's characterizations of the types. This study and the investigations cited above suggest that normal-sphere personality inventories are valid tools for vocational planning with the general population. *They should be equally applicable in psychiatric rehabilitation.*

The following sections present observational rating techniques used for situational assessment in the evaluative workshop and traditional psychometric tests and inventories that address stable vocationally relevant traits. The workshop evaluation serves to identify critical deficits in the individual's work-personality composition in a vocational adjustment workshop. Psychometric tests and inventories assess vocational traits that are not generally susceptible to modification—that is, abilities, interests, and temperamental characteristics—in order to provide a foundation for optimizing the correspondence between the individual and the job. The appropriate "treatments" used with stable vocational traits include self-appraisal, vocational counseling, and occupational exploration. Three techniques related to rehabilitation but too highly specialized for consideration here are assessment of job-seeking skills (see Mathews, Whang, and Fawcett 1980), work-sample evaluation systems (see Botterbusch 1982), and functional rehabilitation diagnosis (see Anthony, Cohen, and Nemec 1986).

Situational Assessment

The evaluative workshop is the most appropriate setting for appraisal of the psychiatrically impaired person's work habits, attitudes, and behaviors. Evaluative workshops simulate the typical work environment in the competitive job market. Clients perform various types of repetitive assembly-line tasks for which they are paid modest piece rates. Professionally trained work evaluators observe client-workers as they perform different tasks and interact with peers and supervisors. They assess the client's work personality, with deficits identified and carefully described so that an individualized, remedial work-adjustment program can be implemented.

Although the fully controlled setting of the evaluative workshop is usually best for assessing the work personality, some clients can be evaluated through trial employment: such jobs as kitchen help, custodial duties, and grounds maintenance may be substituted for the workshop. The critical consideration in selecting an evaluation setting is whether or not adequate opportunities for observation of relevant work behaviors are available.

For currently institutionalized clients the question arises about whether the situational work evaluation should be conducted on the hospital grounds or at a site in the community? Common sense suggests that an evaluative workshop located off the hospital grounds, requiring travel to and from "work," would provide more valid and generalizable assessment results. In fact, experimental evidence suggests strongly that work therapy programs conducted within the confines of the hospital setting tend to foster institutional dependency (Barbee, Berry, and Micek 1969) and that community-based work-adjustment programs for chronic psychiatric patients do not (Soloff 1967). With patients who are too disturbed to leave the hospital grounds, however, it may be desirable to initiate the work-evaluation process within the institution and later move to a community location when the patient improves. Readers interested in the actual conduct of situational work appraisals are referred to relevant articles in Bolton and Cook (1980).

One important advantage of the evaluative workshop setting that is often overlooked is that the work context can be modified experimentally. Gellman (1957) suggests the following dimensions for evaluative manipulation: (a) supervisory attitudes, which may vary from benign to strict; (b) co-worker relationships, which may vary from working alone to being a group leader; (c) work pressure, which may vary from nominal to severe; and (d) work rewards, such as praise or disapproval. In addition, type and level of work as well as emphasis on quantity or quality may be manipulated.

Regardless of the nature of the setting and its location, and the work assessment strategy used, any situational work evaluation should include a structured observational rating form. Numerous vocational rating scales have been constructed (see Bolton 1985a; Roessler and Bolton 1983), and most of these instruments fulfill the designated purpose. The most recently developed instrument, the Work Personality Profile (WPP) (Bolton and Roessler 1986) consists of fifty-eight items that assess eleven dimensions of work behavior that are directly relevant to employment success: (1) acceptance of work role, (2) ability to profit from instruction or correction, (3) work persistence, (4) work tolerance, (5) amount of supervision required, (6) extent trainee seeks assistance from supervisor, (7) degree of comfort or anxiety with supervisor, (8) appropriateness of personal relations with supervisor, (9) teamwork, (10) ability to socialize with co-workers, and (11) social communication skills. Each item is rated on a four-point scale ranging from employability strength (4) to employability deficit (1); completion of the WPP takes between five and ten minutes.

In conjunction with other relevant information, the results of the WPP can serve as a basis for the development of remedial work-adjustment programs for clients, and the use of the WPP at regular intervals can provide measurements of improvement in targeted employability deficits. Appraisal of the work personality can begin in an institutional setting because positive changes in rudimentary work behaviors are anticipated and repeated measurements are an important facet of the evaluation process. By contrast, assessment of stable vocational traits should *not* be initiated until psychiatrically impaired clients have reached the point in their rehabilitation programs that measures of aptitudes, interests, and personality will be valid estimates of future functioning. This decision must rely primarily on the judgment of psychiatrists, psychologists, and social workers.

Psychometric Assessment

Three classes of occupationally relevant traits should be measured in conjunction with a comprehensive vocational assessment: general abilities, vocational interests, and temperamental characteristics.

General Abilities

The General Aptitude Test Battery (GATB) (U.S. Department of Labor 1982) is the most thoroughly researched occupational aptitude test in existence. First published in 1947 by the U.S. Employment Service (USES), it measures nine ability factors with eight pencil-and-paper and four apparatus tests. The nine aptitudes measured are general learning ability (G), verbal aptitude (V), numerical aptitude (N), spatial aptitude (S), form perception (P), clerical perception (Q), motor coordination (K), finger dexterity (F), and manual dexterity (M). The entire battery, which is available through licensing agreements with the USES, can be administered to small groups of examinees in about 2½ hours.

Data concerning the GATB's reliability, longitudinal stability, and validity against occupational performance were summarized earlier. At the present time an individual's GATB aptitude profile can be compared with sixty-six occupational aptitude patterns (OAPs), which consist of minimally acceptable scores for the most salient aptitudes for sixty-six groups of occupations encompassing all jobs in the U.S. economy. Thus, an individual's GATB profile leads directly to the identification of job families for which she or he possesses requisite abilities for vocational success. In the near future the procedures for translating GATB protocols into occupations for which the examinee qualified will be improved using Hunter's research on validity generalization and his demonstration (Hunter 1983) that the GATB actually measures just three constructs—cognitive (GVN), perceptual (SPQ), and psychomotor (KFM) abilities, the first two being essentially redundant for predicting occupational performance. The new translation procedure will probably involve the generation of expected performance levels for each of the sixty-six OAP work groups and a listing of all jobs for which the examinee is moderately well qualified.

In addition to its excellent psychometric characteristics and straightforward translation into suitable occupational areas for the examinee, the major advantage of the GATB is that it is coordinated with all of the U.S. Department of Labor's occupational information resources, including the *Guide for Occupational Exploration* (*GOE*), the *Dictionary of Occupational Titles* (*DOT*), and the *Occupational Outlook Handbook* (*OOH*).

Vocational Interests

For the very reasons just mentioned—excellent psychometric characteristics and availability of extensive occupational resources—the U.S. Employment Service Interest Inventory (USES-II) (U.S Department of Labor 1981) is probably the best instrument to use with vocational rehabilitation clients. Especially significant is the fact that the twelve interest areas assessed by the USES-II are the primary organizing basis for the occupational information presented in the *GOE*. Furthermore, because of the extreme heterogeneity of the occupations within each of the twelve areas with respect to aptitude, occupations are clustered within interest areas by aptitude requirements, that is, OAPs. Thus, each of the sixty-six OAP work groups is characterized by a unique combination of interest preference *and* minimal occupational aptitude requirements.

The USES-II consists of 162 items to which the examinee responds using a three-choice format: like (L), dislike (D), or not sure (?). Administration to individuals or groups can be accomplished by a psychometric aide or a trained secretary in fifteen to twenty minutes. The twelve interest scales of the USES-II are (1) artistic, (2) scientific, (3) plants and animals, (4) protective, (5) mechanical, (6) industrial, (7) business detail, (8) selling, (9) accommodating, (10) humanitarian, (11) leading-influencing, and (12) physical performing. Recent psychometric studies of the vocational interests of handicapped persons concluded that the USES-II is an appropriate choice for use with this population (Brookings and Bolton 1986; 1987). Further information about the USES-II is available in Bolton (1985c).

Temperamental Characteristics

Form E of the Sixteen Personality Factor Questionnaire (16 PF-E) is a simplified version of the well-known personality inventory of the same name (see Bolton 1978; Wholeben 1985). The 16 PF-E was designed for use with persons of limited educational and cultural background. In particular, 16

PF-E is appropriate for completion by individuals whose reading skills are as low as third-grade level. A forced-choice response format, in which all 128 items are phrased as simple questions consisting of two options separated by the conjunction *or*, is used. The inventory can be administered by audiotape cassette if circumstances warrant this approach. A large normative sample of rehabilitation clients is available for interpretation of the 16 PF-E personality profile (Institute for Personality and Ability Testing 1985).

The 16 PF-E measures sixteen temperamental traits that constitute the domain of normal personality functioning: warmth (A), intelligence (B), stability (C), dominance (E), impulsivity (F), conformity (G), boldness (H), sensitivity (I), suspiciousness (L), imagination (M), shrewdness (N), insecurity (O), radicalism (Q1), self-sufficiency (Q2), self-discipline (Q3), and tension (Q4). Disregarding factor B (intelligence), which is essentially outside the personality sphere, the 16 PF primary scales organize statistically into five second-stratum dimensions: (I) extraversion, (II) anxiety, (III) sensitivity, (IV) independence, and (V) discipline. The mean reliability for these secondary scales is .77, and the mean stability (uncorrected for attenuation) for a sample of rehabilitation clients retested after six years was .58 (Bolton 1979). Although the 16 PF focuses on assessment of normal personality traits, the resulting profile does penetrate the pathological domain with two second-stratum vectors: (a) anxiety and depression and (b) sociopathic tendency (see Bolton and Dana 1987).

Other Instruments

The three instruments described above are, in my judgment, the best all-around choices for use in assessing stable vocational traits of psychiatrically impaired clients. But there are many other instruments that might be applicable in certain settings. For example, the Comprehensive Ability Battery (CAB) measures twenty primary abilities with occupational relevance that span the full range of human capabilities. Furthermore, the CAB is unique among multifactor ability tests in that it is the only battery encompassing a theory of ability structure, development, and action (see Bolton 1984). Many vocational theorists would argue that a measure of motivation is essential in vocational assessment. For a review of several instruments appropriate for use with rehabilitation clients, see Bolton (1980). Finally, there are some clients for whom a preliminary vocational appraisal preceding the more comprehensive assessment might be useful; for this purpose the Preliminary Diagnostic Questionnaire (PDQ) (Moriarty 1981), which measures employment-related skills, knowledge, and attitudes in eight areas using a structured interview format, is unique. Sources of additional information about potentially useful instruments are Anthony and Farkas (1982, pp. 22–31) and several chapters in the *Handbook of Measurement and Evaluation in Rehabilitation* (Bolton 1986).

Vocational Diagnosis

The culminating step in the appraisal process is the "interpretation" of test results and other diagnostic information. Interpretation of vocational assessment data includes a synthesis of the evidence into a cohesive portrait of the client and into plans for vocational rehabilitation. Many articles about the vocational diagnostic and planning process have been published (see Bolton and Cook, 1980). A fundamental principle is that information should be considered in proportion to its established validity against vocational criteria. This generally means that psychiatric symptomatology and similar information should be regarded as minimally relevant in vocational planning, while work-related capabilities and characteristics should receive much greater weight. Still, vocational diagnosis in the individual case must consider all types of information as elements of a comprehensive, integrated description of a unique person. Hence, the final determination of the relevance and relative importance of any single piece of data is a matter of the evaluator's clinical judgment.

The most directly applicable framework for organizing work-personality assessment data for psychiatrically impaired clients observed in simulated work settings is the typology of five dominant patterns of vocational maladaption developed by Neff (1985, pp. 219–25). The work personality is a semiautonomous component of the total personality composed of habits, attitudes, and behaviors that are susceptible to modification. Derived from an in-depth analysis of case reports from an evaluative workshop, each type emphasizes a predominant theme of work psychopathology. Greatly condensed, the five types of maladaption are

1. Deficient work motivation. Clients have failed to internalize the "work ethic"; they are indifferent to the productive role; work is not a central need in their personalities.

2. Fear and anxiety. Clients are characterized by low self-esteem; they are overwhelmed by anxiety in the work setting; they are overly sensitive to criticism, and their performance deteriorates under close supervision.

3. Hostility and aggression. Clients use anger and aggression as defensive tactics; their capacities for interpersonal relationships are poor; they exhibit quick tempers and poor self-control.

4. Dependency. Clients have excessive needs for emotional support; they are overly compliant to authority; their immature behavior necessitates continuous supervisory monitoring.

5. Social naivete. Clients are characterized by underdeveloped work personalities; they have never had the opportunity to learn to work; their ignorance or naivete is the result of a highly protected upbringing.

Neff stressed that the five maladaptive types are not pure categories and that most clients represent mixtures or composites of two or three of them. Still, the typology provides a useful scheme for integrating observations recorded on the Work Personality Profile (WPP) into vocational diagnoses of psychiatrically impaired clients. In fact, the fifty-eight items and eleven scales of the WPP are readily organized into Neff's typology of primary work psychopathologies. It should also be apparent that the profile of stable temperamental traits generated by 16 PF-E can further diagnostic understanding of the client's work personality by providing a broader perspective in which to view maladaptive work behaviors.

Translation of information about the client's occupationally relevant traits into implications for vocational planning utilizes the person-environment correspondence model as conceptualized in the Minnesota Theory of Work Adjustment (Dawis 1986), the U.S. Employment Service's Counselee Assessment/Occupational Exploration System (Droege 1986), and Holland's (1984) typology of vocational environments. As suggested previously, the optimal operational scheme for use in vocational rehabilitation is the USES's assessment and exploration system, which is fully embodied in the *Guide for Occupational Exploration* (*GOE*) (U.S. Department of Labor 1979). Using the client's profiles of nine aptitude scores from the GATB and twelve interest scores from the USES-II, the evaluator can generate a list of job families for which the client possesses minimal requisite aptitudes and relatively high interest. Careful exploration of the jobs or types of jobs that the individual qualifies for can proceed following the step-by-step procedures outlined in the *GOE*.

Conversion of the individual's GATB and USES-II profiles into an ordered list of suitable job families and representative jobs can be easily accomplished by computer. Test-scoring organizations currently market computer-generated reports that summarize an examinee's interest and aptitude levels for the sixty-six work groups (job families) in the *GOE*. The reports include graphic presentations of interest and aptitude results, followed by lists of suitable work groups and sample occupations ordered from high interest and high aptitude combinations to average areas. The *Occupational Report* (Bolton 1987a) was developed for use in vocational rehabilitation settings.

The single outstanding weakness of the USES's assessment and occupational exploration system is the absence of any provision for integrating the counselee's temperamental predispositions into the vocational counseling process. However, recent research developments make this desirable addition not only possible but feasible. Using the client's 16 PF-E profile and the modal 16 PF profiles for Holland's six occupational types (see Bolton 1985b), a vector of six similarity coefficients can be calculated. This is accomplished by the *Vocational Personality Report* (Bolton 1987b). Because Holland's typology is congruent with the twelve occupational areas of the *GOE* (see Jones 1980), the client's profile of temperamental traits can be integrated with the results of the GATB and USES-II in the vocational exploration process.

Holland's six occupational types were given earlier. Personality-trait characterizations selected from Holland's (1984, pp. 19–23) descriptions to correspond maximally with 16 PF scales that differentiate the six types are as follows:

1. Realistic: conforming, hard-headed, practical, inflexible, uninsightful;

2. Investigative: independent, intellectual, precise, rational, reserved;

3. Artistic: emotional, imaginative, introspective, nonconforming, sensitive;

4. Social: cooperative, friendly, helpful, responsible, warm;

5. Enterprising: agreeable, ambitious, energetic, extroverted, sociable;

6. Conventional: conforming, conscientious, efficient, obedient, practical.

A final issue that merits attention concerns the client's role in the interpretation of vocational assessment information. Many professionals would argue that the very nature of psychiatric disablement precludes any client involvement in the test interpretation process. However, a very good case can be made for sharing responsibility for the entire appraisal sequence with the client. Vash (1981, ch. 10; 1984) has suggested several principles and strategies for making the client a partner in rehabilitation evaluation. First, explaining the purpose of various tests and assessment techniques to clients serves to engage them as active participants in the evaluative process. Second, sharing the results of tests, inventories, and observational ratings, as well as written reports with clients gives them some responsibility for acting upon the results. Third, clients are life-long experts on themselves, and even if they have experienced some adjustment difficulties, they can bring a wealth of self-knowledge to bear on the interpretation of assessment data. Vash recommends that clients be active participants in the interpretive process and that they be given personal copies of all written assessment reports.

References

Anthony, W. A. 1982. *The vocational functioning of the severely psychiatrically disabled: A table of research results.* Boston: Boston University, Center for Rehabilitation Research and Training in Mental Health.

Anthony, W. A.; Cohen, M.; and Nemec, P. 1986. Assessment in psychiatric rehabilitation. In Bolton 1986.

Anthony, W. A., and Farkas, M. 1982. A client-outcome planning model for assessing psychiatric rehabilitation interventions. *Schizophrenia Bulletin, 8*, 18–38.

Anthony, W. A., and Jansen, M. A. 1984. Predicting the vocational capacity of the chronically mentally ill. *American Psychologist, 39*, 537–44.

Barbee, M. S.; Berry, K. L.; and Micek, L. A. 1969. Relationship of work therapy to psychiatric length of stay and readmission. *Journal of Consulting and Clinical Psychology, 33*, 735–38.

Bolton, B. 1978. The sixteen personality factor questionnaire. In *The eighth mental measurements yearbook*, ed. O. K. Buros, pp. 1078–80. Highland Park, N.J.: Gryphon.

———. 1979. Longitudinal stability of the primary and secondary dimensions of the 16 PF-E. *Multivariate Experimental Clinical Research, 4*, 67–71.

———. 1980. Rehabilitation needs. In *Encyclopedia of clinical assessment*, ed. R. Woody, pp. 1068–76. San Francisco: Jossey-Bass.

———. 1984. Comprehensive ability battery. In *Test critiques*, ed. D. J. Keyser and R. C. Sweetland, 1:214–25. Kansas City, Mo.: Test Corporation of America.

———. 1985a. Measurement in rehabilitation. In *Annual review of rehabilitation*, ed. E. L. Pan, S. S. Newman, T. E. Backer, and C. L. Vash, 4:115–44. New York: Springer.

———. 1985b. Discriminant analysis of Holland's occupational types using the Sixteen Personality Factor Questionnaire. *Journal of Vocational Behavior, 27* 210–17.

———. 1985c. United States Employment Service interest inventory. In *Test critiques*, ed. D. J. Keyser and R. C. Sweetland, 3:673–81. Kansas City, Mo.: Test Corporation of America.

———, ed. 1986. *Handbook of measurement and evaluation in rehabilitation*. 2nd ed. Baltimore: Paul H. Brookes.

———. 1987a. *Manual for the Occupational Report*. Fayetteville, Ark.: Arkansas Research and Training Center in Vocational Rehabilitation.

———. 1987b. *Manual for the Vocational Personality Report*. Fayetteville, Ark.: Arkansas Research and Training Center in Vocational Rehabilitation.

Bolton, B., and Cook, D. W., eds. 1980. *Rehabilitation client assessment*. Austin, Tex.: Pro-Ed.

Bolton, B., and Dana, R. H. 1987. Multivariate relationships between normal personality functioning and objectively measured psychopathology. *Journal of Social and Clinical Psychology*, in press.

Bolton, B., and Roessler, R. T. 1986. *Manual for the Work Personality Profile*. Fayetteville, Ark.: Arkansas Research and Training Center in Vocational Rehabilitation.

Botterbusch, K. F. 1982. Commercial vocational evaluation systems. In *Vocational adjustment of disabled persons*, ed. B. Bolton, pp. 93–125. Austin, Tex.: Pro-Ed.

Brookings, J. B., and Bolton, B. 1986. Vocational interest dimensions of adult handicapped persons. *Measurement and Evaluation in Counseling and Development, 18*, 168–75.

———. 1987. *Confirmatory parcel analysis of the USES Interest Inventory*. Paper presented at the meeting of the American Psychological Association, New York City, August.

Campbell, D. P. 1971. *Handbook for the strong vocational interest blank*. Stanford, Calif.: Stanford University Press.

Cohen, B. F., and Anthony, W. A. 1984. Functional assessment in psychiatric rehabilitation. In *Functional assessment in rehabilitation*, ed. A. S. Halpern and M. J. Fuhrer, pp. 79–100. Baltimore: Paul H. Brookes.

Costa, P. T., Jr., and McCrae, R. R. 1985. Concurrent validation after twenty years: The implications of personality stability for its assessment. In *Advances in personality assessment*, ed. J. N. Butcher and C. D. Spielberger, 4:31–54. Hillsdale, N.J.: Erlbaum.

Dawis, R. V. 1986. The Minnesota theory of work adjustment. In Bolton 1986.

Droege, R. C. 1986. The USES testing program. In Bolton 1986.

Gellman, W. G. 1953. Components of vocational adjustment. *Personnel and Guidance Journal, 31*, 536–39.

————. 1957. Vocational evaluation of the emotionally handicapped. *Journal of Rehabilitation. 23,* 9–10, 13, 32.

Hansen, J. I. 1984. The measurement of vocational interests. In *Handbook of counseling psychology,* ed. S. Brown and R. Lent, pp. 99–136. New York: Wiley and Sons.

Hershenson, D. B. 1981. Work adjustment, disability, and the three R's of vocational rehabilitation: A conceptual model. *Rehabilitation Counseling Bulletin, 25,* 91–97.

Holland, J. L. 1984. *Making vocational choices: A theory of vocational personalities and work environments.* Englewood Cliffs, N.J.: Prentice-Hall.

Hunter, J. E. 1983. *The dimensionality of the General Aptitude Test Battery (GATB) and the dominance of general factors over specific factors in the prediction of job performance.* Washington, D.C.: U.S. Employment Service, U.S. Department of Labor.

Hunter, J. E., and Hunter, R. F. 1984. Validity and utility of alternative predictors of job performance. *Psychological Bulletin, 96,* 72–98.

Institute for Personality and Ability Testing. 1985. *Manual for Form E of the 16 PF.* Champaign, Ill.: Institute for Personality and Ability Testing.

Jones, L. K. 1980. Holland's typology and the new Guide for Occupational Exploration: Bridging the gap. *Vocational Guidance Quarterly, 29,* 70–76.

Mathews, M.; Whang, P.; and Fawcett, S. 1980. Development and validation of an occupational skills assessment instrument. *Behavioral Assessment, 2,* 71–85.

Moriarty, J. 1981. *Preliminary diagnostic questionnaire.* Morgantown, W. V.: University of West Virginia Rehabilitation Research and Training Center.

Neff, W. S. 1985. *Work and human behavior.* 3d ed. Hawthorne, N.Y.: Aldine.

Patterson, C. H. 1962. Evaluation of the rehabilitation potential of the mentally ill patient. *Rehabilitation Literature, 23,* 162–72.

Roessler, R. T., and Bolton, B. 1983. Assessment and enhancement of functional vocational capacities: A five-year research strategy. *Vocational Evaluation and Work Adjustment Bulletin* (monograph).

Schuerger, J. M.; Tait, E.; and Tavernelli, M. 1982. Temporal stability of personality by questionnaire. *Journal of Personality and Social Psychology, 43,* 176–82.

Showler, W. K., and Droege, R. C. 1969. Stability of aptitude scores for adults. *Educational and Psychological Measurement, 29,* 681–85.

Soloff, A. 1967. *A work-therapy research center.* Chicago: Jewish Vocational Service.

Tyler, L. 1965. *The psychology of human differences.* 3d ed. New York: Appleton-Century-Crofts.

U.S. Department of Labor. 1979. *Guide for occupational exploration.* Washington, D.C.: U.S. Government Printing Office.

————. 1981. *USES interest inventory.* Washington, D.C.: U.S. Government Printing Office.

————. 1982. *Manual for the General Aptitude Test Battery.* Washington, D.C.: U.S. Government Printing Office.

Vash, C. L. 1981. *The psychology of disability.* New York: Springer.

————. 1984. Evaluation from the client's point of view. In *Functional assessment in rehabilitation,* ed. A. S. Halpern and M. J. Fuhrer pp. 253–67. Baltimore: Paul H. Brookes.

Wholeben, B. E. 1985. The Sixteen Personality Factor Questionnaire. In *Test critiques,* ed. D. J. Keyser and R. C. Sweetland 4:595–605. Kansas City, Mo.: Test Corporation of America.

12

The Role of Psychotropic Medication in Vocational Rehabilitation

JOHN M. KANE

In this chapter on the psychopharmacology of severe mental illness, Kane not only gives the details of medication management, but also discusses it in the context of the recovery and rehabilitation processes. He lists the most frequently used psychotropic medications and their usual dosages, and describes their usefulness as well as their adverse effects, limitations, and management difficulties. The role of each member of the treatment team is described in relation to medication and particularly in identifying the early signs of relapse. Kane stresses the ways in which drug treatment and vocational rehabilitation affect each other.

In the treatmeat of persons with prolonged mental illness an integrated approach involving vocational rehabilitation, psychosocial strategies, and appropriate medication management is critical in assuring optimal outcome. This chapter focuses on psychopharmacologic treatment, with particular emphasis on the recovery process and long-term treatment strategies.

Persons with schizophrenia constitute the largest population for whom this subject is of critical important; however, persons with other conditions, such as the major affective disorders (e.g., bipolar disorder and major depression), schizoaffective disorder, and some personality disorders (e.g., schizotypal and borderline), may also receive concurrent vocational rehabilitation and drug treatment.

Tables 12.1, 12.2, and 12.3 summarize the major psychotropic drugs in use today and provide some guidelines as to usual therapeutic doses. Dosages outside these guidelines are sometimes used in special circumstances but should be employed only after careful evaluation and consideration of alternate approaches.

Before we examine issues relevant to specific conditions, it is useful to review some general principles with regard to the indications for medication and the process of evaluating psychotropic drug effects. Although we

Table 12.1
Frequently Used Antipsychotics and Their Dosage Relationships

Name			Range of total daily dose	
Generic	Representative brand	Relative potency[a]	Outpatient (mg/day)	Inpatient (mg/day)
Phenothiazines				
Chlorpromazine	Thorazine	100	50–400	200–1,600
Thioridazine	Mellaril	100	50–400	200–800
Mesoridazine	Serentil	50	25–200	100–400
Acetophenazine	Tindal	20	40–80	60–100
Prochlorperazine	Compazine	15	20–60	60–200
Perphenazine	Trilafon	10	8–24	12–64
Trifluoperazine	Stelazine	5	4–10	10–60
Triflupromazine	Vesprin	25	20–100	30–150
Fluphenazine	Prolixin	2	1–5	2–60
Fluphenazine decanoate	Prolixin	.06	6–100	6–100[b]
Thioxanthene				
Thiothixene	Navane	5	6–30	10–120
Chlorprothixene	Taractan	100	50–400	50–600
Butyrophenones				
Haloperiodol	Haldol	2	2–6	4–100
Dibenzoxazepines				
Loxapine	Loxitane	10	15–60	4–160
Dihydroindolone				
Molindone	Moban	10	15–60	40–225

NOTE: Approximate relative potency of antipsychotic-agent dosage may vary with individual responses to the antipsychotic agent employed.

[a]Estimates of relative potency. Relative potency may not be the same in the higher dosage ranges as it is in the lower.

[b]Dosage requirements for fluphenazine decanoate vary widely and may be given at intervals of up to 3–4 weeks.

tend to think of a particular class of drugs or a particular treatment strategy in relation to a specific condition (e.g., antipsychotic drugs and schizophrenia), it is essential to recognize that patients diagnosed as having schizophrenia vary enormously in the nature of their illness, in terms of onset, course, response to treatment, personality, premorbid social and vocational adjustment, responsivity to stress, and so on. It remains a major problem that we still cannot predict with relative certainty the outcomes of our interventions. Therefore, the treatment plan must be tailored to specific patients even though general guidelines may apply to patients in general. Ongoing evaluation of all of the factors alluded to above becomes necessary to maximize the potential benefits of specific treatments.

In my view, everyone involved in the treatment of patients who are receiving medication should have some familiarity with the rationale, goals, and potential adverse effects of drug treatment, since medication interacts in a variety of ways with all other treatment modalities. In addition, the

Table 12.2
Frequently Used Antidepressants and Their Usual Oral Dosage Range

Generic name	Representative brand name	Oral dosage range
Antidepressants		
Amitriptyline	Elavil, Endep	150–300
Amoxapine	Asendin	150–600
Desipramine	Norpramin, Pertofrane	150–300
Doxepin	Sinequan	150–300
Imipramine	Tofranil, Presamine	150–300
Maprotiline	Ludiomil	150–300
Nortriptyline	Aventyl, Pamelor	75–200
Protriptyline	Vivactil	15–60
Trazodone	Desyril	150–600
Trimipramine	Surmontil	150–300
Mao Inhibitors		
Phenelzine	Nardil	30–90
Tranylcypromine	Parnate	20–60
Isocarboxazid	Marplan	10–40
Combination Antidepressant-Tranquilizer		
Perphenazine plus amitriptyline	Triavil, Etrafon	Consult prescribing information
Chlordiazepoxide plus amitriptyline	Limbitrol	
Benactyzine plus meprobamate	Deprol	

physician prescribing medication should have the benefit of feedback from all the individuals who have ongoing contact with the patient in order to evaluate treatment response.

Schizophrenia

Despite the impact of antipsychotic or neuroleptic medication in controlling and preventing the recurrence of delusions, hallucinations, thought disorder, and other major signs and symptoms of schizophrenia, many patients are left with a variety of significant impairments, particularly in social and vocational adjustment. This highlights the importance of familiarity with the extent of the potential benefits and limitations of medication treatment as well as the interactions between various treatment modalities and medication.

We generally divide pharmacologic treatment for illnesses that involve exacerbations and remissions into three phases: acute, continuation, and maintenance treatment.

The acute treatment phase usually involves an attempt to alleviate the more florid signs and symptoms: in the case of schizophrenia, delusions, hallucinations, suspiciousness, and disordered thinking. In general, medication can be dramatically effective in achieving these goals; this has been established in numerous double-blind comparisons between active medi-

Table 12.3
Frequently Used Minor Tranquilizers and Antiparkinsonian Agents and Their Usual Oral Dosage Range

Generic name	Representative brand name	Oral dosage range
Benzodiazepines		
Chlorazepate	Tranzene	15–60
Chlordiazepoxide	Librium	15–10
Diazepam	Valium	6–40
Flurazepam	Dalmane	15–30
Halazepam	Paxipam	80–160
Lorazepam	Ativan	1–10
Oxazepam	Serax	30–120
Prazepam	Centrax	20–60
Temazepam	Restoril	15–30
Triazolam	Halcion	0.25–0.5
Glycerol derivatives		
Meprobamate	Equanil, Miltown, SK Bamate	1,200–1,400
Tybamate	Tybatran	1,250–3,000
Sedating antihistamines		
Hydroxyzine	Vistaril, Atarax	75–400
Antiparkinsonian agents		
Amantadine	Symmetrel	100–300
Benztropine	Cogentin	1–6
Biperiden	Akineton	2–6
Diphenhydramine	Benadryl	25–100
Ethopropazine	Parsidol	50–600
Orphenadrine	Disipal, Norflex	300
Procyclidine	Kemadrin	5–20
Trihexyphenidyl	Artane	5–15

cation and placebos (Klein and Davis 1969). At the same time, however, a substantial proportion of patients may improve only partially, and some fewer cases may not improve at all. The reasons for this variation in treatment response are not well understood, and we are generally not able to predict response in a given patient. We consider issues such as compliance, dosage, and duration of treatment and reevaluate the diagnosis in a patient who fails to show the expected response. Although the focus in this chapter is largely on long-term treatment during the rehabilitation phase, the response during the acute phase to some extent determines the goals and objectives as well as the choice of specific strategies for subsequent treatment. For example, the partial responder who continues to manifest some delusions and hallucinations may be a poorer risk for medication discontinuation or substantial dosage reduction than a patient who has responded more fully. (It may seem paradoxical that the individual who has benefited less from medication may become worse when it is stopped, whereas the individual who benefited most may be able to do without it temporarily. This will be discussed further subsequently.)

If a patient fully recovers or improves substantially, the continuation phase of treatment begins at the point of maximum improvement. This point may occur after several weeks or even months of treatment. The conceptual assumption underlying continuation treatment is that in an illness with remissions and exacerbations an episode that goes untreated might have a finite length. Although this model may be more obviously relevant to affective illness, it is useful in thinking about the treatment of some schizophrenic patients as well. The medication that helped to alleviate the signs and symptoms of an acute episode appears to be necessary to maintain that improvement for at least as long as the episode would have lasted had it gone untreated. Once this period has passed, then a recurrence of symptoms would be considered a "new" episode rather than a reemergence of the original episode. The point at which continuation treatment ends is the point at which preventive treatment begins, the goal of which is the prevention of a new episode.

The patients who respond only partially to medication during the acute phase may, in effect, remain indefinitely in the continuation phase. The treatment strategy remains the continued use of medication to partially control existing psychotic symptoms. A cessation of medication would be more likely to lead to increased symptomatology than it would among patients who have achieved full remission and are ready to enter the prevention phase.

As a rule, it takes several weeks (at least 4–6) to achieve the full benefit that antipsychotics can provide. In this era of decreasing length of hospital stay, it is likely that some continued treatment of the acute episode will occur outside of the hospital. For those patients who do not fully recover, some psychopharmacologists would recommend a trial on higher-than-standard doses, switching to another class of neuroleptic or use of injectable medication. In addition, the patient should be carefully evaluated for side effects which interfere with therapeutic drug response. These side effects can include, for example, akathesia—a subjective sense of restlessness, "crawling under the skin," or inability to sit still—which in the psychotic patient may contribute to anxiety, agitation, paranoid ideation, or bizarre behavior. Akinesia is another behaviorally manifested neurologic side effect of antipsychotic medication which results in a slowing of movements, lack of spontaneity and facial expression, and even reduction in motivation. These side effects can generally be controlled by a reduction in neuroleptic dosage or by the use of antiparkinsonian drugs (see Table 12.4).

Yet, despite several alternative treatments, some patients continue to experience a moderate or severe degree of hallucinations, delusions, or thought disorder. There comes a time when the clinicians and family members need to accept the limitations of pharmacologic or somatic treatment, even though it is difficult to know when to abandon the search for

Table 12.4
Adverse Effects of Neuroleptics

Central nervous system	Autonomic
Dystonia	Dry mouth
Parkinsonism	Constipation
Akathisia	Urinary retention
Acute dyskinesia	Tachycardia
Tardive dyskinesia	Blurred vision
Seizures	Glaucoma (acute narrow angle)
Cognitive dysfunction	Disturbance in temperature regulation
Sedation	Postural hypotension
Disturbance in temperature regulation	Ejaculation disturbance
Neuroleptic malignant syndrome	Paralytic ileus
Tardive dystonia	
Weight gain	

an ideal treatment effect (e.g. the addition of lithium, the use of electroconvulsive therapy, high doses of benzodiazepines). Some clinicians have described improvement when these patients are taken off all medication. In my experience, however, these medications usually are beneficial. Any improvement following drug withdrawal is frequently due to reduction in side effects and is temporary.

Fortunately, the majority of persons with schizophrenia do respond reasonably well to antipsychotic drugs, and for them a number of considerations are relevant to long-term medication treatment and rehabilitation. Medication dosage may be reduced after recovery from the acute episode and after four to eight weeks of stable remission. In the absence of full remission, medication dosages may be lowered with the achievement of maximal response in those patients who continue to have mild psychotic symptoms.

Some reviews of the literature (Klein and Davis 1969) have suggested that 400 milligrams per day of chlorpromazine (or an equivalent dose of another antipsychotic) is the minimum dose necessary for acute treatment of the average patient; however, individual dosage requirements vary enormously. It is likely that, on average, dosage can be reduced for maintenance to 50 percent of that required during the acute treatment phase.

Adverse Effects of Antipsychotic Drugs

In recent years increasing attention has been given to exploring the feasibility and potential advantages of alternative maintenance strategies designed to provide an optimal balance between benefits and risks (Kane 1984). Reduction of cumulative neuroleptic exposure has been a major focus, with the hope of reducing the risk of tardive dyskinesia. Tardive dyskinesia is an involuntary movement disorder usually involving the facial region and/or the extremities. This condition is seen to varying degrees in approximately 20 percent of patients undergoing long-term treatment with neuroleptic drugs (Kane and Smith 1982). Fortunately, the majority of cases are relatively mild and nonprogressive. However, some individuals develop a severe and disabling form of the disorder. This adverse effect has been a major impetus for developing treatment strategies that reduce the dosage of neuroleptic medication. Other adverse effects can be of clinical significance during the long-term treatment. Table 12.4 provides a summary of these adverse effects. I would place particular emphasis on those side effects which might interfere with social and vocational rehabilitation. Although neuroleptic medication plays an important role in the treatment of schizophrenia, optimal outcome depends upon thoughtful application of several treatment modalities.

Schizophrenia has an enormous impact on social and vocational adjustment because of the primary symptoms of the illness and because of its appearance in late adolescence or early adulthood, when it interferes with stages of maturation, individuation, separation, and the pursuit of education and vocational development. As a consequence, vocational rehabilitation is critical in restoring patients to the maximum possible level of adjustment and productivity. After the resolution of an acute psychotic episode or at least following sufficient improvement in psychotic symptoms to allow the patient to concentrate and participate in rehabilitation, this becomes a major focus of treatment. Although medication may have a variety of beneficial effects, this stage of treatment requires careful attention to adverse effects of neuroleptics and other factors which may influence medication dosage requirements. The importance of ongoing communication between all members of the treatment team becomes particularly critical as the rehabilitative process begins.

Drowsiness, restlessness, an excessively dry mouth, psychomotor retardation, and so on may be tolerated to some extent during the initial inpatient treatment of a psychotic episode, but these side effects may represent significant impediments to vocational rehabilitation. The physician prescribing the medication and the rehabilitation therapist must work closely to provide the necessary ongoing assessment and appropriate adjustment of medication. As a rule, most of the side effects that could interfere with patient functioning can be controlled with adjustment of dosage or dosage schedule or change in type of medication. Patients vary enormously in their sensitivity or response to a variety of side effects, and no blanket rules or guidelines apply. For example, drowsiness is frequently a problem with neuroleptic drugs, particularly the so-called low potency drugs, such as chlorpromazine or thioridazine. These effects can be minimized by giving all the medication at night (so that the sedative effects are most pronounced during the time the patient is asleep), by reducing dosage, or by switching to another medication which is less sedating. Akathesia and akinesia can continue to be a problem during the maintenance phase of treatment, though their manifestation may at times be subtle (Rifkin et al. 1978). Dosage reduction or the use of antiparkinsonian agents can improve some patients' ability to sit still or increase their spontaneity and motivation. Consideration of adverse effects has also contributed to our desire to establish the minimum dosages required to prevent relapse and to identify patients who may safely be able to discontinue medication for months at a time.

Benefits of Maintenance Neuroleptics

Table 12.5 is a summary of clinical trials comparing maintenance neuroleptic treatment to placebo treatment under double-blind conditions. Only studies with a duration of at least nine months are included. The effect of pharmacologic treatment is extremely dramatic and consistent across studies in reducing the risk of psychotic relapse and rehospitalization. However, not all patients receiving placebos relapse within a one- to two-year period, and some patients relapse despite continued medication. Considerable attention has been given to attempts to understanding this heterogeneity of outcome and to develop predictors to identify patients for whom particular drug treatment strategies are appropriate. In addi-

Table 12.5
Maintenance Pharmacotherapy in Schizophrenia: Placebo-Controlled Trials

Author	N	Duration of trial	Treatment	Outcome (relapse)
Trochinsky, Aaronson, & Stone 1962	43	1 year	Drug	4%
			Placebo	63%
Engelhardt et al. 1963	446	4 years	Thorazine	1 yr. 15%, 4 yrs. 20%
			Placebo	1 yr. 30%, 4 yrs. 31%
Leff & Wing 1971	35	1 year	Drug	35%
			Placebo	80%
Hirsch et al. 1973	81	9 months	Prolixin decanoate	8%
			Placebo	66%
Hogarty et al. 1976	374	2 years	Drug	1 yr. 31%, 2 yrs. 48%
			Placebo	1 yr. 68%, 2 yrs. 80%
Chien 1975	47	1 year	Prolixin[a]	12%
			Prolixin[b]	37%
			Placebo	86%
Rifkin et al. 1977	73	1 year	Drug	5%
			Placebo	75%
Kane et al. 1982	28	1 year	Drug	0%
			Placebo	41%
Odejide & Aderounmu 1982	70	1 year	Prolixin decanoate	19%
			Placebo	56%

[a]Doctor-regulated interval
[b]Patient-regulated interval

tion, much research in recent years has focused on studying interactions between pharmacotherapy and other factors which influence long-term outcome, such as psychosocial and vocational therapies, premorbid adjustment, family environment, and stressful life events. These will be discussed in more detail subsequently.

Medications remain an important element of treatment even among those patients who have done well on neuroleptic treatment for periods exceeding two years. There remains a substantial risk of relapse if medication is completely discontinued. For example, Cheung (1981) studied patients who had been in good remission for three to five years and found that 62 percent of the subjects withdrawn from neuroleptics (under double-blind conditions) relapsed within eighteen months, as compared to 13 percent of the patients who remained on antipsychotic medication. Similarly, Hogarty et al. (1976) reported a 65 percent relapse rate following discontinuation of neuroleptics for patients who had been in good remission for at least two years.

These studies strongly suggest that the overwhelming majority of persons with schizophrenia will experience a psychotic relapse at some point following the discontinuation of neuroleptic treatment. The interval at which this occurs varies considerably, but the modal time frame appears to be three to seven months for those patients in reasonable remission at the point medication is discontinued. Strategies designed to reduce cumulative neuroleptic exposure must be alert to the high likelihood of relapse. Careful clinical monitoring is required in order to make these approaches successful.

Alternative Pharmacologic Strategies

One maintenance strategy involves substantial dosage reduction and has been referred to as the "low-dose" strategy. The intent is to give a much lower dose than was used in treating an acute episode. Patients are carefully observed for signs of relapse, and dosages are increased, preferably on a temporary basis, when necessary. Recent studies suggest that doses of fluphenazine decanoate (a long-acting injectable neuroleptic) as low as 5 to 10 milligrams given every other week are sufficient to maintain remission in a substantial proportion of individuals with schizophrenia (Kane et al. 1983; Marder et al. 1984). Long-acting injectable drugs have been used in many long-term treatment trials in recent years to eliminate noncompliance as a potential factor in outcome variability. When oral medications are prescribed, the physician is often uncertain whether or not patients who relapse did so because they had taken their medications erratically. Individuals who are becoming ill may stop medication, and it is often unclear as to which came first—the relapse or the noncompliance. In addition, in titrating dosage downward, injectable administration provides better control of dosage within a narrow range and more predictable absorption and metabolism.

The utilization of low-dose treatment has been shown to reduce side effects, improve subjective well-being, and lead to some gains in psychosocial adjustment. However, the risk of relapse is increased, and careful clinical monitoring is necessary (Kane et al. 1983; Marder et al. 1984).

A second maintenance strategy involves so-called targeted or intermittent drug treatment (Herz 1984; Carpenter and Heinrichs 1984). This approach involves the complete discontinuation of medication followed by careful observation for early signs of relapse (referred to as prodromal signs) with immediate reinstitution of medication, again, one hopes, on a temporary basis. This strategy follows from the observation that many patients do not relapse for several months following medication discontinuation; therefore, continued drug treatment could be viewed as unnecessary. In addition, many individuals have characteristic patterns of relapse. If families, clinicians, and patients are aware of these early signs, then a potential relapse can be treated quickly before it becomes severe enough to lead to significant psychosocial or vocational disruption.

Prodromal Signs of Relapse

The negative side of these strategies is that the risk of relapse is increased, and for a small proportion of individuals who do relapse, the episode may not be controlled as quickly or fully as we would like. In addition, both of these strategies depend upon early detection of clinical worsening. Therefore, they are most applicable to patients who maintain some degree of insight and who have a psychosocial and clinical support system which is observant and responsive. A major focus in these strategies is to educate patients and families about the importance of detecting early signs of relapse and about how to respond to them appropriately.

These treatment approaches have also led to several other important considerations. First of all, what are "prodromal" signs and symptoms? Herz (1984) and others have observed that some patients show a pattern of signs or symptoms during the early stages of a relapse which are consistent from one episode to another. A careful history-taking and recognition of these patterns are extremely useful in detecting a relapse. These early manifestations may not be of a psychotic nature and may include anxiety, insomnia, and hostility. However, since some individuals with schizophrenia may experience anxiety or insomnia which are not precursors of a psychotic relapse but a transient response to a stressful situation, it may be difficult to make this distinction. Clinicians with a conservative view allow for temporary increase or reinstitution of medication if such symptoms occur. Clearly, the better the treatment team knows the patient, the more likely a correct assessment will be made. Some patients experience an increase in suspiciousness, hallucinations, delusions, or other psychotic symptoms as the first signs of impending relapse, but even here, a change in these areas of psychopathology does not automatically mean that a relapse is occurring.

The rehabilitation therapist plays a critical role in identifying and responding to potential prodromal signs and distinguishing them from expectable responses to changes in vocational activity responsibility, level of expectation, and the like. The patient is likely to experience anxiety when starting a new job or returning to an old job after a psychotic episode. The therapist should understand and respond to a recurrence of symptoms in that context instead of assuming that a relapse is imminent. Similarly, by recognizing that a potentially anxiety-provoking situation is about to occur, the clinical team can try to prevent an excessive increase in anxiety by providing more supportive therapeutic contacts and a temporary dosage adjustment. This is the kind of situation where close cooperation among members of the treatment team is critical.

The Role of Stress

Despite its intuitive appeal, the association between stress and schizophrenic relapse is not clear-cut. The literature remains inconsistent, and clinicians have observed that some individuals with schizophrenia handle apparently very stressful situations with ease while reacting badly to seemingly minor events. Given this anomaly, should medications be used as a prophylactic measure when a patient is to undergo a particularly stressful event? My own view is that such measures may be warranted when working within a low-dosage or intermittent dosage protocol because of the greater risk of relapse under these conditions. Some clinicians use antianxiety agents as a treatment for prodromal signs such as anxiety or insomnia, or as a preventive measure prior to a known stressor. It is important to recognize, however, that some individuals have a paradoxical reaction to benzodiazepines and may become more hostile or irritable following their use. Although the use of benzodiazepines seems reasonable in this context, the efficacy of this approach has not been well-studied.

Herz (1984) has reported that 70 percent of patients and 93 percent of family members indicated that they noticed some changes prior to a psychotic episode that led them to recognize the onset of a decompensation. This underscores the family's potential contribution to treatment strategies that involve the recognition of prodromal signs. The most common signs reported by patients and families were tension and nervousness, diminished appetite, difficulty concentrating, difficulty sleeping, restlessness, reduced enjoyment, preoccupation with one or two things, and depression. Many of these symptoms are also seen in anxious states and/or depression, and it is important to consider the differential diagnosis in this situation, since depression or anxiety disorders may occur in individuals with schizophrenia and may not be a sign of relapse.

Differential diagnosis is further complicated by the multifaceted nature of schizophrenia. Potential adverse effects of the drugs used to treat this condition can make it difficult at times to distinguish between some schizophrenic symptomatology and drug reactions. This is particularly true for "negative symptoms." Much attention has been given in recent years to the concept of "negative symptoms" in schizophrenia, which refers to blunted affect, emotional withdrawal, reduced motivation and pleasure capacity, psychomotor retardation, and so on. Many clinicians have suggested that these symptoms are not responsive to neuroleptics and to some extent represent a residual deficit which many persons with schizophrenia experience even in the absence of more florid symptoms (e.g., delusions, hallucinations). It appears, however, that these phenomena are more complex. Patterns of symptoms may differ in response to pharmacotherapy at different stages of the illness. For example, during a relapse or acute exacerbation, the psychomotor retardation, apathy, and withdrawal may respond substantially to neuroleptic treatment. When these symptoms are present during the maintenance phase of treatment, neuroleptics may have a worsening effect, often mediated by neurologic side effects (particularly akinesia), which can lead to diminished affect, reduced spontaneity, psychomotor retardation, and so on.

When such symptoms are seen during the maintenance phase of treatment, a trial of antiparkinsonian drugs or a reduction in the dosage of the neuroleptic may be helpful in making the differential diagnosis. Another consideration is that the patient is, in fact, depressed or demoralized. Depression and demoralization represent different though to some degree overlapping phenomena, and each has its own treatment implications. Major depressive disorder is not responsive to environmental manipulation. The patient's pleasure capacity is reduced, and other vegetative signs—disturbances of appetite, sleep, concentration, and energy—are apparent and may respond to antidepressant medication. Demoralization, on the other hand, represents a realistic feeling of discouragement, helplessness, and hopelessness in response to a bad situation. The latter is not at all an unreasonable response to the recognition that one has a schizophrenic illness. Rehabilitative and other psychosocial strategies are necessary to help overcome this problem. Clearly, however, these various possibilities need to be considered in the management and rehabilitation of such individuals.

Those members of the treatment team working with the patient on a day-to-day basis are in a position to observe the patient's reactions to successes and failures as well as to reinforcement and discouragements and are therefore in an ideal position to distinguish between phenomena such as depression and demoralization. The success of rehabilitation in general will depend heavily on the team's ability to deal effectively with different aspects of the illness and stages of recovery.

There are a variety of other factors which should be considered in the context of pharmacologic treatment because they have been found to be related to severity of illness and relapse proneness. I have alluded to stress as a possible precipitant of relapse or exacerbation in some patients receiving low-dose or intermittent treatment. One type of stress which has received increasing attention in recent years has been family attitude and response to the patient. Several studies have suggested that overinvolved and critical or rejecting attitudes on the part of the family—referred to in some studies as "expressed emotion"—are associated with higher relapse rates among patients living in this environment (Leff and Vaughn 1980; Vaughn et al. 1984). Therefore, this influence should be taken into consideration in planning medication and rehabilitative strategies.

Another factor is the level of psychosocial and vocational adjustment which the patient achieved prior to the onset of the illness. Research has suggested that the poorer the premorbid adjustment, the poorer the outcome. The level of psychosocial adjustment has also been shown to influence relapse rates among patients who are withdrawn from medication following recovery from a first episode of schizophrenic illness. Those patients with better premorbid adjustment were less likely to relapse within the first year of follow-up (Kane et al. 1982).

Personality undoubtedly plays an important role in influencing treatment compliance, treatment response, and long-term outcome; however, this is an area which has not been well-studied. One reason for this is a general lack of consensus as to how to assess personality in a reliable and consistent fashion. This diagnostic problem is more difficult in schizophrenia because of the problem of separating effects of the illness on social skills, ego strengths, and motivation from the influence of the individual's underlying personality. Experienced therapists working with chronically ill patients certainly utilize a knowledge of the patient's apparent personality characteristics in formulating and evaluating treatment approaches. This is particularly important in rehabilitation efforts in helping the therapist to establish realistic goals and reasonable levels of expectations. One of the most difficult aspects of rehabilitation in schizophrenia is making judgments as to the nature and extent of the limitations imposed by the illness and the level of functioning or adaptation which represents the optimum goal of therapeutic efforts. One of the most frequent areas of frustration and uncertainty for relatives of patients with this illness is lack of clarity as to what to expect from the patient and how far the relatives should encourage, expect, or "push" role functioning and vocational adjustment. The rehabilitation worker in conjunction with other members of the treatment team (given all of the information alluded to above) must make judgments and recommendations in this context.

Conclusion

There are a variety of factors which influence long-term outcome in schizophrenia (and other chronic conditions). I have alluded to some of these issues, with particular emphasis on those which have been studied in interaction with medication effects. Given the considerable heterogeneity of outcome in schizophrenia, we still have a long way to go in accurately predicting outcome for a given individual. It is essential that all perspectives be brought to bear in reviewing a patient's history, planning treatment strategies, and evaluating outcome. Schizophrenia is a complex illness which requires thoughtful integration of biologic, psychologic, psychosocial, and rehabilitative issues and treatment approaches.

The treatment team must coordinate long-term treatment strategies including medication, rehabilitation, and family therapy. The team approach is critical in allowing the psychiatrist and the rehabilitation worker to share information and formulate an approach which provides the best clinical management and the greatest hope for the patient's independent social functioning.

References

Carpenter, W. T., Jr., and Heinrichs, D. W. 1984. Intermittent pharmacotherapy of schizophrenia. In Kane 1984, pp. 69–82.

Cheung, H. K. 1981. Schizophrenics fully remitted on neuroleptics for three to five yeras—to stop or continue drugs. *British Journal of Psychiatry, 138,* 490–94.

Chien, C-P. 1975. Drugs and rehabilitation in schizophrenia. In *Drugs in combination with other therapies.* ed. M. Greenblatt, pp. 13–34. New York: Grune and Stratton.

Engelhardt, D. M.; Rosen, B.; Freedman, N.; Mann, D.; and Margolis, R. 1963. Phenothiazines in the prevention of psychiatric hospitalization, II: Duration of treatment exposure. *Journal of the American Medical Association, 186,* 981–83.

Herz, M. I. 1984. Intermittent medication and schizophrenia. In Kane 1984, pp. 51–68.

Hirsch, S. R.; Gaind, R.; Rohde, P. D.; Stevens, B. C.; and Wing, J. K. 1973. Outpatient maintenance of chronic schizophrenic patients with long-acting fluphenazine: Double-blind placebo trial. *British Medical Journal, 1,* 633–37.

Hogarty, G. E., and Goldberg, S. C. 1974. Collaborative study group: Drug and sociotherapy in the aftercare of schizophrenic patients: One-year relapse rates. *Archives of General Psychiatry, 28,* 54–64.

Hogarty, G. E.; Ulrich, R. S.; Mussare, S.; and Aristiquestra, N. 1976. Drug discontinuation among long-term, successfully maintained schizophrenic outpatients. *Diseases of the Nervous System, 37,* 494–500.

Kane, J. M., ed. 1984. *Drug-maintenance strategies in schizophrenia.* Washington, D.C.: American Psychiatric Association.

Kane, J. M., and Smith, J. 1982. Tardive dyskinesia: Prevalence and risk factors. *Archives of General Psychiatry, 39,* 473–81.

Kane, J. M.; Quitkin, F.; Rifkin, A.; et al. 1982. Fluphenazine vs. placebo in patients with remitted acute first-episode schizophrenia. *Archives of General Psychiatry, 39,* 70–73.

Kane, J. M.; Rifkin, A; Woerner, M.; et al. Low-dose neuroleptic treatment of outpatient schizophrenics, I: Preliminary results for relapse rates. *Archives of General Psychiatry, 40*, 893–96.

Klein, D., and Davis, J. 1969. *Diagnosis and drug treatment of psychiatric disorder.* Baltimore: Williams and Wilkins.

Leff, J. P., and Vaughn, C. E. 1980. The interaction of life events and relative's expressed emotion in schizophrenia and depressive neurosis. *British Journal of Psychiatry, 136*, 146–53.

Leff, J. P., and Wing, J. K. 1971. Trial of maintenance therapy in schizophrenia. *British Medical Journal, 3*, 559–604.

Marder, S. R.; Van Putton, T.; Mintz, J.; et al. 1984. Costs and benefits of two doses of fluphenazine. *Archives of General Psychiatry, 41*, 1025–29.

Odejide, O. A., and Aderounmu, A. F. 1982. Double-blind placebo substitution: Withdrawal of fluphenazine decanoate in schizophrenic patients. *Journal of Clinical Psychiatry, 43*, 195–96.

Rifkin, A.; Quitkin, F.; Kane, J. M.; et al. 1978. Are prophylactic antiparkinsonian drugs necessary? A controlled study of procyclidine withdrawal. *Archives of General Psychiatry, 35*, 483–89.

Rifkin, A.; Quitkin, F.; Rabiner, C. J.; and Klein, D. F. 1977. Fluphenzine decanoate, fluphenazine hydrochloride given orally, and placebo in remitted schizophrenics. *Archives of General Psychiatry, 34*, 43–47.

Troshinsky, C. H.; Aaronson, H. G.; and Stone, R. K. 1962. Maintenance phenothiazine in the aftercare of schizophrenic patients. *Pennsylvania Psychiatry Quarterly, 2*, 11–15.

Vaughn, C. E.; Snyder, K. S.; Jones, S.; et al. 1984. Family factors in schizophrenic relapse: A replication. *Schizophrenia Bulletin, 8*, 425–26.

13

Ego Functioning and Vocational Rehabilitation

JEAN A. CIARDIELLO, MYRA E. KLEIN, and SHAWN SOBKOWSKI

Several authors have stressed the importance of improving ego functioning in the vocational rehabilitation process. Ciardiello, Klein, and Sobkowski use Bellak's Ego Function Scale to study the relationships among specific ego functions and employment in thirty schizophrenic subjects. Three ego function factors are identified and correlate significantly with measures of psychiatric symptomatology, and social and vocational functioning. The implications of these findings are discussed with specific suggestions for vocational rehabilitation program development.

Despite the vocational rehabilitation efforts of the past twenty years, reports in the literature have shown that as many as two-thirds of discharged chronic mental patients remain unemployed (Evje et al. 1972). In 1965, the research unit of the Veterans Administration conducted one of the most extensive studies of the vocational rehabilitation of the chronically mentally ill. Over 3,600 schizophrenic patients under 60 years of age who had been discharged from hospitals six months earlier were questioned. Two-thirds reported working one month or less, and only 14 percent had worked five months or more (VA 1965). Addressing a similar question experimentally, Griffiths (1974) tested the effectiveness of vocational rehabilitation by randomly assigning fifty-six schizophrenic subjects to treatment and control groups. After fifteen months, assessments revealed no significant differences between those who had participated in the vocational rehabilitation program and those who had not. On the basis of these results, Griffiths concluded that rehabilitation had no detectable effects on schizophrenic subjects. Even within sheltered workshops, schizophrenic clients were two to three times less likely to be placed in competitive employment than were individuals with other disabilities (Ciardiello 1981a). The Na-

This chapter first appeared in *The Broad Scope of Ego Function Assessment*, ed. L. Bellak and R. Goldsmith (New York: John Wiley & Sons, 1984), and is reprinted by permission of John Wiley and Sons.

tional Institute of Handicapped Research (1979) concluded that "although mentally disabled clients make up the largest number of cases eligible for vocational rehabilitation services, they have the least probability of success before and after rehabilitation" (p. 1).

While it is clear that rehabilitation programs serving schizophrenic clients have had a great deal of difficulty meeting their vocational objectives, the reasons for this lack of success are unclear. Several variables have been identified as predictive of rehabilitation outcome. Watts and Po-Kwan (1976) and Griffiths (1974) found that low self-esteem was one of the best predictors of vocational rehabilitation outcome, being invariably associated with unemployment in former psychiatric patients. A fear of losing disability benefits (Gunn 1975), motivation to work (Searls, Wilson, and Miskimins 1971; Griffiths, Hodgson, and Hallam 1974), realism in vocational choice (Patterson 1957; Searls, Wilson, and Miskimins 1971), an inconsistency between aptitude patterns and available employment opportunities (Ciardiello 1981a), and certain biographical data have also been cited as significant variables in the vocational rehabilitation of schizophrenic persons.

Past failures to rehabilitate schizophrenic clients and the results of rehabilitation outcome research underscore the need to understand more about the ways in which the schizophrenic disability impairs vocational functioning and frustrates the efforts of rehabilitation programs to return disabled persons to the work force. A better understanding of the vocational functioning of schizophrenic persons has important implications for the rehabilitation process. If critical variables can be identified, an assessment strategy can be devised to determine which clients are most likely to benefit from specific program interventions and which interventions are most likely to facilitate their vocational success.

Ego Functioning

In general terms, Freud conceptualized ego functioning as reflected in an individual's ability to love and to work. According to Freud's structural theory of personality, the ego is the central integrating core of the personality, mediating between the inner demands of the id and superego and outer demands from the environment. Therefore, successful work selection and performance can be seen as requiring a complex set of ego functions which effectively integrate the self and the world of work.

Bellak and Loeb (1969), Federn (1952) and many others who are psychoanalytically oriented view schizophrenia as primarily an ego dysfunction. When early ego development has been seriously impaired, the result is often a schizophrenic syndrome which is characterized by regressive and restitutional symptoms which often include depersonalization, passivity, disordered thought, delusions, and hallucinations. Although these symptoms can be controlled to some extent in some patients with the use of chemotherapy, the important functions of the ego rarely escape severe impairments. The changing realities of the work world often place strenuous demands on the ego to achieve high levels of adaptive, integrative, and autonomous functioning; this presents a challenge to the normal ego, and it seems likely that the impaired ego of the schizophrenic person would experience a great deal of difficulty coping with vocational demands (Ciardiello and Bingham 1982).

Hartmann (1964) noted that although ego weaknesses are characteristic of schizophrenic patients, specific ego functions are differentially affected. The vocational difficulties of schizophrenic persons can be clarified by relating specific ego functions to their roles in work selection and performance. For instance, flexibility and adaptability is important in work because even the most routine jobs do not remain unchanged over time. Supervisors come and go, machinery is modernized, schedules change, new products are assembled, and the reactions and requests of customers vary. Rigid adherence to former thought patterns and failure to adapt to the requirements of a new job situation can seriously hinder work performance. Thus, adaptive regression in the service of the ego (ARISE) can have important implications for vocational functioning, particularly in variable work environments. Individuals whose ARISE capability is poor would be more likely to succeed in a work environment in which there were few changes and least likely to succeed in variable work settings. A low ARISE capacity would also suggest that the person would have difficulty making realistic vocational choices which took into account new information about themselves or an occupational alternative. Similarly, other specific deficits in ego functioning have some predictable vocational consequences. In brief, inadequate reality testing often results in delusions and/or hallucinations which can make it almost impossible for the individual to concentrate on work tasks. Poor judgment is likely to lead to inappropriate responses to supervisors and co-workers and inaccurate estimations of the time and resources needed to complete a work assignment. The ability to follow directions, benefit from feedback, and work cooperatively with others is often impaired by exaggerated or inadequate boundaries resulting from disturbances in the individual's sense of reality of the world and of the self. Various dimensions of autonomous functioning—attention, concentration, memory, learning, perception, motor functioning, language skills, habit patterns, and intention—are the essential aspects of work itself. The remaining ego functions—object relations, impulse control, thought processes, defensive functioning, stimulus barrier, synthetic functioning, and mastery-competence—also can be seen to have important and often obvious effects on work performance and selection.

When the employment difficulties of schizophrenic individuals are viewed in terms of specific ego functioning patterns, a clearer and more comprehensive theoretical picture of their vocational strengths and weaknesses begins to emerge. However, there are several important empirical questions which are unanswered: (*a*) Do schizophrenic persons who are employed have higher levels of ego functioning than those who are unemployed? (*b*) Are certain ego functions more important than others in the successful vocational rehabilitation of schizophrenic individuals? (*c*) Do schizophrenic individuals with higher levels of ego functioning report less psychiatric symptomotology and higher levels of general and vocational functioning than individuals exhibiting lower levels of ego functioning? These questions were investigated in the following preliminary study of ego functioning and the vocational rehabilitation of schizophrenic clients.

Procedure

As part of a three-year research project focusing on the vocational assessment and rehabilitation of the chronically mentally ill, thirty schizophrenic clients enrolled in a psychosocial rehabilitation program were interviewed for three or four hours over several sessions by specially trained, masters-level psychologists. All of the subjects had been diagnosed as schizophrenic (by clinical records and a reevaluating clinician); the predominant subtypes were chronic undifferentiated (57%) and paranoid (33%). Of the subjects, 40 percent were female and 60 percent male; the mean age was 32 years; 90 percent were white and 10 percent were black; 63 percent had had some paid work experience (usually program-assisted) during the six months prior to the interview, and 43 percent were employed for some time during the month of the assessment.

In part, the interview consisted of a detailed employment history, Bellak's (1973) Ego Functioning Scale, the SCL-90 (Deragotis 1977), and the Katz Social Adjustment Scale (Katz and Lyerly 1963). The Ego Functioning Scale is a semi-structured interview developed by Bellak, Hurvich, and Gediman (1973) for the clinical assessment of ego functions. Each subject was given four global ratings from 1 to 7 (with half points) for each of the twelve dimensions of ego functioning. Scoring was done from the recorded interviews; and current, characteristic, highest, and lowest levels of ego functioning were rated for each dimension. The SCL-90 is a ninety-item, self-report symptom inventory developed by the Clinical Psychometrics Research Unit of Johns Hopkins University to measure the psychological symptom patterns of psychiatric and medical patients. The Katz Social Adjustment Scale was developed in conjunction with the forerunner of the SCL-90 to assess those aspects of general functioning in the "normal" adult world which did not fall within the traditional notion of psychiatric symptoms. The two Katz scales used were the Activities of Daily Living (ADL) and Leisure Time Activities (LTA) scales. The reliability and validity of each of these instruments for schizophrenic subjects are well documented. In addition, psychometric monitoring of these instruments during the course of the project, supported their reliability and validity for research purposes (Ciardiello and Turner 1980).

The data were analyzed using regression techniques to test the relationships among the variables of interest, and a discriminant function analysis was used to determine if current ego function ratings could be used to classify schizophrenic subjects as presently employed or unemployed.

Results and Discussion

Scores for thirty schizophrenic subjects on each of the twelve dimensions of characteristic ego functioning ranged from 2 to 6, with most scores falling between 4 and 5, a grand mean of 4.2, and a standard deviation of 1. Compared to Bellak's (1973) group of fifty schizophrenic subjects, the present sample showed lower overall levels of ego functioning and less variability in their scores. Intercorrelations among the twelve scales were significant in almost every instance and higher than those reported by Bellak, Hurvich, and Gediman (1973). These differences probably reflected the fact that Bellak's sample consisted of acute schizophrenic inpatients, while the subjects in the present investigation were chronic outpatients attending a rehabilitation day program.

High scale-score intercorrelations indicated that each of the ego function scales was not operating independently. In order to identify the independent dimensions of ego functioning for chronic schizophrenic subjects, the twelve scale scores were factor analyzed using a varimax rotation and the principal components method. Although the sample size was small, it met Cattell's (1966) recommended criteria of a 2.5 subject to variable ratio (30:12). Results of the factor analysis are reported in Table 13.1. We identified three factors which explained 79 percent of the variance in the ego function scores. The first factor explained 62 percent of the variance and consisted of eight of the twelve scales. Factor I overlapped factor III by sharing loadings for the reality testing, judgment, sense of reality and autonomous functioning scales; factors II and III shared the defensive functioning scale; and factors I and II overlapped on ARISE. The scales shared by factors I and III supported the notion of Rapaport (1951) and others that reality testing, judgment and sense of reality can be considered aspects of autonomous functioning. The overlap in scales can also be attributed to the chronicity of the sample; greater differentiation of ego functions would be expected in individuals who had not suffered from severe and chronic ego impairments.

Examining the factor structures, the three conceptual dimensions of ego functioning are not evident unless the factors are viewed in terms of their general functional consequences. Which factor or set of ego functions re-

Table 13.1
Factor Analysis of Characteristic Ego Function Scores for Thirty Schizophrenic Clients

Ego function factor	Factor loadings	Eigen values	% explained variance
I.			
Reality testing	.698	7.45	62
Judgment	.696		
Sense of reality	.546		
Thought processes	.815		
ARISE	.594		
Autonomous functioning	.676		
Synthetic functioning	.767		
Mastery-competence	.825		
II.			
Regulation and control	.801	1.25	10
ARISE	.517		
Defensive functioning	.536		
Stimulus barrier	.803		
III.			
Reality testing	.616	.82	7
Judgment	.627		
Sense of reality	.684		
Object relations	.802		
Defensive functioning	.746		
Autonomous functioning	.408		

NOTE: Loadings of .400 or greater were used to determine factor inclusion.

flects a schizophrenic individual's ability to love, and which factor is related to his or her ability to work? The ego functions in factor I combined reality orientation and autonomous, adaptive, and integrative functions, as well as mastery-competence, which are essential for survival in the work world. While factor III included reality orientation and autonomous functioning, it also included object relations and defensive functioning. Thus, factor III included the ego functions which seem to be related to successful social adjustment.

The second factor was made up of regulation and control of impulses, affects, and drives; ARISE; defensive functioning; and stimulus barrier. The common element which seems to link this set of ego functions is that they can provide protection against threats to the individual from within and from without. Some of these adaptions and defenses include the person's ability to tolerate anxiety, depression, and frustration and to regulate sexual impulses, and the ability to use defense mechanisms adaptively, instead of becoming uncontrollably psychotic. In essence, factor II ego functions work together to deal with internal and external threats so that they do not result in psychiatric symptoms.

Summarizing the face validity of these three ego functioning factors for schizophrenic clients, factor I included ego functions related to vocational functioning, factor II consisted of defensive ego functions which inhibit the formation of psychiatric symptoms, and factor III was made up of ego functions which appear to have important roles in social adjustment. In order to test the face validity of these factors and to determine their construct and concurrent validity, factor scores were used to discriminate employed and unemployed schizophrenic clients; and ego function factor scores were correlated with measures of psychiatric symptom distress (SCL-90) and social adjustment (Katz).

As expected, ego function factor I was successful in correctly classifying 84 percent of the schizophrenic subjects as employed for any length of time during the six months prior to the assessment. Wilks' Lambda for the discriminant function analysis was .60 and was significant at the .0002 level. Current ego functioning scores for individual scales were also used to discriminate between schizophrenic subjects who had any paid work experience during the month of the assessment. Two specific ego function scores were found to achieve greater than chance discriminations. Autonomous functioning (Wilks' Lambda = .70, $p < .002$) and ARISE (Wilks' Lambda = .63, $p < .002$) correctly classified as currently employed or unemployed a total of 70 percent of the cases. The results of these three discriminant function analyses are reported in Table 13.2.

Since the major ego functions were considered by Bellak, Hurvich, and Gediman (1973) to be autonomous functions of the ego, it is not surprising that autonomous functioning was found to be an important variable in work performance. In addition, autonomous ego functions such as habit patterns, skills, routines, interests, learning, intentionality, and motility have central roles in work, and as Bellak, Hurvich, and Gediman (1973) noted, impaired autonomous functioning may result in difficulty in carrying out one's usual job or in the complete inability to work.

The importance of ARISE in work performance has been previously illustrated; however, there are two aspects of ARISE which may make it particularly relevant in understanding the vocational adjustment of chronic schizophrenic clients. Using the broad, adaptive sense of ARISE, this ego function not only permits greater flexibility in meeting the demands of a job, but also gives the individual creative alternative strategies to deal with

Table 13.2
Discriminant Function Analysis Using Ego Functioning Scores to Discriminate the Employment Status of Thirty Schizophrenic Clients

Significant ego function variable	Wilks' Lambda	Sig.	Rao's V	Sig.	Change in V	Sig.
Factor I	.60	.0002	18.48	.00001	18.48	.00001
Autonomous functioning	.70	.002	11.89	.001	11.89	.001
ARISE	.63	.002	16.14	.001	4.25	.039

the schizophrenic disability itself, so that it is less likely to interfere with vocational functioning. In other words, the individual with a high ARISE score is not only better able to adapt to the demands of work but is also better able to adjust to the disabling effects of schizophrenia. A related idea suggested by Bellak, Hurvich, and Gediman (1973) was that adaptive regressions in the service of the ego may also serve to maintain a flexibility of ego functions themselves, so that autonomous ego functioning is not disrupted under stress. Ego impairments tend to be more discrete when the structure of the ego is less rigid and there are a number of different ways and ego functions available to meet the demands of everyday life. This type of successful adjustment to mental illness and ego adaptability is exemplified by a schizophrenic worker whose sense of reality warns him that his impulse control is very poor on a given day. Good judgment tells him that if he goes to work, he will become uncontrollably angry with his boss and that the consequences may be unemployment and/or hospitalization. He demonstrates successful functioning in seeing absence from work as an adaptive way to deal with poor impulse control and requesting that his supervisor allow him to take a vacation day. In this case ARISE is useful in his adjustment to work and in preventing his anger from overrunning his other ego functions resulting in further decompensation.

Turning to factor II, previous studies (Ciardiello and Turner 1980; Ciardiello, Klein, and Sobkowski 1981) failed to demonstrate significant relationships between psychiatric symptomotology and vocational functioning. These findings were consistent with the finding of the present study that seven of the nine SCL-90 subscales were correlated significantly with ego function factor II and only two subscales (paranoid ideation and psychoticism) were correlated significantly with factor I. For chronic schizophrenic subjects, vocational functioning was a separate dimension of ego functioning independent of the ability to deal with internal and external threats without symptom formation. The correlation matrix in Table 13.3 illustrates the significant negative relationships between ego function factor II and SCL-90 subscales; correlation coefficients ranged from $-.45$ for the anxiety scale to $-.29$ for psychoticism.

Psychoticism ($-.29$), interpersonal sensitivity ($-.29$), and the Katz Social Adjustment Scale ($-.40$) correlated significantly with ego function factor III. Since this was a chronic schizophrenic sample, it is not surprising that psychoticism was related to each of the three ego function factors. The significant correlations with the interpersonal scale of the SCL-90 and the Katz Social Adjustment Scale supported the hypothesis that factor III reflected those aspects of ego functioning which are important in the social adjustment of chronic schizophrenic clients. Although factor III was found to be functionally independent of the other factors, it overlapped on four ego functions (reality testing, judgment, sense of reality, and autonomous functioning) with factor I. Again, this finding is consistent with the signifi-

Table 13.3
Correlations between Ego Function Scores and the SCL-90/Katz for Twenty-Nine
Schizophrenic Clients

SCL-90/Katz scales	Ego function factor I	Ego function factor II	Ego function factor III
SCL-90			
Somatization	−.27	−.22	.06
Obsessive-compulsive	−.23	−.36	−.18
Interpersonal sensitivity	−.18	−.38	−.29
Depression	−.18	−.43	−.24
Anxiety	−.22	−.45	−.28
Hostility	−.21	−.40	−.09
Phobic anxiety	−.21	−.41	−.08
Paranoid ideation	−.33	−.23	−.20
Psychoticism	−.29	−.29	−.29
KATZ			
Activities of Daily Living (ADL)	−.01	−.00	.40

NOTE: Italicized values are significant at the .05 level.

cant relationship between employment status and scores on the Katz ADL scale (Ciardiello 1981b). Therefore, social and vocational functioning in schizophrenic clients have certain ego functions in common, as well as ego functions which appear to be unique to each.

In general, signficant relationships were found between ego function factor I and employment status; factor II and SCL-90 scales; and factor III and the Katz Social Adjustment Scale. Although there was some overlap in ego functions, the three factors were found to be functionally independent. These findings suggest that chronic schizophrenic clients use a set of ego functions in work different from those needed to maintain mental health. Possibly this differential use of ego functions explains previous findings that some schizophrenic clients reported considerable psychiatric symptomotology, but remained employed. Since factors I and III shared several ego functions, the different roles of these functions in the social and vocational rehabilitation of schizophrenic clients were less clear. However, if the three factors identified in this study are found to be reliable and valid in other studies with chronic schizophrenic subjects, then perhaps the factor overlap can be viewed as reflecting the multipurpose nature of ego functions and possibly some compensatory functioning which results from chronic ego impairment.

Implications for Rehabilitation

Three different sets of ego functions have been identified as having important and differential impacts on the mental health and functioning of chronic schizophrenic clients. If these three characteristic ego function factors are found and validated by others studying comparable subjects, there are several ways that ego function assessment can be useful in the rehabilitation process.

Assessing a client's ego strengths and deficits using Bellak's Ego Functioning Scale generates a profile which can be used in individual rehabilitation planning. Program interventions can be focused to address specific ego function deficits, particularly those which are interfering with the ability to work. Bellak, Hurvich, and Gediman (1973) outlined strategies for improving each of the twelve ego functions. Bellak and Black (1960) have emphasized that the ego functions of psychotic persons in the community can be substantially improved by devising interventions and experiences which make maximal use of ego strengths to remediate ego deficits. For instance, an autonomous function, like an interest in automobile mechanics, can be used to improve object relations by meeting others with the same interest and working together to repair a car.

According to the results of the present study, several ego functions (factor I) were related to successful vocational functioning. Higher levels of autonomous functioning and ARISE were found to be associated with employment for most schizophrenic clients. Therefore, these two ego functions have particular importance in the vocational rehabilitation process and should be the focus of program interventions geared to returning clients to the work force. Along with factor I scores, clients' scores on the autonomous functioning and ARISE scales can also be used as measures of work readiness.

In addition to identifying the ego functioning patterns of clients, vocational counselors can also analyze jobs in terms of the varying degrees to which specific ego functions are required. It seems likely that schizophrenic clients have a greater chance to achieve vocational success in those jobs which place demands on their ego strengths rather than their weaknesses. Therefore, congruence between the ego-functioning profiles of jobs and clients is an important consideration in work selection. Similarly, vocational rehabilitation programs which offer sheltered employment are often able to structure jobs so that they are consistent with an individual's pattern of ego functioning. For instance, a schizophrenic client with poor object relations, some impairment in autonomous functioning, and good judgment and reality testing can probably be successfully employed as a night security person at a warehouse.

Ego function assessments can also serve as a guide to the selection of prevocational activities which will improve ego functioning and work readiness. Whether clients are work ready or not, program interventions which improve certain sets of ego functions can be expected to improve clients' mental health, social functioning, and ability to engage in the activities of daily living. Gains in ego functioning not only improve clients' chances to achieve vocational success but also enhance functioning in other life roles and, thus, improve the general quality of their lives.

Lastly, ego function assessment can be used to evaluate the progress of individual clients in achieving rehabilitation goals. On a program level, results of the ego function assessment can be used to evaluate the outcome and impact of rehabilitation programs. Ego function assessment will also have an important role in future research which evaluates the relative effectiveness of rehabilitation strategies to improve the ego functions of schizophrenic clients. In addition, a reliable and valid assessment of ego functions offers a comprehensive way to conceptualize the vocational difficulties of schizophrenic clients and an effective strategy to evaluate the solutions offered by rehabilitation programs.

References

Bellak, L., and Black, B. 1960. The rehabilitation of psychotics in the community. *American Journal of Orthopsychiatry, 30,* 346–55.

Bellak, L.; Hurvich, M.; and Gediman, H. 1973. *Ego functions in schizophrenics, neurotics, and normals: A systematic study of conceptual, diagnostic, and therapeutic aspects.* New York: Wiley and Sons.

Bellak, L., and Loeb, I. 1969. *The schizophrenic syndrome.* New York: Grune and Stratton.

Cattell, R. B. 1966. The meaning and strategic use of factor analysis. In *Handbook of multivariate experimental psychology,* ed. R. B. Cattell. Chicago: Rand McNally.

Ciardiello, J. A. 1981a. Job-placement success of schizophrenic clients in sheltered workshop programs. *Vocational Evaluation and Work Adjustment Bulletin, 14* (3), 125–28.

———. 1981b. *A path model to predict the employment status of psychiatrically disabled clients.* Ph.D. diss., Rutgers, The State University.

Ciardiello, J. A., and Bingham, W. C. 1982. The career maturity of schizophrenic clients. *Rehabilitation Counseling Bulletin, 26,* 3–9.

Ciardiello, J. A.; Klein, M. E.; and Sobkowski, S. 1981. *Final report of the vocational rehabilitation project, Part I* (SREG 116). Trenton, N.J.: Department of Education, Division of Vocational Education and Career Preparation.

Ciardiello, J. A., and Turner, F. D. 1980. *Final report of the vocational assessment project* (SREG 808). Trenton, N.J.: Department of Education, Division of Vocational Education and Career Preparation.

Deragotis, L. R. 1977. *SCL-90 revised version manual, I.* Baltimore: Johns Hopkins University School of Medicine, Clinical Psychometrics Research Unit.

Evje, M.; Bellander, I.; Gibby, M.; and Palmer, I. S. 1972. Evaluating protected hospital employment of chronic psychiatric patients. *Hospital and Community Psychiatry, 23,* 24–28.

Federn, P. 1952. *Ego psychology and the psychoses.* New York: Basic Books.

Griffiths, R. D. 1974. Rehabilitation of chronic psychotic patients: An assessment of their psychological handicap, an evaluation of the effectiveness of rehabilitation, and observations of the factors which predict outcome. *Psychological Medicine, 4,* 316–25.

Griffiths, R. D.; Hodgson, R.; and Hallam, R. 1974. Structured interview for the assessment of work-related attitudes in psychiatric patients: Preliminary findings. *Psychological Medicine, 4,* 326–33.

Gunn, R. L. 1975. Special problems in work adjustment of the mentally ill. In *Modification of behavior of the mentally ill: Applied principles,* ed. R. E. Hardy and J. G. Cull. Springfield, Ill.: Charles C. Thomas.

Hartmann, H., ed. 1964. Comments on the psychoanalytic theory of the ego (1950). In *Essays on ego psychology,* ed. H. Hartmann. New York: International Universities Press.

Katz, M. M., and Lyerly, S. B. 1963. Methods for measuring adjustment and social behavior in the community, I: Rationale, description, discriminative validity, and scale development. *Psychological Reports*, 13(2), 503–35.

National Institute of Handicapped Research, Department of Health, Education, and Welfare. 1979. Post-employment services aid mentally disabled clients. *Rehabilitation Brief: Bringing Rehabilitation into Effective Focus*, 6(2), 1.

Patterson, C. H. 1957. Interests and the emotionally disturbed client. *Educational and Psychological Measurements*, 17, 264–80.

Rapaport, D. 1951. The autonomy of the ego. *Bulletin of the Menninger Clinic*, 15, 113–23.

Searls, D. J.; Wilson, L. T.; and Miskimins, R. W. 1971. Development of a measure of unemployability among restored psychiatric patients. *Journal of Applied Psychology*, 55, 223–25.

Veterans Administration. 1965. To work again, to live again: The vocational rehabilitation of homebound veterans. VA pamphlet no. 21-65-1. Washington, D.C.: Veterans Administration, Department of Veterans Benefits.

Watts, F. N., and Po-Kwan, Y. 1976. The structure of attitudes in psychiatric rehabilitation. *Journal of Occupational Psychology*, 49, 39–44.

14

The Human Dimension of the Vocational Rehabilitation Process

Dennis J. McCrory

Much of the rehabilitation literature is concerned with the technical aspects of the process. McCrory emphasizes the important factors involved in the human dimension of vocational rehabilitation. He offers a number of well-chosen cases to illustrate typical complications and difficulties in the course of rehabilitation. When vocational counselors have a long-term perspective, they can better understand stress points and the difficulties involved in attaining vocational goals.

The Vocational Rehabilitation Process

While many professionals play their part in rehabilitation, the "expert" in vocational rehabilitation is the vocational rehabilitation counselor. He may have received graduate training in a rehabilitation program or may have acquired his knowledge and skills in a career in human services with special on-the-job training (Creasey and McCarthy 1981). Traditionally his practice has taken place in a state-federal vocational rehabilitation agency or in a rehabilitation facility. More recently he may work in a psychiatric hospital or a community mental health center. Most recently he may have a private practice. He usually has a variety of skills, including assessment, planning, counseling, coordinating, and placement, but preeminent are his understanding of the world of work, a knowledge of community resources and opportunities, and an ability to get things moving. Havens (1965) has identified four features that are crucial for a successful vocational rehabilitation counselor in psychiatric work: the abilities to like one's clients, to be objective, to be interested in helping, and to be able to work through resistances and develop client motivation.

Yet rehabilitation counselors are often undervalued. Lamb and Mackota (1975) asked whether vocational rehabilitation counseling was considered a "second-class profession." Olshansky (1980) made a plea to allow the rehabilitation profession "a seat at the table" in the community planning for people with chronic mental illness. Smith, Zimney, and Lindberg, (1981) examined why psychiatric patients were infrequently referred for vocational counseling and found that psychiatrists were often unfamiliar with vocational rehabilitation services or believed that rehabilitation could not be helpful for their patients. Mental health professionals, with the exception of occupational therapists, typically have had little exposure to rehabilitation counselors in their training or practice. Educational efforts are being made (Talbott 1978, 1984; McCrory and Marrone 1984). However, trust and confidence grow best through working together. This is just beginning to happen.

Vocational rehabilitation services have usually been considered late, if at all, in the treatment process. By then, the client has accepted the "chronic patient" role, and he and his family have adapted their expectations to his impaired state. It is often extremely difficult at this point to persuade them to engage in a rehabilitation process of indefinite duration and uncertain outcome. Lovejoy (1982) and an anonymous patient (Anonymous 1980), in first-person accounts, have written compellingly about the negative impact of diminished expectations on the person with prolonged mental illness.

Gruenberg (1967) has described "the social breakdown syndrome." A person with major psychiatric illness has to cope not only with the impairment itself, but with its impact on his life structure, the way he sees himself, and the changed expectations of those around him. Some patients may recover from their acute psychosis and return to full functioning in a timely fashion. For others, the psychosis may leave a residual disability, a loss of self-confidence, and an attitude among significant others that he is permanently and totally handicapped even though his psychiatric prognosis may be much more positive. Consider, for example, a person with a bipolar disorder who becomes excited as he thinks of returning to work, even as his wife becomes frightened that he is becoming psychotic again and discourages his thinking about work. Or consider a teenager, fully recovered from his paranoid psychosis, whose mother can't believe that he can hold a job at a gas station "after what he's been through" and encourages him to quit lest he get sick again. Social-breakdown syndromes need not become chronic and are often reversible. Treatment, education for patients and their families, and, in particular, timely rehabilitation programming can prevent or interrupt this downward spiral. But, sadly, a rehabilitation intervention may come too late, after altered expectations have become resistant to change. Clinicians and mental health programs may actually contribute to this (Perl et al. 1980).

Moreover, rehabilitation counselors themselves can be seriously challenged to imagine how some people with prolonged and severe psychiatric illness can benefit from their help. There are a number of assessment methods (Anthony 1979; Marsh et al. 1980; McCarthy 1981) for establishing the "rehabilitation diagnosis": these deal with client strengths, interests, needs, and environmental supports, demands, and opportunities. Marrone and associates (1984) have stated that positive indicators—such as cooperation with a treatment plan, stated interest in work, previously gratifying work experiences, and keeping counseling appointments—may balance length of illness or current serious impairments in a rehabilitation evaluation. A counselor is also better able to help seriously impaired patients when the community has a network of programs, particularly day treatment with a prevocational emphasis, crisis intervention services, and transitional employment (Beard, Schmidt, and Smith 1963).

Olshansky (1972) has emphasized the ups and downs of the vocational rehabilitation process, just as Breier and Strauss (1983) and Kanter (1985) have portrayed the vicissitudes of patients' clinical courses. I have come to see the process as cyclical, like a tilted helix. I have called it the "rehabilitation cycle," in which the client may grow, regress, grow, plateau, grow some more, regress (not quite as far as previously), and so on. Regressions may be minor: increased discomfort, irritability, difficulty in concentrating, brief periods of insomnia. They may be major: psychosis, loss of control, suicidal behavior, rehospitalization. Yet, failure to reach a particular goal or a relapse with brief hospitalization need not be devastating experiences. In the context of the rehabilitation alliance they may prove to be valuable learning experiences that lead to more careful planning and support. Plateaus may also be seen in a positive light as opportunities to build self-confidence.

Consider the following examples of the rehabilitation process in action. Note the variety of clinical courses and the very individualized nature of the rehabilitation process.

Jeff is a 28-year-old single man. He has been working as a labeler in a garment factory for eight years. Diagnosed as an autistic child at age 1½, he was additionally found to be mildly retarded after he started school. He began psychotherapy for his avoidant, rigid, and dependent personality at age 10. He began to take busses to appointments at 11, and perform household chores at 12. He was in self-contained classrooms through his school career. In high school he was introduced to work. In his junior year he was referred to the local DVR office, which led to a comprehensive work evaluation in a sheltered workshop that summer and after graduation a six-month period of vocational adjustment training. He decided he liked factory work and was placed at his current job. Two years later Jeff wanted to be independent of his family and applied to a DMH-sponsored residential program to learn independent living skills. After a three-year wait he began a two-year training program in which he learned to budget, shop, cook, housekeep, and get along with rooommates. He also joined a clubhouse program, where he participates in evening and weekend social functions.

Laura is 60. She is married with four grown children. She works as a housekeeper for an elderly couple and is preparing for her husband's retirement. A foster child, she developed a personality disorder and an inclination to depressions with psychotic features. She was hospitalized many times with multiple courses of shock treatment until she made a long-term relationship with a therapist who supported her as her children grew up and left home. She began to do office work but frequently changed jobs. Following a brief hospitalization for an overdose with her antidepressants, Laura was referred for vocational counseling. It became clear that she suffered from a lack of self-confidence and that office work challenged her capacity to sit at a desk, attend to multiple small details, and socialize with staff. Counseling was pursued for a year. Her counselor supported her confidence, explored vocational options with her, and strengthened her job-seeking skills. She did try another office job before she chose to become a professional housecleaner, a job which she held for two years. She then decided the pace was too hectic, and left to find her current job one year ago.

Greg is 50 years old. He works as a hotel-function room manager and is about to remarry. A very successful businessman with an M.B.A., he ran into trouble during his midlife transition. He started drinking, lost his first wife, went into bankruptcy, and had his first manic episode. He was unable to resume his previous level of responsibility, panicked, unsuccessfully tried a number of entry-level jobs, and suffered four more hospitalizations before he was stabilized on lithium. He decided to remain unemployed and live on disability insurance benefits. Three years later his insurance company referred him to a private rehabilitation group. Initially suspicious of his counselor, Greg agreed to share his vocational history. Over the next eighteen months he rewrote his resume, gathered references, explored vocational options, held simulated interviews, and rebuilt his confidence to the point of negotiating a financial understanding with his insurer. He conducted a search for a position where he could use his human relations and management skills without the same level of responsibility that he had held before. His therapist supported this plan and after a brief search he found his current position, which he has held for the past year.

Ned is 25. He works on a maintenance crew and lives in a cooperative apartment. A very shy boy, the "baby" of his family, he had his first schizophrenic episode at age 16. He unsuccessfully tried to return to school and held a number of short-term jobs. He tried to become more active socially, but mostly he stayed at home, where he developed an elaborate fantasy life, became overwhelmed, and eventually needed rehospitalization. He quickly recompensated, but even with medication and psychotherapy, he could not tolerate the thought of "what am I going to do with myself." He resisted numerous attempts to refer him for vocational rehabilitation counseling and was hospitalized three more times. When a quarterway house opened, Ned and his family agreed to try it. He spent six months learning to live away from his family and went from a day treatment program to a work-adjustment training program at a sheltered workshop. He moved to a community residence. Some months later he began a training program in maintenance work and then joined a maintenance crew. Finally, he moved into a cooperative apartment. He and his family are pleased with his work, and enjoy visits together.

Phil is 32 years old and is preparing to enter graduate school. He had a series of psychotic reactions following his graduation from college, before he joined a psychosocial clubhouse. After a year of working in the day-activity program, he chose to enter the transitional employment (TE) program. After one unsuccessful attempt, he was able to work at three TE's. He then took a clerical job, which he held for two years before he took a staff position at the clubhouse for three years. He developed his confidence, moved away from his parents, and became active socially. He decided that he wished to resume his education, and he has just been accepted into a highly regarded language program.

These cases illustrate a number of considerations. Rehabilitation is hard work and can take a long time and a number of steps and cycles. In each case there was persistence, despite prolonged psychiatric illness and chronic social breakdown syndromes, to proceed through a sequence of treatment and rehabilitation services which acted as stepping stones, ladders, or ramps toward more consistent and often higher levels of adaptation. These steps were planned and supported by clients, families, therapists, and rehabilitation counselors, who were able to build a rehabilitation alliance. These cases also represent successful outcomes as judged by clients, families, and caregivers. Jeff, Laura, Greg, Ned and Phil can function consistently, socialize, and be productive. Support is available. There are opportunities for further growth. They are getting on with their lives.

Transitions, Transitional Stress, and Crises

The rehabilitation process is a series of transitions at several levels. There are changes in relationships and activities. There are changes in places where these relationships and activities take place. There are changes in the person, in the way he sees himself and other people see him, in his level of skill, independence, ambition, and personality integration. Because change involves discomfort and heightened stress, growth and success require the mastery of uncomfortable states. In the case of people with prolonged mental illness, growth also requires learning to master their "pathological inclinations."

Erikson (1959, 1963) proposed the epigenetic theory of development. As we master one step, we prepare the basis for the next step. If we do not fully master one step, we are not fully prepared for the next step and are vulnerable to failure. We "become" over time, building our identity and capacities to master life's challenges. Each state has a "crisis," at which, after a "decisive encounter" with the environment, we have incorporated, or not incorporated, the ability and the self-confidence to deal with the expectations of that developmental stage. It is often at such crisis points that our patients/clients have succumbed to "transitional stress," resolving the crisis unsuccessfully with an impaired self and lack of confidence. Thus, in addition to having difficulty meeting their own expectations as well as those of the environment, they must also deal with the stress of failure and falling behind and the acknowledgement that they are somehow "different" but must carry on.

In some ways the patient role is a protection from this painful acknowledgement. If one remains a patient, then somehow one is not accountable for this failure. If one accepts the sick role, then one need not accept the responsibility to face life's challenges before getting well. But, this self-protection is a trap.

Erikson focused particularly on the "occupational identity." Historically, people have defined themselves by the work they do. The chronic mental patient has defined himself and has been defined, perhaps unwittingly, in the occupation of patient. For some patients, as Margolin (1963) has pointed out, failure is a desirable outcome, a compromise between their own wishes for automony and their unwillingness to meet parental expectations. While this may be true for some of our clients, many do not seek failure but encounter it because of their inability to find a way out of the dilemma of the sick role.

The rehabilitation process is intended to be such a way to help clients reduce their impairment, compensate for their disability, adapt to the environment. Yet even with accurate assessment, realistic planning, a rehabilitation alliance, and adequate opportunities, the process is hazardous and stressful—paradoxically, even more so as it succeeds.

Some people experience this heightened stress when they begin a step in the process— "initiation stress," as I have termed it. Some experience it as they are completing a step— "termination stress." We are all familiar with the pains of starting and ending. A more subtle stress is "actualization stress," the suffering many of us know as we grow and change. This is the basis of the "rehabilitation crisis" (McCrory et al. 1980). As the client becomes more functional and potentially more independent, he can become very uncomfortable with his changed state and the dual implication of losing his supports at the same time that expectations are heightened. Thus, the more firmly one has accepted and been accepted in the impaired role, the more change one goes through to become functional and independent. The more ungratifying one has found the role as an ordinary person, the more conflict successful rehabilitation efforts will engender. For example, in the case histories previously mentioned, Laura's suicide attempt took place just days after she said to her therapist that she felt better than she had in twenty years. After she had said that, the unspoken thought occurred to her that she must therefore say goodbye to him. The rehabilitation crisis need not be overwhelming, if it is anticipated and acknowledged and support is given by the rehabilitation team at these times of transition. Consider the following.

> Tom is 29. Having been a "chronic patient" for six years, he was referred to a sheltered workshop two years ago. His attendance, punctuality, productivity, and overall appearance and behavior slowly improved to the point where transitional employment (TE) was recommended by his counselor. Within a week he became irritable, then assaultive, then psychotic, and required hospitalization. He had stopped his medication. He quickly recovered once the medicine was reinstituted. He reentered the program, he was again recommended for TE, and a similar regression occurred. His therapist and his counselor thought they recognized a pattern and shared it with Tom. Two months later he again approached TE, and they reminded him of this pattern. He said that, indeed, he felt very nervous. He had begun to believe that he could actually return to work, and he imagined that he would have to take over the family business. He did not want that, but neither did he want to disappoint his family, who had stuck by him for many years. His therapist acknowledged this dilemma, and Tom agreed to increase his medicine. He took off a few days and discussed the problem with his family, who, surprisingly, supported the idea that he make his own choice. He returned to the shop and began his TE successfully. Three months later he again suffered heightened stress as it was clear that he was mastering this step. At his request he was hospitalized for several days. He is now beginning interest and aptitude testing to prepare for vocational skill training, and is much more comfortable at his job and with the thought of working.

Many unexpected and unexplained regressions in the context of successful programming can be explained, and often prevented, by an awareness of this phenomenon: at times of transition there is heightened stress. When this stress is acknowledged and anticipated, a client need not leave a program if he becomes more symptomatic. He often will respond to clarification and additional support by family and caregivers. In the rehabilitation alliance, however, he may need a "time out," a "mental health leave," or, as in Tom's case, a brief hospitalization. Team communication is crucial at these times, both for clinical understanding and planning, as well as to prevent the danger of covert team disagreements.

If there are additional stresses operant at the same time—such as a personal disappointment, a significant family event, or a change in staff—the process of transition may need to be slowed down or interrupted so that the client can deal with these other matters before the cumulative stress becomes overwhelming. I call this a "coping crisis."

Unforturnately, it often happens that rather than additional support being offered during times of transition, support is actually reduced in the belief that the client is doing well. The following case illustrates this point.

Mike is 29. He had been a patient for eight years and a client at a workshop for three years. Initially he was withdrawn and preoccupied with grandiose fantasies. Whenever under stress, he would stay home and become engrossed in his compensatory fantasy life. At the workshop he slowly became more involved and energetic and became a steady worker. He terminated his therapy. He completed TE, whereupon he left the shop, terminating also with his counselor. He got a job in a warehouse and came by the workshop during his first week, looking wonderful. He was complimented by his counselor, his former colleagues, and his supervisors. That weekend Mike made a serious suicide attempt.

I call this an "acute impoverishment crisis." While Mike was to all appearances successful, during this time of heightened stress he felt all alone. He had achieved work, but at the cost of his sense of connection with people who cared about him. He now faced a situation where he expected himself to cope, with neither old defenses nor supports. Prevention would have required maintaining these relationships. Mike's roles as patient and client had provided him with people in his life. Now, although he was working, his work had lost its social meaning.

Such impoverishment crises can occur in a variety of ways. Consider the case of Joe:

Joe, a 23-year-old schizoid man had worked in a warehouse job after graduation from a special education program. He became bored, quit, and applied for rehabilitation services. His counselor referred him to a workshop, where he proved a good worker, and then placed him in another solitary job. He worked there for five months, then left again. He reapplied for services, and this time his counselor referred him to a psychosocial rehabilitation clubhouse. He did well and began a TE in a mailroom. At his next counseling session he said he did not like his TE because there were no people around and he felt lonely. It became clear that he had quit his jobs because he had unmet social needs. He was encouraged to attend the evening social program and was reassured that he could still be a club member even after he returned to work. He continued his TE and began to attend the evening program.

This is a "delayed impoverishment crisis." People cannot indefinitely tolerate loneliness, emptiness, and lack of meaning. Such a situation gets to them, and they become overwhelmed. This is an invisible stress. Nothing unusual has happened to be recognized as a stressor. And this is just the point: "nothing" is happening. We must be careful, lest by helping a client to function more independently we cause him or her to lose something of great value in the bargain. Activities such as membership in a social club, an active alumni group of a residential program, or a recreational program can continue to support his or her social identity as he or she is losing the social opportunities and supports of the patient/client role. Additionally, continued participation in these programs presents us with the opportunity to recognize early signs of regression and to give additional support during the ups and downs of ordinary life that so many of our clients find hard to master.

The last crisis I wish to mention is the "planning crisis." At times our plan may be a mistake: the gradient of change is too great, the timing for implementation is poor, the team does not fully support it, something unexpected occurs, the client is not ready for this step. When this happens, and the client becomes overwhelmed, we must recognize the inappropriateness of the plan, not just the exacerbation of the client's psychopathology. A new plan needs to be formulated, after a "time out." At other times a plan may indeed be correct, but something extrinsic to the programming takes place, such as a funding shortage, no timely openings at the next step when the client is ready, no jobs. Again, acknowledgement, support, and replanning are indicated to preserve the rehabilitation alliance.

I have found that an awareness of these various types of crisis can make the vicissitudes of a client's course more understandable, predictable, and treatable, and often more avoidable over time.

References

Adler, G. 1970. The psychotherapy of schizophrenia: Semrad's contributions to current psychoanalytic concepts. *Schizophrenia Bulletin, 5*, 130–37.

Anderson, T. P. 1975. An alternative frame of reference for rehabilitation: The helping process versus the medical model. *Archives of Physical Medicine Rehabilitation, 56*, 101–4.

Anonymous. 1980. First-person account: After the funny farm. *Schizophrenia Bulletin, 6*, 544–46.

Anthony, W. A. 1979. The rehabilitation approach to diagnosis. *New Directions for Mental Health Services, 2*, 25–36.

Anthony, W. A.; Buell, G. T.; Sharratt, S.; and Althoff, M. E. 1972. The efficacy of psychiatric rehabilitation. *Psychological Bulletin, 78*, 447–56.

Anthony, W. A.; Cohen, M. D.; and Vitale, R. 1978. The measurement of rehabilitation outcome. *Schizophrenia Bulletin, 4*, 365–81.

Beard, J. H.; Malamud, T. J.; and Rossman, E. 1978. Psychiatric rehabilitation and long-term hospital rates: The findings of two research studies. *Schizophrenia Bulletin, 4*, 622–35.

Beard, J. H; Schmidt, J. R.; and Smith, M. 1963. The use of transitional employment in the rehabilitation of the psychiatric patient. *Journal of Nervous and Mental Diseases, 13*, 507–14.

Beigler, J. S. 1952. Therapeutic ambition: Handicap for counselors. *Journal of Rehabilitation, 18*, 9–11.

Bray, G. P. 1980. Team strategies for family involvement in rehabilitation. *Journal of Rehabilitation, 46*, 20–23.

Breier, A., and Strauss, J. S. 1983. Self-control in psychotic disorders. *Archives of General Psychiatry, 40*, 1141–45.

Chittick, R. S.; Brooks, G. W.; Irons, F. S.; and Dreane, W. N. 1961. *The Vermont story* (out of print). Burlington, Vt.: Queen City Printers.

Climo, L. 1983. Helping some state hospital mental patients make small but necessary changes: Transference openings from countertransference traps. *Community Mental Health Journal, 19*, 413–20.

Creasey, D. E., and McCarthy, T. P. 1981. Training vocational rehabilitation counselors who work with chronic mental patients. *American Journal of Psychiatry, 138*, 1102–6.

Cubelli, G. E. 1970. Some dynamics of the rehabilitation process. *Rehabilitation Literature, 31*, 200–203.

Erikson, E. H. 1959. Identity and the life cycle. *Psychological Issues*, monograph no. 1. New York: International Universities Press.

Erikson, E. H. 1963. *Childhood and society*. New York: Norton.

Foreman, S. A., and Marmar, C. R. 1985. Therapist actions that address initially poor therapeutic alliances in psychotherapy. *American Journal of Psychiatry, 142*, 922–26.

Fox, R. P. 1973. Therapeutic environments: A view of nondyadic treatment situations. *Archives of General Psychiatry, 29*, 514–17.

Gendel, M. H., and Reiser, D. E. 1981. Institutional countertransference. *American Journal of Psychiatry, 138*, 508–11.

Gruenberg, E. M. 1967. The social breakdown syndrome: Some origins. *American Journal of Psychiatry, 123*, 1481–89.

Gruenberg, E. M 1974. Benefits of short-term hospitalization. In *Strategic interventions in schizophrenia*, ed. R. Cancro, M. Fox, and L. Shapiro, pp. 251–69. New York: Behavioral Publications.

Harding, C. M.; Brooks, G. W.; Ashikaga, T.; and Strauss, J. S. 1987. The Vermont longitudinal study of persons with severe mental illness, I: Methodology, study sample, and overall current status. *American Journal of Psychiatry, 144*, 718–26.

Harris, M.; Bergman, H. C.; and Greenwood, V. 1982. Integrating hospital and community systems for treating revolving-door patients. *Hospital and Community Psychiatry, 33*, 225–27.

Hatfield, A. B. 1979. The family as partner in the treatment of mental illness. *Hospital and Community Psychiatry, 30*, 338–40.

Havens, L. L. 1965. Skills and personality required to effectively counsel the emotionally ill. In *Vocational rehabilitation counselling specialization: Cause and effect*, ed. W. M. Holbert. Georgia Division of Vocational Rehabilitation, Atlanta.

Jacobs, D. H.; Rogoff, J.; Donnelly, K.; Birnbaum, B.; and Russion, R. 1982. The neglected alliance: The inpatient unit as a consultant to referring therapists. *Hospital and Community Psychiatry, 33*, 377–81.

Kanter, J. 1985. The process of change in the long-term mentally ill: A naturalistic perspective. *Psychosocial Rehabilitation Journal, 9*, 55–69.

Lamb, H. R. 1969. Community-based treatment of long-term schizophrenic patients. In *Progress in community mental health*, ed. L. Bellak and H. H. Barton, vol. 3. New York: Grune and Stratton.

———. 1979. Staff burnout in work with long-term patients. *Hospital and Community Psychiatry, 30*, 396–98.

Lamb, H. R., and Mackota, C. 1969. Vocational rehabilitation services. In *Handbook of community mental health practice*, ed. H R. Lamb, S. Heath, and J. J. Downing, pp. 200–16. San Francisco: Jossey-Bass.

———. 1975. Vocational rehabilitation counseling: A "second-class" profession? *Journal of Rehabilitation, 38*, 21–23, 39.

Lovejoy, M. 1982. Expectations and the recovery process. *Schizophrenia Bulletin, 8*, 605–9.

McCarthy, T. P. 1981. *Rehabilitation diagnosis*. Presented as part of a course entitled "Psychiatric Rehabilitation, Principle and Practice" at the annual conference of the American Psychiatric Rehabilitation Association, New Orleans.

McCrory, D. J.; Connolly, P. S.; Hanson-Mayer, T.P.; Sheridan-Landolfi, J. S.; Barone, F. C.;

Blood, A. H.; and Gilson, A. M. 1980. The rehabilitation crisis: The impact of growth. *Journal of Applied Rehabilitation Counseling, 11,* 136–39.

McCrory, D. J., and Marrone, J. A. 1984. The physician and the disabled patient: A challenge to medical education. *Journal of Medical Education, 59,* 429–31.

Margolin, R. J. 1963. The failure syndrome and its prevention. *Journal of the Association for Physical Medicine and Rehabilitation, 17* (3), 77–82.

Marrone, J.; Horgan, J.; Scripture, D.; and Grossman, M. 1984. Serving the severely psychiatrically disabled client within the VR system. *Psychosocial Rehabilitation Journal, 8,* 5–23.

Marsh, S. K.; Konar, V.; Langton, M. S.; and LaRue, A. J. 1980. The functional assessment profile: A rehabilitation model. *Journal of Applied Rehabilitation Counseling, 11,* 140–44.

Olshansky, S. 1972. Eleven myths in vocational rehabilitation. *Journal of Applied Rehabilitation Counseling, 3,* 229–36.

———. 1980. The deinstitutionalization of schizophrenics: A challenge to rehabilitation. *Rehabilitation Literature, 41,* 127–29.

Perl, M.; Hall, R.C.W.; Gardner, E. R.; and Stickney, S. K. 1980. The social breakdown syndrome revisited: Psychotogenic staff-patient relationships. *Psychiatric Opinion, 17,* 23–26.

Peterson, R. 1978. What are the needs of chronic mental patients? In Talbott 1978.

Reider, N. 1953. A type of transference to institutions. *Bulletin of the Menninger Clinic, 17,* 58–63.

Rogers, C. 1967. The conditions of change from a client-center viewpoint. In *Sources of gain in counseling and psychotherapy,* ed. B. Berenson and R. Carkhuff. New York: Holt, Rinehart, and Winston.

Saferstein, S. L. 1967. Institutional transference. *Psychiatric Quarterly, 41,* 551–56.

Sederer, L. 1975. Psychotherapy patient transfer: Secondhand Rose. *American Journal of Psychiatry, 132,* 1057–61.

Smith, D.A.P.; Zimny, G. H.; and Lindbergh, S. S. 1981. How psychiatrists use vocational rehabilitation resources. *Hospital and Community Psychiatry, 32,* 714–16.

Stanton, A. H., and Schwartz, M. D. 1949. The management of a type of institutional participation in mental illness. *Psychiatry, 12,* 13–26.

Sullivan, H. S. 1930. Socio-psychiatric research: Its implications for the schizophrenia problem and for mental hygiene. *American Journal of Psychiatry, 87,* 991–97.

Talbott, J. S. 1978. *The chronic mental patient.* Washington, D.C.: American Psychiatric Association.

———. 1984. *The chronic mental patient: Five years later.* New York: Grune and Stratton.

Zetzel, E. 1956. Current concepts of transference. *International Journal of Psychoanalysis, 37,* 182–96.

———. 1970. Therapeutic alliance in the analysis of hysteria. In *The capacity for emotional growth,* ed. E. R. Zetzel, pp. 182–96. New York: International Universities Press.

15

The Rehabilitation Relationship: The Case for a Personal Rehabilitation

EDWARD R. RYAN

Ryan draws on his own experiences in rehabilitating the seriously mentally ill to stress the personal relationship as the crucial factor. He focuses on the "why" of rehabilitation rather than on the "how to," and advocates a rehabilitation program which encourages the personal interest of the practitioner in the life of the client. The five steps to develop this type of program are consideration, flexibility, creativity, opportunity, and curiosity. Ryan concludes that the optimal conditions for vocational rehabilitation occur in the context of a personal relationship which can prevent both practitioner and client "burnout."

This chapter focuses on the personal relationship as the central experience in the vocational rehabilitation of persons with prolonged mental illness. I am offering this perspective because I have observed it to be the crucial factor in work with a wide variety of seriously disturbed persons, and because I am concerned about the increasing emphasis on technical and impersonal solutions to the problem of mental illness. Let me begin by stating what I mean by *personal rehabilitation:* I refer to change in the client and in his or her vocational status made possible through the quality of the relationship with the rehabilitation worker. All of the dimensions of the rehabilitation—the client's history, the assessment, the retraining, the job opportunity, and the job placement—are referred to the personal interest, decision, energy, and motivation of the particular person who is rehabilitating himself or herself. The client, then, is not just anybody; she or he is a unique person with whom you or I develop a personal rehabilitation relationship. All of our technical knowledge of the rehabilitation process and of prolonged mental illness is only information, and as such it can become dull and hackneyed—with the result that many vocational rehabilitation specialists "burn out" with clients, especially with the mentally ill. Is there anything really interesting or intriguing about trying to place one mentally ill patient after another in a job, when it is done technically, according to preconceptions about mental illness and formulae about the rehabilitation process? And worse, how are we to remain interested when the mentally ill are known to be difficult, unreliable, and strange; when they bring to the rehabilitation relationship ways of being and relating that interfere directly with our best planned "how-to" methods? Is it any wonder that so many rehabilitation specialists try to avoid the mentally ill—or, if they must work with the mentally ill, do a cursory, technical, impersonal, and, ultimately, unsatisfactory job? Why? Because there is no spark of life, no intellectual or emotional challenge, no genuine personal involvement, in rehabilitation by the numbers. Yet the problem is not the rehabilitation process, nor is it the mentally ill. What we are looking for—a real challenge, personal growth, and the fun of being involved for all it is worth—is right in front of us. All that is required is that we remember that each of us is a person and that whatever we do together is personal—for both of us.

Sometimes this involves a real awakening. While psychotherapeutic approaches have traditionally emphasized empathy and the personal relationship, rehabilitation of the mentally ill usually has focused on *how* such a task could be accomplished, with an emphasis on method. The basic assumption underlying the concept of rehabilitation has been that the mentally ill are a subpopulation among us who, because of their illness, are handicapped in their pursuit of productive lives and so must be rehabilitated.

I am offering a different perspective here and making a case for a personal rehabilitation. My emphasis is not on how to but, rather, on *why*— and specifically, on discovering why any person with prolonged mental illness would wish to rehabilitate him or herself. I believe a personal rehabilitation is made possible through seeking an answer to this question. By wanting to know why, our eyes and ears are opened to that person sitting across from us, bizarre as he or she may appear. Our preconceptions about people can give way to curiosity about this person. Our knowledge of the formulae for successful rehabilitation can give way to ignorance about the particular process that will be successful in this case. Our professional distance can give way to personal involvement. Often, our self-assurance will give way to doubt, even fear. The clarity of our definition of our selves, of our clients, and of rehabilitation gives way to confusion. Am I advocating an approach that leads to doubt, fear, and confusion? Yes! In fact, it is important that we begin in this state, for it is the open way. The answers to our questions are not yet available, but we have a new question now: Why would this person be interested in rehabilitation, and how might I be involved?

Compare this way with technical, methodological rehabilitation. Before a mentally ill person is even admitted into our vocational rehabilitation programs, we have begun to discuss "how to" work with him or her. Sometimes we devise elaborate formulations of his or her life without even having met the person; sometimes we relegate this person to a typology and prepare to rehabilitate the type. As we do this, we gradually lose interest, because *we* are not types, and we cannot bear to work in such stereotyped ways. Once we do meet the individual and especially once she or he begins to interfere with our rehabilitation goals, there is usually an endless series of discussions about "how to" rehabilitate the wretch. But in the process, without realizing it, we enter into a routinized, impersonal relationship with that person, which often ends in frustration, despair, or fatigue. We fall back on the abstract idea of the rehabilitation process, and we often blame the client for not achieving that ideal. What was that encounter, then, and *who* was involved? We realize that we had never gotten to know this man or woman personally.

Why should this be? Let's move slowly in answering. Caseload pressure, quotas, the exigencies of funding, difficulty in communication, need to protect our placement opportunities, the bureaucracy—these are well-known and well-worn answers. I would like to suggest another possibility, one that responds more to the personal question involved. I think we devote an enormous amount of attention to rehabilitation goals, and so we become acutely aware of the formidable resistance of the chronically mentally ill client to meeting those goals. This attention to our goals and the client's resistance seems to obfuscate the personal challenge we face, and the potential fun we might enjoy, in relating humanely and therapeutically to that particular person sitting across the desk from us. Perhaps foremost among our reasons for sticking to goals and being vexed by the client's resistance is the fact that mentally ill people often act in weird ways. Though at times fascinating, these thought and behavior patterns are departures from everyday reality and are thus unsettling, or even frightening.

Further, when we receive referrals from mental health professionals, their records may include a measurement and cataloging of these idiosyncratic behaviors. Often the psychiatric treatment described has been focused on reducing these symptoms or on discovering their etiology. At times mental health professionals are called on to prevent psychologically disturbed patients from seriously hurting themselves or others. So it is only natural that psychiatric referrals will often highlight symptoms. However, this predominant attention to symptoms often overshadows the person. Similarly, when we encounter such a person who is acting strangely, we are likely to send him or her back to the referral source for more treatment or to undertake a "how to" technique.

Over the past twelve years I have participated in a series of programs for the rehabilitation of the mentally ill. After thousands of experiences with these clients I have come to believe that the question is not how to rehabilitate, but rather, why would this particular person, acting or thinking so strangely, wish to change the course of his or her life, and how will I be involved personally in answering that question? For despite all that has been written about effective rehabilitation programming and public policy, rehabilitation is personal. It happens in one person at a time, and for personal reasons.

In our rehabilitation efforts we often become ensnared in the dilemma of *the person versus the program.* We urge our client to get involved in the program. Yet, we know that mere participation in any program does not have an automatic rehabilitative effect and that not every person who joins a program must conform with its standards to become rehabilitated. Though belief in a program may be important for the maintenance of morale, security, and hope, such a belief is relevant only when program participation is consistent with why any particular client wishes to change the course of his or her life. Program procedures, rules, and beliefs cannot consider the personal life of the client, and why he or she may wish to change, or remain unchanged. Only other persons can do that; only we can do that.

Our experiences with our clients can guide us toward developing a rehabilitation program that encourages the interest of the staff in the lives of the clients. The development of such a program involves five steps: consideration, flexibility, creativity, opportunity, and curiosity. The first step, consideration, refers to our careful consideration of the conditions we believe any person would find conducive to taking stock of his or her life. Among these we might include safety, friendliness, honesty, trust, and humor. These are not prescriptions; they are suggestions. I hope they will stimulate you to consider what conditions you need or have needed in order to reflect honestly on your life. Once you establish a set of conditions, you must remain flexible. Not everyone with whom you work, and perhaps only a few mentally ill persons, will need or want the conditions we have selected. This flexibility cannot be built into a program formula; it can exist when the "program" allows for, expects, and encourages the personal flexibility of the staff.

The optimal rehabilitation conditions for any particular client will be discovered in the context of a personal relationship with that client. When a rehabilitation program is founded on consideration and flexibility, there will be an enormous energy liberated within ourselves and within our clients to accomplish the third step: creating an environment in which each of us can become personally engaged in vocational rehabilitation. Naturally such an environment will be continuously changing, as persons, interests, and relationships change. Through involvement, opportunities arise for personal rehabilitation of clients and personal transformation of staff. When the creative energy of all participants is regarded as necessary to develop new opportunities, these opportunities will be discovered. When this discovery occurs in the context of personal relationships, the opportunities will fit personal interests. Our interest in consistency, or our desire for stability, or our pride in accomplishment, may pull us toward reifying a process into policies and procedures. While this may be inevitable at times, it is important to remain curious and maintain an open inquiry into why this person might decide to pursue rehabilitation goals while that person might not. When we do fall into a set way of doing things or reify a cherished belief, perhaps we might keep available a part of our energy to check ourselves, to inquire into our ways, and to keep it personal.

In other words, the most challenging part of developing a personal rehabilitation is that it inevitably becomes personal for us, the rehabilitation therapists. We look in the mirror and ask a parallel question to that we have been asking about the client: Why should I—a so-called "staff member"—wish to transform my own life, and what parts might the persons I meet in a rehabilitation setting—the clients and other staff members—play in that decision and in that process? Once rehabilitation develops from being merely a program, whether in our institutions or in our minds, to being a personal interaction, our own resistance to transformation, as represented in a rigid adherence to program procedures, is no longer necessary.

This does not mean that we cease to be professionals or that all of our knowledge, experience, and training evaporates. We remain professionals: personal rehabilitation is our vocation, and we maintain the boundaries of that professional relationship with the client. So, for example, we do not become the client's personal friend, though we may be friendly. We do not become the client's lover, though we may tolerate the romantic, sexual, and affectionate feelings that arise in any personal relationship. We do not become the client's antagonist, though we may tolerate the hateful, critical, and antagonistic feelings that also arise in any personal relationship. We do not become the client's savior, though we may tolerate his or her idealization of us in the process of his or her regaining self-esteem. We do not become the client's detractor, though we do not back away from constructive criticism. We do not try to do the rehabilitation for the client, though we may be his or her advocate and cheerleader at times.

We have been trained in how to rehabilitate, but the art of rehabilitation involves transforming all of our training and knowledge into a personal rehabilitative relationship, so that *the client* discovers how to rehabilitate himself or herself. In reflecting on our commonality with our clients, their families, and our staff fellows, we remember why we have wished to make changes in our own lives and how difficult such a process can be. We remember our aspirations and our limitations. The reciprocal interplay between our openness to experiences with our clients in the present and memories of our own efforts to change evolves into our empathy—our interest in knowing the client as he or she really is personally; our compassion—the emotional awareness of the commonality between us; and eventually, our love—the heartfelt interest in this particular individual and the warm, caring commitment to his or her welfare. This interest transforms the how-to knowledge into a personal commitment.

Perhaps an anecdote will illustrate this spontaneous kind of self-rehabilitation. A man in his late thirties came to our program for rehabilitation. He had been unemployed for several years. He had been in several psychiatric treatments, both inpatient and outpatient, since his early twenties, including psychiatric, psychosocial, substance abuse, alcoholism, and behavior-modification approaches. Despite all of these experiences, he remained a hard-drinking, drug-using, reckless, violent, difficult, and at times psychotic person. Because he was an intelligent man, several attempts at rehabilitation over the years had resulted in a series of job placements. But his disruptive, arrogant, threatening, and overbearing behavior had consistently resulted in prompt terminations. Though he said he wanted to work and live a more stable life, he also communicated that he was a chronically mentally ill person incapable of working.

He began to work with a woman staff member who was quiet, emotionally honest, and socially inhibited. Before long, he was acting in psychotic and threatening ways and treating her in a demeaning way publicly. At first she was frightened and fell back on a controlling strategy of anonymity—that is, she would become a nonperson, thus not offended, and he would also become a nonperson, thus no more than a specimen exhibiting a panoply of pathology. Though this was a "safe" response she found it unsatisfying and disturbing, so she summoned up her courage and tried to get to know him personally. She allowed herself to be aware of this client's insults and of the painful memories she had of having been insulted as a child. She saw more clearly how her own social inhibition was the result of this early, harsh criticism. She remembered her efforts to be more open and the helplessness she felt to live beyond criticism. She realized that her own self-criticism was no more than an identification with those who had been so critical of her. She went through the painful mourning of these experiences and emerged freer to express her own thoughts and emotions.

She decided to reveal her pain and anger directly to the client. Her nondefensive openness shocked him. At first he refused to accept the integrity of her invitation to a truly personal relationship. He tried to dismiss her and her feelings in the same arrogant manner he had relied on for years. Again she responded directly—and personally. Though he could not admit it for a while, he was moved by her emotional honesty, her personal vulnerability, and her compassion. Privately he began to reconsider his arrogance and cruelty. Remarkably, he began to take stock of his life—not because she had used a how-to technique to control him, but because in her relationship with him she had lived out the reality of what it is to be personal. Thus she had spoken *directly* to why he might wish to revive a previously lost way of being and relating. For the first time in a long time, he apologized and felt freer to reveal himself to her candidly. She became his first confidante. Though this vocational rehabilitation was to take a rocky road until he finally found his vocational niche, he was able to stick with it because he could rely on her. Each came to mean a great deal to the other. The personal vulnerability they allowed and revealed was mutually confirmed. It thus became a shared awareness of their common vulnerability and the route to rehabilitative freedom for this client. In this context, self-help is other-help without control or egoism.

Our efforts and thoughts have been restricted to a false dichotomy between a transforming personal relationship and a successful vocational rehabilitation. Some "clinicians" are still loathe to think of themselves as doing rehabilitation, and "rehabilitation specialists" are not interested in doing therapy. Over the years I have seen sensitive rehabilitation specialists question their creativity because what they were doing seemed too much like therapy. Conversely, I have observed equally sensitive psychotherapists question their effective participation in rehabilitation activities because they worried that what they were doing was somehow no longer psychotherapy. We suffer from the restrictions we invented. In all healing, the personal relationship is important. In psychosocial rehabilitation of the mentally ill this is central: therapy and rehabilitation are one.

It is always a great experience when personal connections are made. Once we can know the persons, regardless of their unusual behaviors, they will recover from being apathetic mental patients. This transformation inspires hope. People who are chronically mentally ill are like people who have been shipwrecked and, after years of being cast about, have been tossed up on the beach—exhausted, terrified, without food or water. When we walk toward them at the initial interview, it is as if we lived on that island and went down to the beach for a walk, only to be surprised by these bedraggled and desperate strangers. To them we appear to be strange people in war paint and feathers. As we approach them, they become even more terrified. When we see that they are like us, only shipwrecked, we are able to offer them a drink of water and some personal comfort. Once they can trust us, their own considerable energy will get them through the how-to of rehabilitation. But it will be the hope they derive from our personal involvement that will make their commitment possible.

Of course, there is usually a great disparity in resources and skills between us and our clients. As we become personally committed to such a client, we begin to think about resources in new and often upsetting ways. We may discover that the client, despite his or her limitations, has capacities to support himself, other clients, and us. We may feel the pressure within ourselves to exert professional (status) power, so as to reassure ourselves that we are in charge of the rehabilitation. This kind of power-wielding usually eclipses the initiative of the client. Therefore, an important transformation for us is the recognition that the client is the primary force in rehabilitation. Sometimes all we have to do, once the client is connected with us personally, is stand back and watch the client rehabilitate him or herself.

Each step we take personally with our clients inevitably allows us to release our denial of the disorder among us. Gradually we allow ourselves to live within the disorder, accepting what it is, openly, and being ourselves personally in the midst of it all. Eventually we find ourselves working for the prevention of the conditions in which mental illness develops and continues. As we assist our clients in rehabilitating themselves, we become involved in changing the conditions in which we live. Often prevention, like rehabilitation, has been conceived as a how-to activity, with great attention to instituting programs of prevention. Prevention in that context is not a personal participation in changing conditions toward greater mental health. In personal rehabilitation we become involved in prevention for personal reasons. What begins as tertiary prevention—helping a client to prevent further breakdown—evolves through personal commitment into primary prevention—our involvement in creating resource availability that prevents mental illness as a social outcome.

I have presented the personal approach to vocational rehabilitation as a way of liberating our empathy, compassion, and kindness in our work with persons with prolonged mental illness and, thus, as a way of creating a basis of interest, motivation, and energy for the challenging rehabilitative process. The personal approach may be considered an alternative to the mechanical how-to approach, but it is often the choice of this alternative that makes the how-to process possible. When considering the impasse that so often arises in the vocational rehabilitation of the mentally ill, perhaps it is worth reflecting on an ancient Zen koan. A koan is a riddle presented by a teacher to a student to assist the student in his or her own movement toward enlightenment about the way things really are.

It seems that there was once a very revered monk who practiced a virtuous life of devotion and service and who was known as a holy man. After years of service, the monk decided to go on a pilgrimage to a far-off shrine, as a sign of his devotion. In preparing himself for the journey, he vowed that he would never take a step back once he had set out, whatever the conditions he might encounter. And so he walked for miles and miles, over days and weeks, through all terrains and all kinds of weather. One day he came to a deep chasm in the forest across which was strung a rope bridge. The bridge was quite primitive, made of a single woven rope to walk on and two side ropes to guide oneself by hand. It was a very precarious crossing, to be sure. The monk walked slowly and steadily across the bridge, taking care not to fall. When he came to the middle of the bridge he met another monk coming in the opposite direction. This monk was also on a pilgrimage and had also made a sacred vow not to take a single step backwards. There they were. Your job, says the teacher to the student, is to help them.

It is a terrible dilemma. The student contemplates the situation over time, and the teacher reminds him or her of how desperate the monks were and how much they needed help. Finally, the student may discover the solution to this impossible dilemma. The answer is simply this: There is no bridge and there are no monks; but this is an example of the kind of negative and destructive stories we allow ourselves and others to put into our minds that cause us such unhappiness. So, too, in rehabilitation, there are many stories we can tell ourselves about the client, the situation, and ourselves that can makes us very unhappy. But these stories are as illusory as the monks on the bridge, and the personal relationship we create with our clients may just be the reality in which our kindness and energy can be liberated.

IV

CONCLUSION

In the first of the two concluding chapters Bond and Boyer do a thorough review of the research literature and examine the reported success of vocational rehabilitation programs. The last chapter summarizes and integrates the main themes of the book, emphasizing both the positive and negative aspects of vocational rehabilitation since deinstitutionalization. Ciardiello uses the past to make some recommendations about the future of vocational rehabilitation in the United States.

16

Rehabilitation Programs and Outcomes

GARY R. BOND and SARA L. BOYER

Bond and Boyer examine the reported success of vocational rehabilitation programs in returning chronically mentally ill clients to paid employment. They present the methodological limitations of the twenty-one studies cited and classify results by type of program. These types include hospital-based programs, sheltered work, assertive case management, psychosocial rehabilitation, supported employment, rehabilitation counseling, job clubs, remedial education, occupational training, and post-employment services. Although Bond and Boyer conclude that none of the twenty-one programs helped clients sustain competitive employment over time, they were more optimistic when outcome criteria and type of program were qualified. They make several recommendations to improve future outcome research.

This chapter examines the effectiveness of various types of vocational programs in helping psychiatrically disabled clients achieve employment. The focus is on vocational outcomes, though recognizing that quality of life, self-esteem, and other aspects of community adjustment are important in both the conception and the evaluation of many programs. Employment, however, is the "bottom line." Programs serving clients variously described as "mentally ill," "emotionally disturbed," "psychiatrically disabled," "psychotic," "former psychiatric patients," or with other diverse and often vague labels are included. At present, the field lacks a common vocabulary to describe the level of disability for those who are mentally ill. There is no counterpart, for example, to the intelligence testing used to classify the mentally retarded. Therefore, the definitional problem has been sidestepped.

Anthony, Buell, Sharatt, and Althoff (1972) concluded that psychiatric rehabilitation programs have little impact on rates of competitive employment. Since then, evaluation studies have continued to report modest outcomes. However, progress has been made in the development of well-articulated community-based programs, as this review makes clear.

Our review is based on two sources: the published psychological and rehabilitation literature, with particular emphasis on the past ten years, and unpublished presentations from national conferences sponsored by the International Association of Psychosocial Rehabilitation Services.

The published literature does not do justice to the wide range of vocational programming offered across the United States and elsewhere. For example, even though one survey found 119 transitional employment programs in operation in 1984 (Fountain House 1984), only three controlled evaluations have been published (Beard et al. 1963; Bond and Dincin 1986; Dincin and Witheridge 1982). Such innovations as client-employing businesses (Carroll and Levye 1985) are familiar to practitioners, yet they are barely mentioned in the literature. A number of unpublished evaluations have been conducted over the past decade which, if unearthed, might add to our knowledge. Since practitioners are more inclined temperamentally to *doing* than to *evaluating,* more information is shared within professional networks than is documented in the literature.

Our literature search included an examination of *Psychological Abstracts* and *Index Medicus* between 1975 and 1985 under such headings as "Vocational rehabilitation," "Mental disorders," "Psychosis," "Schizophrenia," "Psychosocial rehabilitation," "Occupational adjustment," and "Psychiatric patients." We also consulted literature reviews conducted by others (Anthony et al. 1972; Anthony, Cohen, and Vitalo 1978; Hursh and Anthony 1983; Jacobs, Donahoe, and Falloon 1985; Kunce 1970; Rubin and Roessler 1978; Spooner, Algozzine, and Saxon 1980) and the annotated bibliography prepared by Klein (1984).

We excluded programs without an explicit vocational focus from this review, since the available evidence suggests they have little impact on employment. In fact, comprehensive day programs may on occasion inhibit clients from seeking work. Three studies illustrate these assertions.

Hogarty, Goldberg, and Schooler (1974) found that medications and major-role therapy (a one-to-one counseling model using a "problem-solving method to respond to the interpersonal, personal, social, and rehabilitation needs"), had no effect on the "performance of major role." Similarly, Mosher and Menn (1978) in their evaluation of an intensive therapeutic community found no differences in number of patients employed or attending school full- or part-time, although the experimental group did achieve a higher average occupational level. Vitale and Steinbach (1965), in a nonexperimental study, found that only 17 percent of clients achieved employment while at a day center offering an organized program of psychotherapeutic, social, recreational, and medication services, compared with 57 percent of those in a less intensive mental hygiene clinic.

Simply keeping clients out of the hospital is not sufficient to improve their vocational functioning. General training in problem solving, skills, and socialization, and help in residential needs, do not automatically lead to better vocational functioning. More specific vocational programming must be provided.

Unlike Anthony's landmark reviews (Anthony et al. 1972; 1978), this review makes no attempt to establish baseline rates against which to measure the efficacy of programs. We found that results varied widely as a function of such factors as the selectivity of samples and definitions of outcome. Therefore, we took a different tack and focused on controlled and quasi-controlled studies.

A Continuum of Vocational Rehabilitation Programs

There has been surprisingly little attention given in the literature to classifying psychiatric vocational programs. Spooner, Algozzine, and Saxon (1980) classified programs into four types: community, rehabilitation unit, operant technology, and medication regimens, a typology that mixes location of treatment with intervention methodology. Anthony and associates (1972) distinguished between inpatient and outpatient treatment and delineated four subtypes of outpatient treatment: drug maintenance, aftercare, planned follow-up counseling, and transitional facilities. Their schema did not include important subtypes, such as sheltered workshops, or more recent developments, such as the job club. Some authors have focused on counseling stages in the rehabilitation process. Rubin and Roessler (1978) identified these as client evaluation, plan development, work-adjustment training, and placement. Anthony (1980) identified three stages: work adjustment, career counseling, and career placement. These schemes did not differentiate types of work-adjustment training, which is a principal distinguishing feature among programs.

Table 16.1 classifies approaches according to the degree to which work experiences are provided in normalized community employment. As with any typology, it is an oversimplification; for example, counseling is listed as a separate program even though counseling occurs in each of the preceding program types.

Table 16.2 is a compilation of the basic findings from twenty-one studies. Each study met the following criteria: (a) inclusion of a control or quasi-control group; (b) inclusion of some specific form of vocational rehabilitation in the experimental program; (c) program specifically designed for the mentally ill, or at least with separate statistics provided on psychiatric subsamples; and (d) vocational outcome data provided. The publication dates range from 1963 to 1986, with a median date of 1972. All but two of these studies used random assignment. Also, the percentage of clients contacted at initial follow-up exceeded 90 percent, except in studies by Bell and Ryan (1984) (79%), Meltzoff and Blumenthal (1966)

(86%), and Lamb and Goertzel (1972) (76%). The follow-up rates declined as the length of the follow-up period increased.

Not all were methodologically rigorous, however. The major shortcomings were insufficient details on treatment conditions, vague description of outcome measures, and insufficient details on dropouts. Also, four studies had fewer than forty subjects and might be excluded because of lack of statistical power.

Hospital-Based Programs

Interest in hospital-based vocational programs has waned in the past two decades as hospital stays have decreased in duration. The exceptions appear to be in the Veterans Administration (VA) system (Bell and Ryan 1984; Kuldau and Dirks, 1977; Ryan and Bell 1985) and in programs in Europe and Canada (Barkley, Pixley, and Walker 1976; Mezquita-Blanco 1984). Studies reporting follow-up statistics include Barkley, Pixley, and Walker 1976; Brown 1970; Cheney and Kish 1970; Ekdawi 1972; Hoffman 1965; Johnson and Lee 1965; Katz-Garris et al. 1983; Llorens, Levy, and Rubin 1964; Mezquita 1973; Miskimins, Cole, and Oetting 1968; Programs for patient-workers 1976; Schwartz 1976; Walker and Asci 1971; and Watson and Maddigan 1972.

The early literature on hospital-based vocational programs often took the stance that productive activity helped increase self-esteem and general functioning and that therefore work activities within the hospital were therapeutic and could accelerate discharge. Kunce (1970) criticized the "work as therapy" principle, citing studies of hospital work programs and discharge rates. In one randomized study, Barbee, Berry, and Micek (1969) found that patients in hospital work programs remained hospitalized significantly longer. Because experimental patients were also significantly more likely to return to the hospital where the study was being conducted, Barbee, Berry, and Micek believed that such programs could create an "institutional dependency." They noted three sources of secondary gain for participation: wages for work; supportive, nondemanding supervisors; and socializing among coworkers. Certain kinds of patients may be more likely to develop dependency. For example, Watson and Maddigan (1972) found that for short-term patients, a work therapy program actually increased the number of days in the community during the follow-up period, but this was not true for the long-term patients. The purpose of the work program is also important. Hartlage's (1967) survey examined the reasons hospital administrators gave for providing work programs. Those programs which were intended mainly to keep patients active had the lowest discharge rates.

As shown in Table 16.3, the evidence for institutional dependency is not uniform, but the burden of proof is on those who believe hospital work

Table 16.1
A Continuum of Vocational Rehabilitation

1. *Hospital-based programs.* Vocational preparation for inpatients, including
   a. Work duties within the hospital (Barbee, Berry, and Micek 1969).
   b. Community jobs while living in the hospital (Walker et al. 1969).
2. *Sheltered work.* Unskilled work, usually in a segregated setting, in which pay is usually below minimum wage (Lamb 1971), including
   a. Comprehensive rehabilitation centers for the general disabled population (Ciardiello 1981).
   b. Long-term psychiatric workshops (Wilder 1976).
   c. Sheltered enclaves (Fairweather et al. 1969).
3. *Assertive case management.* Clients actively assisted in problems of everyday living (housing, income support, finding employment) (Stein and Test 1980).
4. *Psychosocial rehabilitation.* The Fountain House model (Beard, Propst, and Malamud 1982; Dincin 1975), offering graded vocational opportunities, such as
   a. *Prevocational training:* Unpaid work in a rehabilitation center intended to teach good work habits.
   b. *Transitional employment:* Under an agreement between a rehabilitation center and an employer, work by clients in temporary part-time, entry-level community jobs.
      i. *Group placements:* TE positions in which a group of clients work at the same work site under the supervision of a rehabilitation staff worker.
      ii. *Individual placements:* Advanced TE positions for clients capable of working as regular part-time employees.
   c. *Volunteer placements:* Meaningful community work for which clients are not compensated. Used both as preparation for paid work and as a long-term vocational alternative (Keys 1982; Lang, Richman, and Trout 1984).
5. *Supported employment.* Permanent employment in community jobs under agreements between rehabilitation programs and employers (Black 1985; Pati and Morrison 1982).
6. *Counseling and Education.*
   a. *Rehabilitation counseling:* Assessment of skills, empathic understanding, skill-training, and career development (Anthony 1980).
   b. *Job clubs:* A systematic behavioral program to help clients develop job leads and obtain work (Azrin and Philip 1979).
   c. *Remedial education:* Tutoring clients in preparation for G.E.D. (Bond et al. 1984).
   d. *Occupational training:* Preparation for jobs in demand in the labor market (Johnson and Patterson 1957).
   e. *Postemployment services:* Continued supportive services for clients who are employed in the community (Sands and Radin 1978).

can accelerate discharge. Dependency may, in fact, extend to community settings, as will be discussed later.

Most reviewers have concluded that there is no relationship between successful adjustment to work programs within the hospital and posthospital employment. Walker and McCourt (1965) examined posthospital employment rates for 211 veterans, 53 percent of whom had been active in paid or unpaid hospital work programs. Six months after discharge, only 23 percent were employed. Moreover, there was no correlation between hospital work status and employment in the community.

The bulk of evidence suggests that there are better alternatives than

Table 16.2
Controlled Studies of Vocational Programs for the Mentally Ill

Study	Subjects	Group Experimental	Group Control	Follow-up Period	Outcome Sheltered/TEP jobs	Outcome Competitive employment while in program	Outcome Employment after leaving program	Comments
Hospital-Based Programs								
Becker (1967)	RA, inpatients (mainly veterans)	Intensive social/vocational program (N = 25)	Custodial care (N = 25)	8 mos.	E > C		E = C	Results did not replicate when program expanded
Bell & Ryan (1984)	Non., VA inpatients	In-hospital job placement (N = 28)	Two psycho-dynamic wards (N = 59)	6–18 mos.			E > C	Retrospective comparison; method details incomplete
Kuldau & Dirks (1977)	RA, VA inpatients	Day hospital, community housing, sheltered work (N = 41)	Rapid discharge, industrial therapy (N = 48)	18 mos.			E > C	Sample partitioned on work history; those with below-ave. history did poorly in both programs
Ryan & Bell (1985)	RA, VA inpatients	In-hospital & community job placements (N = 32)	Traditional intensive inpatient treatment (N = 26)	6 mos.		E = C		For duration and earnings, E > C
Walker & McCourt (1965)	Non., male VA inpatients	Active in vocational program (N = 112)	Not active in vocational program (N = 49)	6 mos.			E = C	Post hoc comparison; treatment and selection factors confounded

236

Walker et al. (1969)	RA, successful workers in hospital jobs	Community placement for paid job (N = 14)	Hospital job placement (N = 14)	6 mos.	E > C	E = C	
Sheltered/Segregated Programs							
Griffiths (1974)	RA, outpatients (2 yrs. as inpatient before)	Sheltered workshop (N = 14)	Aftercare (N = 14)	15–29 mos. (ave. = 18 mos.)	E = C		Incomplete details on treatment & methods
Fairweather et al. (1969)	RBA, male inpatients moved to community	Lodge (N = 75)	Aftercare (N = 75)	Every 6 mos. to 3⅓ yrs.	E > C	E = C	Examined median percent employed full-time; unusual data analysis
Weinberg & Lustig (1968)	RA, outpatients	Sheltered workshop (N = 20)	Vocational counseling (N = 18)	2 yrs.		E = C	Few details
Community Programs							
Beard et al. (1963)	Rot., community referrals	PSR program with TEP (N = 274)	Waiting list (N = 78)	3, 6, 9, 12 mos.		E = C	Not all subjects received TEP; few vocational details
Bond & Dincin (1986)	RA, community and hospital referrals	PSR program with accelerated TEP (N = 62)	PSR program with gradual TEP (N = 63)	9 & 15 mos.	E > C	E = C	Statistical trend favors E's; work-experienced did better in E condition

continued

ABBREVIATIONS: C = control group; E = experimental group; FT = full time; Non. = nonexperimental; PSR = psychosocial rehabilitation; RA = random assignment; RBA = randomized block assignment; Rot. = rotating assignment; TEP = transitional employment program; VA = Veterans Administration.

Table 16.2 *continued*

Study	Subjects	Group Experimental	Control	Follow-up Period	Outcome Sheltered/ TEP jobs	Competitive employment while in program	Employment after leaving program	Comments
Dincin & Witheridge (1982)	RA, community and hospital referrals	PSR program (N = 50)	Social club (N = 43)	9 mos.		E = C		Outcome is comparison on paid jobs including TEP; C's earned more than E's
Field et al. (n.d.)	RA, community and hospital referrals	Assertive case management + job developer but no sheltered workshops (N = 18)	Assertive case management + sheltered workshops (N = 18)	4, 8, 14, 18 mos.	E = C	E = C	E = C	Both groups improved over premeasures
Lamb & Goertzel (1972)	RA, hospital referrals	Halfway house/ high expectation program (N = 48)	Family care/low expectation program (N = 43)	6, 12, 18, 24 mos.	E > C	E = C		E's had higher hospital use initially
Marx, Test, & Stein (1973)	RA, inpatients at state hospital	Assertive case management (N = 65)	C1 = regular ward (N = 20); C2 = research ward (N = 20)	5 mos.	C2 > E C2 > C1	E > C1 E > C2		E and C2 had similar percentage employed when sheltered and competitive employment combined

Study	Sample/Assignment	Experimental group	Control group	Follow-up		Outcome	Comments
Meltzoff & Blumenthal (1966)	RA, male outpatients at VA center	Day treatment with vocational component (N = 33)	Psychotherapy and medication (N = 36)	18 mos.	E > C	E = C	30% of E's versus 14% of C's had job starts (p < .10)
Stein & Test (1980)	RA, clients seeking admission to hospital	Assertive case management (N = 57)	Hospitalized short-term (N = 59)	4, 8, 12 mos.	E > C	E = C	On some measures (FT employment & earnings) E > C for competitive employment
Wolkon, Karmen, & Tanaka (1971)	RA, hospital referrals	PSR program (N = 108)	Aftercare (N = 207)	12, 18, 24, 30 mos.		E = C	68% dropout rate prior to entry; vocational program unclear
Counseling/Job Club							
Azrin & Philip (1979)	RA, community & hospital referrals (not all mentally ill)	Job club (N = 19)	Vocational lecture (N = 6)	2–6 mos.		E > C	Outcome was obtaining job; 32% of sample found at 6 mos.; dropouts not included
Briggs & Yater (1966)	RA, hospital referrals	Vocational counseling (N = 74)	No treatment (N = 60)	Variable ave. = 13 mos.		E = C	
Purvis & Miskimins (1970)	RA, outpatients	E1 = group counseling (N = 52); E2 = individual counseling (N = 47)	No treatment (N = 50)	Not stated		E = C	Outcome measure was 3 mos. or more of employment

ABBREVIATIONS: C = control group; E = experimental group; FT = full time; Non. = nonexperimental; PSR = psychosocial rehabilitation; RA = random assignment; RBA = randomized block assignment; Rot. = rotating assignment; TEP = transitional employment program; VA = Veterans Administration.

Table 16.3
Studies Examining the Institutional Dependency Hypothesis

View of hypothesis	Study	Description of study	Findings
Favor	Barbee, Berry, & Micek (1969)	Inpatients randomly assigned to hospital-based work therapy or no-work control	Patients in work program remained hospitalized longer
Favor	Bond & Dincin (1986)	Psychosocial program participants randomly assigned to gradual or accelerated vocational program	After 15 months, 35% of gradual group on prevocational work crews versus 15% of accelerated group
Favor	Hartlage (1967)	Survey of psychiatric hospitals	Hospitals using work therapy "to keep patients active" reported lowest discharge rate
Neutral	Johnson & Lee (1965)	Inpatients matched on demographics, assigned to work therapy or no work control	No differences in hospital release time or subsequent community adjustment
Favor	Mezquita (1973)	Correlational study of patients in hospital-based work therapy	Patients with maximum salaries remained in rehabilitation unit longer
Favor	Vitale & Steinbach (1965)	Matched clients assigned to mental hygiene clinic or to more intensive day treatment	Mental hygiene group spent less time in clinic and more were employed
Oppose	Watson & Maddigan (1972)	Inpatients randomly assigned to paid work program or no work control	Long-term patients unaffected by work program in terms of days in community. Short-term patients in work program had more days in community.

work programs located within a hospital. Kuldau and Dirks (1977) showed that inpatients who were provided with an employment service, community housing, and day treatment had significantly better employment outcomes than a control group which was offered unpaid hospital work. Similarly, Ryan and Bell (1985) have shown that providing VA inpatients with vocational training and community jobs leads to somewhat better employment outcomes at six months than does a traditional intensive inpatient program. Marx, Test, and Stein (1973) showed that inpatients who were discharged and provided intensive case management had better employment outcomes than patients who received progressive inpatient treatment including paid hospital work. On the basis of studies of industrial therapy in British hospitals, Davies (1972) concluded that work programs within the hospital "do not subject patients to the same demands and pressures they are likely to meet in normal factories."

Sheltered Work

A widely used option for psychiatric clients is the sheltered workshop. This approach includes both rehabilitation centers serving a general disabled population (Bellak and Black 1960; Ciardiello 1981; Estroff 1981; Gellman 1957; Lamb et al. 1971; Olshansky 1973; Richardson and Krieger 1976) and workshops specifically designed for psychiatric clients (Cohen 1976; Evje et al. 1972; Gold Award 1980; Gray 1980; Price, Rance, and Pribnow 1979; Roomy 1984; Wilder 1976). Several British programs (Acharya et al. 1982; Davies 1972; Early 1975; Stevens 1973) appear also to include sheltered workshops, although because of differences in British laws regarding employment of the disabled and British psychiatric services, direct comparisons are difficult. Some workshops are time-limited, while others are intended to be permanent placements. Sometimes the workshop is seen as a setting in which to assess whether a client is prepared to go on to competitive employment (Gellman 1957; Salkind 1971a). Sometimes the workshop is expressly intended as a long-term placement (Wilder 1976). We found only two controlled evaluations of the effects of sheltered workshops on competitive employment rates (Griffiths 1974; Weinberg and Lustig 1968). While neither found significant results, both studies were limited by their small sample size. Sheltered employment has also been used as an outcome variable in a number of studies (Lamb and Goertzel 1972; Marx, Test, and Stein 1973; Stein and Test 1980). Sheltered work has been seen, then, both as an end in itself and as a means to an end.

Most observers agree that sheltered work is an appropriate terminal goal for a segment of the mentally ill population, as is the case for other disabilities. But even when the workshop experience is intended to be temporary, there is a tendency for clients to remain indefinitely. Two surveys document this point. Greenleigh Associates' (1975) national sheltered workshop survey found that only 10 percent of workshop clients were placed annually in competitive employment. Rudrud, Ziarnik, Bernstein, and Ferrara (1984) cited a survey indicating that only 3 percent of clients in sheltered employment for at least two years ever continued on to competitive employment. While Olshansky (1973) argued that most clients who are referred to workshops require permanent sheltered work, it is also plausible that, once placed, clients develop an institutional dependency which may make it difficult for them to consider more independent alternatives.

A more specific drawback of traditional sheltered workshops is that psychiatric clients apparently have poorer outcomes than clients with other disabilities. Studies by Ciardiello (1981), Olshansky (Olshansky 1973; Olshansky and Beach 1974, 1975), and Dalton and Latz (1978) found that, at least in comparison to the mentally retarded, the mentally ill are less successful. Gellman (1957) reported that the emotionally disturbed "presented the most difficult problems." Whitehead (1977) found that mentally ill clients earned an average of $0.45 per hour in workshops, compared with $1.05 per hour for other disabled persons.

A compilation of results from studies with comparisons among two or more disability groups is given in Table 16.4. Generally these investigators have compared the success rates for disability groups with no attempt to control for severity of disability. On a conceptual level one can question the meaningfulness of cross-disability comparisons, but as a practical matter, programs are vitally concerned with how well certain disability groups will do in their setting. While these results are somewhat mixed, there is a general consensus that psychiatric clients are more difficult to place than those with other disabilities (Dunn 1981).

Some authors have suggested that since traditional workshops are designed for the physically disabled and the mentally retarded, they are not well suited to the mentally ill (Ciardiello 1981; Newman 1970). In a participant-observer study, Estroff (1981) found that mentally ill clients disliked sheltered workshops, not only because of the low pay and monotonous work, but also because of the stigma of being in a work setting with mentally retarded persons.

Adaptations of sheltered programs that take into consideration the strengths and weaknesses of the mentally ill may fare better. In this regard, more research on career development needs to be conducted (Lustig, Lam, and Leahy 1986). Ciardiello (1981) found that schizophrenic clients did significantly poorer than the general working population on a battery of tests measuring finger dexterity and the ability to assemble parts—that is, the very kinds of skills required in an industrial workshop. Wilson and Rasch (1982) found that the placements which psychiatric clients held longest usually involved working with things rather than with people or data. In an early study, Johnson and Patterson (1957) reported that World War II veterans classified as psychotic did poorly when compared to physically disabled veterans in skilled and semiskilled work. Probably through intuition and trial and error, rehabilitation programs for the mentally ill have selected sheltered and transitional work programs which avoid a high level of interpersonal skills and fine motor coordination. So, for example, janitorial services, housekeeping, and stock work are popular choices. (These are also, of course, low-status positions.) Studies need to be conducted to test these intuitions.

More detailed investigations of where and when work is done are also needed. Dincin (personal communication) has speculated that the choice of service occupations, such as janitorial work and housekeeping, may be

Table 16.4

Employment Rates for the Mentally Ill and for Other Disability Groups

Study	Program type	Comparison groups	Employment criterion	Percentage employed				
				Mentally ill	Neurotic	Mentally retarded	Physically disabled	Other
Barkley, Pixley, & Walker (1976)	Hospital-based	Mentally retarded, personality disorder, organic brain syndrome	Full-time employment > 3 months	14		10		9
Miskimins, Cole, & Oetting (1968)	Hospital-based	Alcoholic	Employed at time of study and employment > 6 months	47				47
Acharya et al. (1982)	Sheltered	Affective disorder, neurosis, personality disorder, organic	Open employment	73	43[a]			43[a]
Ciardiello (1981)	Sheltered	Other (physically disabled or mentally retarded)	Successful completion of sheltered workshop	16		37[b]	37[b]	
Olshansky (1973), Olshansky & Beach (1974, 1975)	Sheltered	Mentally retarded, physically disabled	Competitive employment	25		40	26	
Azrin & Philip (1979)	Job club	Physically disabled	Obtained full-time employment	90			92	
Pumo, Sehl, & Cogan (1966)	Job club	Orthopedic, mentally retarded, blind, epileptic	Obtained employment	64		67	64	75
Dalton & Latz (1978)	Occupational training	Mentally retarded, other nervous system disorders, orthopedic	Placed in employment	57	72	70 (mod.) 82 (mild)	60–78	
Johnson & Patterson (1957)	Occupational training	Neurotics, physically disabled	Obtained employment or completed training	39	56		62	

[a]Combined figure for neurotic, personality disorders, and organic brain syndrome.
[b]Combined figure for mentally retarded and physically disabled.

unwise when these jobs must be done at night, because they may have the unintended side effect of disrupting circadian rhythms. Rotating shift work is difficult even for normal workers (Rose 1984). Since mental illness is often accompanied by odd sleep patterns, shift work may be especially disruptive.

The traditional sheltered workshop typically attracts factory contract work and is done in a segregated setting. One alternative to this is the client-employing business. Carroll and Levye (1985) have described their experiences with two such businesses, a greenhouse and a bakery. Another variation on this model is the formation of a nonprofit corporation affiliated with a rehabilitation agency which seeks out subcontracts in the community for such jobs as yard work, janitorial services, and warehouse work. Thresholds, for example, has provided jobs through Thresholds Rehabilitation, Inc., for its members over the past several years (Forman and Hills-Cooper 1986).

The requirements for running a business and the rehabilitation needs of clients do not always coincide (Salkind 1971b). Proponents argue that the normalizing influence of the demands of a small business is healthy because it shifts clients' attention from personal problems to the concrete demands of production (Carroll and Levye 1985). However, client-employing businesses may tend to evaluate their success in terms of profits rather than clients served.

Client-employing businesses require leadership from individuals with an entrepreneural bent and tremendous energy. It is unlikely that such businesses are a viable alternative for more than a fraction of the mentally ill population.

The logical extension of the sheltered workshop is the segregated society or lodge, as formulated by Fairweather, Sanders, Maynard, Cressler, and Bleck (1969), in which clients not only work in a protected setting but also live together. A related "enclave" approach has been developed in England (Early 1975). Adaptations of the lodge model have been reported throughout the United States (Fairweather 1980). Fairweather (personal communication, 1986) states that there are over one hundred lodges currently in operation, noting a recent unpublished study conducted by the Texas Department of Mental Health. Since the promising initial research of Fairweather and his associates (1969), however, there have been no further published controlled evaluations.

A recent program evaluation of "small-group work therapy," an Arkansas program modeled after the lodge, examined employment success for fifty active members, who had averaged twelve years in the program (Faulkner et al. 1986). Ten percent were competitively employed, and 50 percent were employed under a handicapped worker's certificate. Altogether, 550 patients were treated in the program over a fourteen-year period. While about one-third of the initial group of 121 entrants into the program have gone on to more independent settings, there are no follow-up employment data.

Assertive Case Management

Stein and Test's (1980) Training in Community Living (TCL) program (known now as the Program for Assertive Community Treatment, or PACT) is based on the premise that clients must be helped specifically and concretely in the tasks of everyday living, including employment. Unlike the earlier hospital-based programs, which often assumed that transfer of training would naturally occur when the client was returned to the community, TCL staff help clients find jobs, take them to work if necessary, and go to extraordinary lengths to help them succeed.

The TCL model was preceded at Mendota State Hospital by a program following similar principles for inpatients (Marx, Test, and Stein 1973). Even earlier, some of these same general principles were used in the de-institutionalization of state hospital patients in Vermont (Brown 1970).

The effectiveness of assertive case management was supported in both of two well-designed, carefully executed studies (Marx, Test, and Stein 1973; Stein and Test 1980). Another study of long-term treatment of young schizophrenics, now in progress (Test, Knoedler, and Allness 1985), is expected to further replicate many of the basic findings. However, these studies have not supported the hypothesis that TCL prepares clients to continue functioning at the same level after the case management is discontinued.

Because of their disenchantment with sheltered workshops, the staff at TCL began developing their own vocational alternatives in the late 1970s. A study was designed to evaluate the relative effectiveness of their program for clients, who were provided with indigenous work training sites established by TCL staff, as compared with clients receiving TCL services and also assigned to sheltered workshops. They found no vocational differences between groups. Both approaches increased competitive employment. Employment outcomes deteriorated after service was discontinued (Field et al. n.d.).

Currently PACT is staffed with vocational rehabilitation counselors and has developed an extensive network of job sites. Among active members, 30–40 percent are employed at any given time, and another 40 percent are involved in prevocational activities (Knoedler 1986).

There have been a number of replications of the PACT model, although most have not emphasized vocational goals. One program, Harbinger, located in Grand Rapids, Michigan, attempts to place clients in community businesses. A controlled evaluation of ninety-one clients admitted over a thirty-month period found that 26 percent of Harbinger clients and 18 percent of controls were involved in some type of work, a nonsignificant difference (Mulder 1982).

The chief drawback of the PACT approach is that it brokers services, rather than offering them directly. Staff members are dependent on the availability and cooperation of community resources in providing intermediate vocational placements. The next type of program to be reviewed, the psychosocial rehabilitation program, shares with PACT a similar attitude regarding active outreach and concrete help, but differs in the way vocational programming is provided.

Psychosocial Rehabilitation

"Psychosocial rehabilitation" (PSR) is a philosophy which emphasizes pragmatic goals such as prevention of rehospitalization, competitive employment, and independent living (Dincin 1975). Those served by PSR are referred to as "members" to stress their need to be involved in a total program of rehabilitation, including social, recreational, and residential opportunities. Services are not compartmentalized into different service agencies. In the vocational program the emphasis is on teaching proper work habits and attitudes rather than on training in the skills needed for a specific occupation. Most members are then placed in entry-level jobs rather than in skilled positions, regardless of their prior work history. The goal is to provide success experiences and to avoid the past pattern of repeated failures characteristic of many members.

Fountain House pioneered the use of the transitional employment program (TEP) for the psychiatric population and is the oldest and largest of PSR agencies (Bean and Beard 1975; Beard, Propst, and Malamud 1982; Beard et al. 1964; Lanoil 1982). In a recent survey Rutman (1986) found that of 157 agencies who had sent staff to Fountain House for training, 105 currently had TEPs.

The vocational program at Thresholds is a good example of the PSR model (Bond and Dincin 1986). It consists of a series of graded work experiences. The prevocational program consists of morning work crews which work on various chores necessary for the maintenance of the program (e.g., housekeeping, food preparation) or engage in clerical work (such as mass mailings for Thresholds or other nonprofit agencies). While members are not paid, they are expected to function as regular employees by being punctual, attending regularly, dressing properly, taking instruction, and so forth. Within the TEP there are two major gradations: the group placement, in which a number of members work at a site under the supervision of a Thresholds staff worker, and the individual placement, in which the member works as a regular employee, usually on a time-limited basis.

Paradigmatically, members begin in the prevocational crew, move on to the group placement after three to six months depending on their progress, then move on to individual placement, and finally, move to their own job. Members usually start with a two-day-per-week schedule, gradually increasing their hours to a maximum of twenty hours per week. Members who fail at a placement are given other opportunities; usually they return to the crew before starting a new placement. Volunteer placements—that is, employment in nonpaying jobs in the community—are another alternative for members, either as an intermediate step between the prevocational crew and TEP, or as temporary alternatives when paid placements are not available (Keys 1982; Lang, Richman, and Trout 1984).

An early study by Meltzoff and Blumenthal (1966) described a day treatment program with a vocational component which appears to share the PSR philosophy of gradual introduction of clients into the world of work. The experimental group, which was compared to clients receiving traditional office therapy, was twice as likely to have attempted competitive employment. However, even for the experimental group, the average duration of employment was less than one month over an eighteen-month period.

No differences in employment rates between a control group with no vocational program and a group in a vocational program have been found in studies conducted at Fountain House (Beard et al. 1963), Hill House (Wolkon, Karmen, and Tanaka 1971), or Thresholds (Dincin and Witheridge 1982). However, the Hill House study is not a stringent test of the psychosocial rehabilitation model in that the vocational program appears to have been limited. Wolkon, Karmen, and Tanaka (1971) note that "the major method of intervention is social group work, with individual counseling and transitional work projects provided as needed." None of these three reports documents the extent of transitional employment participation in the experimental condition.

Dincin and Witheridge (1982) found identical employment rates for Thresholds members and a randomly assigned control group not receiving vocational programming. The average earnings from employment were actually greater for the control group. A possible explanation for these null findings is that, like the comprehensive day program in the Vitale and Steinbach (1965) study, psychosocial rehabilitation programs may foster an institutional dependency in the form of the prevocational crews. The crews may provide a warm and supportive environment which may not challenge members to seek jobs, at least in the short term.

The role of prevocational crews has been examined in only a few studies. Growick (1976) found that a work-adjustment program improved work attitudes but did not decrease manifest anxiety. Turkat and Buzzell (1982) examined client movement through their PSR program. Clients typically showed alternating cycles of progress and regression. Members returned more frequently to the prevocational crews than to any other program component. The authors suggest that while transitional employment may be more "glamorous and innovative," prevocational training is more heavily used. In a survey conducted by members in twenty-four psychosocial clubhouses, Malamud and associates (1985) found that only 12 percent of a sample of 1,400 members were in competitive or transitional employment and 46 percent were still involved in prevocational day program activities. In practice, prevocational training seems to be used at least partly to keep clients engaged in a rehabilitation program. A multisite evaluation of prevocational training currently underway in Ohio should increase our understanding of its role (Knicely, personal communication, 1986).

As a follow-up to the earlier Thresholds study, Bond and Dincin (1986) examined whether an accelerated approach to TEP might lead to better vocational outcomes, drawing on Newman's (1970) concept of "instant placement." The rationale was that the prevocational work crews might actually be creating a disincentive to seeking competitive employment. The study also examined whether an accelerated approach might at the same time precipitate a higher rate of rehospitalization. Lamb and Goertzel (1972) found that a high-expectancy treatment program for patients discharged from a state hospital, while leading to better employment outcomes, also led to an initially higher rehospitalization rate.

Bond and Dincin (1986) found that, after fifteen months, 20 percent of the accelerated subjects were in competitive employment, compared with 7 percent of gradual subjects ($p < .10$), and that 15 percent of the accelerated subjects were attending prevocational crews, compared with 35 percent of the gradual subjects (a significant difference). Accelerated subjects had been employed in either TEP or competitive employment for significantly more weeks during the follow-up period than controls. There were no differences between conditions in rehospitalization rates.

Although PSR programs have been shown to reduce rehospitalization (Beard, Malamud, and Rossman 1978; Bond et al. 1984; Dincin and Witheridge 1982), they have not demonstrated their value in increasing competitive employment, despite their vocational emphasis.

A number of studies have suggested that the longer clients attend a vocational program, the better their vocational outcomes (see Table 16.5). The majority have studied PSR programs. Because of the correlational nature of these studies, however, it is unclear how to interpret these findings. One possibility is that the more vocationally prepared and better motivated clients are more likely to continue in such programs. Alternatively, the effects of rehabilitation may be slow and cumulative (Bond et al. 1984; Harding et al. 1985; Test et al. 1985).

Table 16.5
Studies Examining the Attendance-Outcome Hypothesis

Study	Program type	Nature of comparison	Results
Douzinas & Carpenter (1981)	Hospital-based	Completers vs. noncompleters	Completing the vocational program accounted for the largest portion (43%) of the variance in obtaining full-time employment
Evje et al. (1972)	Sheltered	Those competitively employed, those in sheltered employment, and those not employed	Hours spent in program predicted employment outcomes. $\bar{X} = 287$ no employment $\bar{X} = 360$ sheltered $\bar{X} = 521$ competitive
Barry (1982)	Psychosocial	Correlational	$r = 0.46$ between time in program and length of time in competitive employment
Bond (1984)	Psychosocial	Cross-tabulation of time in program and 6-month follow-up status	Linear relationship between time in program and percentage self-supporting. <6 mos. 17% 6–12 mos. 17% 12–24 mos. 33% >24 mos. 44%
Dincin & Kaberon (1979)	Psychosocial	Length of stay for employed vs. unemployed members at termination	Mean days in program $\bar{X} = 172$ for those employed $\bar{X} = 133$ for those unemployed
Roomy (1984)	Psychosocial	Completers vs. noncompleters	Completers of the program were employed more hours than noncompleters
Azrin & Philip (1979)	Job club	Correlational	$r = -0.62$ between percentage of sessions attended and number of days required to find a job
Purvis & Miskimins (1970)	Counseling	Active participants vs. nonparticipants	No relationship between active participation and vocational success

Supported Employment

"Supported employment" is an extension of the concept of TEP to permanent placements in community jobs (Black 1977, 1985). Variations of this model have been more widely used in Europe than in the United States (Bennett 1971). In the United States, state and federal dollars have been rapidly increasing, but most such programs have been funded for the mentally retarded population (Rutman 1986).

A federal program providing supported employment is Projects with Industry, or PWI (Pati and Adkins 1981; Pati and Morrison 1982). One such PWI program, the Midwest Association of Business, Rehabilitation, and Industry, an affiliate of Jewish Vocational Services located in Chicago, serves a mixed disability population. Program statistics showed that 26 percent of their initial clients were mentally ill (Pati and Adkins 1981). In its first two years, JVS-MABRI placed 69 percent of 240 job-ready applicants, of whom 93 percent maintained employment for thirty or more days (Pati and Morrison 1982). Separate statistics for mentally ill clients are not available, although placing them appears to be more difficult and to require more follow-up than with other disabilities. An important question is what proportion of the mentally ill population, and with what preparation, would be appropriate for PWI.

Laws governing supported work are much more favorable in Europe. Bordieri and Comninel (1986) have identified four international approaches: quota systems, government grants, government wage subsidies, and affirmative industries. None of these are without drawbacks, and all but the last would require changes in national policy. The Marriott Corporation is an example of an employer that has sponsored affirmative action for those with psychiatric disabilities.

Rehabilitation Counseling

Wehman (1981) has suggested that verbal counseling is a weak form of intervention which, by itself, is an inappropriate vocational strategy for the severely disabled. Two early studies with the mentally ill (Briggs and Yater 1966; Purvis and Miskimins 1970) support this viewpoint.

Anthony's skill-training model has been examined in the context of training rehabilitation counselors (A Skills-Training Approach, 1980). His assumption is that counselors cannot help clients achieve a higher skill level than the counselors themselves exhibit. Anthony's study demonstrated that counseling skills could be taught and that clients seen by more skilled counselors felt better understood. Psychiatric clients assisted by counselors trained in this program increased their employment rate from 27 percent for the six months prior to the counselors' training to 46 percent at follow-up. Without a control group, however, these findings are difficult to evaluate.

Many of the models which stress counseling processes have been developed in academic settings rather than by practitioners in psychiatric programs (Anthony 1980; Lustig, Lam, and Leahy, 1986; Rubin and Roessler 1978). Some of these models are based on theories of rehabilitation originally developed for other disability populations. The assumption that rehabilitation concepts developed for the physically disabled can be adapted to psychiatrically disabled (Anthony 1982) has not been empirically validated.

Job Clubs

The job club, a structured approach to gaining employment (Azrin and Besalel 1980), was developed by Azrin for the general unemployed population. It has been adopted for use with psychiatric clients with encouraging results (Azrin and Philip 1979; Jacobs et al. 1984; Keith, Engelkes, and Winborn 1977).

Azrin and Philip (1979) randomly assigned a heterogenous sample of job-seekers to their job club or to a lecture control group. Within the subsample of former psychiatric patients, 89 percent of the nineteen assigned to the job club obtained jobs, compared to 33 percent of the six controls. Certain methodological details of this study are bothersome: the criterion for success was obtaining a job, and no data on job retention are reported; only 32 percent of the sample was followed at six months; dropout rate is not reported; only clients who attended the respective programs are included. Also, the distribution of formerly hospitalized clients between the two treatment conditions is skewed.

Keith, Engelkes, and Winborn (1977) obtained results similar to Azrin and Philip's for a heterogeneous disabled population, although they do not give findings for the psychiatric subsample. Subsequent research by Jacobs (Jacobs et al. 1984) casts doubt on Azrin and Philip's (1979) claim that the approach works equally well for all disabled populations. These investigators found that the psychiatric clients required a longer period of time to obtain jobs than the general figures reported by Azrin and Philip. Kramer and Beidel (1982) reported that only 15 percent (6 of 41) of the clients in the job-finding program were employed at one-year follow-up, although their approach did not follow Azrin's principles.

Several authors have made contradictory suggestions for modifications. Dunham (1982) suggests that the group should meet only once per week to avoid undue pressures. Jacobs and associates (1984), on the other hand, feel that the daily approach provided the structure needed by the mentally ill. Kramer and Beidel (1982) suggest that the job club may need to be more intensive than their twenty-hour program to be successful.

Despite these objections, the job club seems to be a promising technique which could be used in conjunction with other vocational programs. Finding a job is part of the process, but it does not address the fact that psychiatric clients have great difficulty retaining jobs. Research needs to include an assessment of who does best in these programs (looking at dropouts and remainers, for example) and information on job retention.

Remedial Educational and Occupational Training

The dual handicaps of mental illness and academic deficits have been found to be strongly associated with vocational difficulties (Katz-Garris

1982; Marengo 1983). At Thresholds as many as half of new admissions score below the ninth-grade level in both reading and mathematics (Bond et al. 1984). For that reason Thresholds has developed a remedial educational program to help members obtain their G.E.D. Basic educational and occupational training is likely to be an important component of vocational preparation, although this area has not been researched.

One study of a comprehensive rehabilitation center serving clients with either physical or behavioral disabilities, however, has found that type of occupational training received did not match type of job obtained (Cook and Brookings 1980). This finding is congruent with the practice in PSR programs of training work habits and not specific vocational skills.

Postemployment Services

If mentally ill clients are able to obtain jobs but have more difficulty than other disabled groups in keeping them (Roessler, Hinman, and Greenwood 1985), then vocational programs should include intensive postemployment services (Sands and Radin 1979). In most PSR programs clients continue to attend weekly employment groups and to see their caseworker for an extended period of time after obtaining competitive employment. There are no published evaluations of follow-up services, even though the literature suggests that success rates decline after treatment is terminated.

Summary: Evaluation Studies

Do psychiatric vocational programs help clients achieve competitive employment? The answer is complicated by the diverse outcome measures used. If the criterion is the competitive employment rate at the end of the follow-up period, then only two studies (Bell and Ryan 1984; Marx, Test, and Stein 1973) yielded significant results. If the criterion is job starts in competitive employment, then four other studies (Azrin and Philip 1979; Kuldau and Dirks 1977; Meltzoff and Blumenthal 1966; Ryan and Bell 1985) might qualify. Compiling the summary judgments given in the competitive employment columns listed in Table 16.2 shows that only four of twenty-one studies showed an overall advantage to experimental subjects on competitive employment. Moreover, these four studies each have methodological limitations. The general conclusion is that none of the approaches discussed in this chapter have demonstrated efficacy in helping clients achieve and maintain competitive employment over any sustained period of time.

In contrast, when the criterion was paid employment (including transitional and sheltered employment), eight of ten studies indicate that when clients are given intensive support and are placed in jobs that are not too demanding, they often function at a level beyond usual expectations. Both intensive support and positive expectations that clients can succeed appear to be important elements. Given the additional finding that employment success is often not maintained after treatment ends (Fairweather et al. 1969; Test, Knoedler, and Allness 1985), then supported work programs may be the best way to increase employment rates.

Directions for Future Research

Standardization of Employment Outcome Criteria

Employment measures are confounded by labor market conditions, and there are certain types of productive activities (such as housework, volunteer work, and schoolwork) which have an ambiguous relationship to employment (Bachrach 1976). Despite their imperfections, employment measures are objective and verifiable, they are consensually validated indicators of adjustment, and they are associated with positive self-regard.

As a reaction to the vocational rehabilitation (VR) system's dependence on an oversimplified definition of successful closure, Reagles, Wright, and Butler (1972) and Hawryluk (1972, 1974) have advocated composite indices of rehabilitation gain. However, such indices are one level of abstraction away from the raw data and as such may obfuscate research findings. The advantage of conventional employment measures is that they can be interpreted directly and also analyzed statistically.

The following suggestions are derived from the literature review. First, the measures should be appropriate and sensitive to the actual effects of vocational programs. Full-time employment, as stipulated by Anthony and associates (1972), may be too stringent as the sole measure of success. Part-time community employment is an appropriate goal for a large segment of the unemployed mentally ill population. On the other hand, combining paid employment, school attendance, volunteer work, and even, in some instances, attendance in a day program into a single category of productive activity, as do some investigators, dilutes the concept of employment beyond useful limits. Paid employment seems to be a suitable compromise and should be a major outcome variable.

Second, the use of multiple outcome measures is recommended, instead of the composite measure discussed above. Despite possible redundancy, this approach makes interstudy comparisons possible. Moreover, using multiple measures generally requires only a modest additional amount of data collection and compilation. Measures should include the percentage of clients in paid employment at the end of evaluation period, the percentage of time employed, and total earnings from employment (Bond and Dincin 1986). Studies should also report the percentage of clients in full-time employment and the percentage of clients employed at any time during the follow-up period. A number of investigators have reported a breakdown of vocational outcomes according to a continuum. Providing such detailed information allows other investigators to draw their own conclusions.

Measures based on employment "at any time" during an evaluation period must be interpreted cautiously because of the difficulty clients have in retaining jobs. Type and level of occupational attainment has been considered by some investigators (e.g., Jacobs et al. 1984). Inclusion of this information in an evaluation study may be useful in advancing our understanding of the client-occupation matching process. In reality, most graduates of psychiatric rehabilitation programs achieve, at best, entry-level jobs, making this point less relevant. In addition, wages may serve as a convenient proxy for occupational attainment.

Job satisfaction has been reported by a number of investigators. Inclusion of a simple scale within an outcome battery may be helpful for understanding job retention (Estroff 1981).

Ideally one would like measures of job performance, but pragmatically it is difficult to build such measures into an evaluation design. Moreover, in the case of paid employment, adequacy of job performance is indirectly, if imperfectly, measured by job retention.

The use of individualized vocational outcome measures, such as Goal Attainment Scaling (Kiresuk and Sherman 1968), is not recommended even though success for one client may be different than for another. Such problems are better addressed through the selection of homogeneous samples and sample stratification.

Adequacy of Follow-up

The length of the follow-up period becomes a critical variable because of the length of time required to achieve rehabilitation gains. Some of the studies reviewed did not have a standardized interval for follow-up, and most of the controlled studies used a follow-up interval of eighteen months or less. A consistent drawback to extending the follow-up period is sample attrition, although a low percentage of lost subjects with longer follow-up is possible (Harding et al. 1985). Dropouts from a program are usually the hardest to locate at follow-up. Because dropouts often have poorer outcomes, studies which have high sample attrition run the risk of biasing results. These should be minimum standards: an eighteen-month follow-up period and 80 percent follow-up rate on the initial sample.

Description of Samples

A major ambiguity in the studies reviewed is the comparability of samples. Lacking valid measures of vocational potential (Anthony and Jansen 1984), investigators have described their samples in only the broadest of terms. Discrepancies in success rates can be explained partly on this basis. For example, because the VR system is mandated to accept cases believed to be rehabilitable, success rates are not comparable to those for samples of unscreened clients discharged from state hospitals.

Beyond basic demographic information (especially age, sex, education, and number of lifetime hospitalizations) studies should report summary information on length of unemployment, longest time continuously employed in community jobs, and source of income. Income source is important because of studies supporting a "disincentive hypothesis" for some forms of government assistance (Berkowitz 1981; Walls 1982). Researchers should carefully document dropout rates throughout every stage of the rehabilitation program. If these suggestions seem obvious, a scan of the literature will demonstrate how incomplete this information often is.

Another issue is equivalence of experimental and control groups when there is sample attrition. High dropout rates defeat the purpose of randomization. One counterstrategy was used by Bond and Dincin (1986), who waited until clients had attended the vocational program for a month before randomizing subjects. In this way they eliminated from their sample clients who were early dropouts from the program.

Stratification of Samples

The value of sample stratification in evaluating vocational programs has now been shown in a number of studies. The general design strategy requires classifying clients on a specific background variable prior to randomization. Logistically, such a design involves little additional effort. The resultant factorial design allows for better control of a potentially confounding variable and for examination of interaction effects.

Three studies used prior work experience to classify clients (Bond and Dincin 1986; Kuldau and Dirks 1977; Ryan and Bell 1985). A simple dichotomy was used in each case; for example, Bond and Dincin defined clients as "work-experienced" if they had been employed continuously for at least one year at any time prior to admission and classified the remainder as "work-inexperienced." All three studies had the same basic results: Clients with better work histories benefited significantly more from the enriched vocational program as compared with the control treatment; clients with poorer work histories did poorly in both conditions.

Meltzoff and Blumenthal (1966) classified clients as either "high adjusted" or "low adjusted," based on ratings on eight psychological dimensions. In the experimental condition, 50 percent of the high adjusted group obtained employment, compared with 19 percent of the low adjusted group. In the control condition, 26 percent of the high adjusted group obtained employment, compared with none of the controls.

Cost-Benefit Issues

Proponents of rehabilitation services have traditionally used economic arguments to justify programs, arguing that taxpayers' money is wisely spent on rehabilitation efforts (Berkowitz and Berkowitz 1983). Few of the studies reviewed, however, included estimates of costs and benefits. The reasons are not difficult to find: measurement of economic variables is complex, and few economists have been involved in mental health research. By general consensus, only one mental health study (Weisbrod, Test, and Stein 1980) qualifies as a comprehensive cost-benefit analysis.

Nevertheless, economic issues of vocational programs should not be ignored. A preliminary effort would include estimates of the following variables for three time frames (before, during, and after treatment): (a) employment earnings, (b) government assistance received by clients, (c) program costs, and (d) hospitalization costs. Given the modest employment outcomes reported in most studies, employment earnings seldom offset program costs in the short term (Bond 1984). Methodologies used with other disabilities which project future earnings (Reagles, Wright, and Butler 1972) require unrealistic assumptions when applied to mentally ill clients, who have difficulties with job retention.

A study by Richardson and Krieger (1976) suggests a compromise methodology for estimating future earnings: the use of data from only the most successful clients in the computation of future benefits. Their approach is based on the assumption that the high-success group may sustain employment over the long term. No completely satisfactory method has yet been proposed which accurately represents long-term benefits. On the available evidence it appears that vocational programs for the mentally ill are difficult to justify on a solely monetary basis.

Conclusion

In this chapter we have suggested a typology of vocational programs for the mentally ill. Whether it adequately represents the field is an empirical question. More surveys like those conducted by Fountain House (1984) and Greenleigh Associates (1975) to identify what proportion of clients are being served in various types of programs are needed. It is likely that most mentally ill clients, in fact, receive no vocational programming at all. A 1983 survey of community mental health centers in Indiana found that 74 percent of the chronically mentally ill clients seen in these centers were unemployed, 2 percent were in volunteer employment, 4 percent were doing sheltered work, 17 percent were competitively employed, and 3 percent were in school or in training (Miller 1985). This same survey identified psychosocial/vocational programming as the second highest priority need (after housing) among eleven possible alternatives.

We have stressed the theme of institutional dependency throughout this chapter. Paradoxically, we have also suggested that clients are most likely to benefit from long-term involvement in rehabilitation programs. The resolution of these two seemingly contradictory sets of findings is this: clients need both to be challenged and to be supported. Extended participation in overly protective environments is stultifying. On the other hand, psychiatric clients need long-term support in retaining jobs; placing them in paid employment is nearer the beginning than the end of that process. They need programs which accommodate their relapses and slow progress.

This review comes at a time when there has been renewed interest in vocational rehabilitation for the mentally ill at both the state and federal levels. While our conclusions are pessimistic, much of the research we reviewed was done during a period of great upheaval related to deinstitutionalization. Whether or not there will be a maturing of the field of psychiatric rehabilitation which will lead to greater success in the vocational arena remains to be seen.

Acknowledgment

Our thanks to Ralph Swindle, Ph.D., South Central Community Mental Health Center, Bloomington, Indiana, for his helpful comments.

References

Acharya, S.; Ekdawi, M. Y.; Gallagher, L.; and Glaister, B. 1982. Day-hospital rehabilitation: A six-year study. *Social Psychiatry, 17,* 1–5.

Anthony, W. A. 1980. *The principles of psychiatric rehabilitation.* Baltimore: University Park Press.

———. 1982. Explaining "psychiatric rehabilitation" by an analogy to "physical restoration." *Psychosocial Rehabilitation Journal, 5,* 61–65.

Anthony, W. A.; Buell, G. J.; Sharratt, S.; and Althoff, M. E. 1972. Efficacy of psychiatric rehabilitation. *Psychological Bulletin, 78,* 447–56.

Anthony, W. A.; Cohen, M. R.; and Vitalo, R. 1978. The measurement of rehabilitation outcome. *Schizophrenia Bulletin, 4,* 365–83.

Anthony, W. A., and Jansen, M. A. 1984. Predicting the vocational capacity of the chronically mentally ill. *American Psychologist, 39,* 537–44.

Azrin, N. H., and Besalel, V. B. 1980. *Job club counselor's manual: A behavioral approach to vocational counseling.* Baltimore: University Park Press.

Azrin, N. H., and Philip, R. A. 1979. The job-club method for job handicapped: A comparative outcome study. *Rehabilitation Counseling Bulletin, 23,* 144–55.

Bachrach, L. L. 1976. A note on some recent studies of released mental hospital patients in the community. *American Journal of Psychiatry, 133,* 73–75.

Barbee, M. S.; Berry, K. L.; and Micek, L. A. 1969. Relationship of work therapy to psychiatric length of stay and readmission. *Journal of Consulting and Clinical Psychology, 33,* 735–38.

Barkley, A. L.; Pixley, F.; and Walker, C. 1976. Industrial therapy: A study of success rates over an eight-year period. *Rehabilitation Literature, 37,* 130–39, 144.

Barry, P. 1982. Correlational study of a psychosocial rehabilitation program. *Vocational Evaluation and Work Adjustment Bulletin, 15,* 112–17.

Bean, B. R., and Beard, J. H. 1975. Placement for persons with psychiatric disability. *Rehabilitation Counseling Bulletin, 18,* 253–58.

Beard, J. H.; Malamud, T. J.; and Rossman, E. 1978. Psychiatric rehabilitation and long-term rehospitalization rates: The findings of two research studies. *Schizophrenia Bulletin,* 4, 622–35.

Beard, J. H.; Pitt, R. B.; Fisher, S. H.; and Goertzel, V. 1963. Evaluating the effectiveness of a psychiatric rehabilitation program. *American Journal of Orthopsychiatry, 33,* 701–12.

Beard, J. H.; Propst, R. N.; and Malamud, T. J. 1982. The Fountain House model of psychiatric rehabilitation. *Psychosocial Rehabilitation Journal, 5,* 47–54.

Beard, J. H.; Schmidt, J. R.; Smith, M. M.; and Dincin, J. 1964. Three aspects of psychiatric rehabilitation at Fountain House. *Mental Hygiene, 48,* 11–21.

Becker, R. E. 1967. An evaluation of a rehabilitation program for chronically hospitalized psychiatric patients. *Social Psychiatry, 2,* 32–38.

Bell, M. D., and Ryan, E. R. 1984. Integrating psychosocial rehabilitation into the hospital psychiatric service. *Hospital and Community Psychiatry, 35,* 1017–28.

Bellak, L., and Black, B. J. 1960. The rehabilitation of psychotics in the community. *American Journal of Orthopsychiatry, 30,* 346–55.

Bennett, D. 1971. The hard-to-employ. *Occupational Mental Health, 1,* 9–12.

Berkowitz, M. 1981. Disincentives and the rehabilitation of disabled persons. *Annual Review of Rehabilitation, 2,* 40–57.

Berkowitz, M., and Berkowitz, E. 1983. *Benefit cost analysis.* Washington, D.C.: National Rehabilitation Information Center.

Black, B. J. 1977. Substitute permanent employment for the deinstitutionalized mentally ill. *Journal of Rehabilitation, 43,* 32–35, 39.

———. 1985. New developments in the use of work for therapy and rehabilitation of mental patients. Paper presented at the meeting of the International Association of Psychosocial Rehabilitation Services, Boston, June.

Bond, G. R. 1984. An economic analysis of psychosocial rehabilitation. *Hospital and Community Psychiatry, 35,* 356–62.

Bond, G. R., and Dincin, J. 1986. Accelerating entry into transitional employment in a psychosocial rehabilitation agency. *Rehabilitation Psychology, 31(3),* 143–55.

Bond, G. R.; Dincin, J.; Setze, P. J.; and Witheridge, T. F. 1984. The effectiveness of psychiatric rehabilitation: A summary of research at Thresholds. *Psychosocial Rehabilitation Journal, 7,* 6–22.

Bordieri, J. E., and Comninel, M. E. 1986. Competitive employment for workers with disabilities: An international perspective. Menomonie, Wis.: University of Wisconsin—Stout. Unpublished paper.

Briggs, P. F., and Yater, A. C. 1966. Counseling and psychometric signs as determinants in the vocational success of discharged psychiatric patients. *Journal of Clinical Psychology, 22,* 100–104.

Brown, J. K. 1970. Mental patients work back into society. *Manpower, 2,* 23–25.

Carroll, C. R., and Levye, R. 1985. Cookie Place and a New Leaf: A profile of two businesses providing supported work for people with psychiatric disabilities. Paper presented at the meeting of the International Association of Psychosocial Rehabilitation Services, Boston, June.

Cheney, T. M., and Kish, G. B. 1970. Job development in a Veterans Administration Hospital. *Vocational Guidance Quarterly, 19,* 61–65.

Ciardiello, J. A. 1981. Job placement success of schizophrenic clients in sheltered workshop programs. *Vocational Evaluation and Work Adjustment Bulletin, 14,* 125–28, 140.

Cohen, L. 1976. A hospital's sheltered workshop as a rehabilitative and supportive resource for discharged patients. *Hospital and Community Psychiatry, 27,* 559–60.

Cook, D. W., and Brookings, J. B. 1980. The relationship of rehabilitation client vocational appraisal to training outcome and employment. *Journal of Applied Rehabilitation Counseling, 11,* 32–35.

Dalton, R. F., Jr., and Latz, A. 1978. Vocational placement: The Pennsylvania Rehabilitation Center. *Rehabilitation Literature, 39,* 336–39.

Davies, M. H. 1972. The rehabilitation of psychiatric patients at an industrial therapy unit outside the hospital. *International Journal of Social Psychiatry, 18,* 120–26.

Dincin, J. 1975. Psychiatric rehabilitation. *Schizophrenia Bulletin, 13,* 131–47.

Dincin, J., and Kaberon, D. A. 1979. *Attendance as a predictor of success in rehabilitation of former psychiatric patients.* Final report to the Chicago Community Trust.

Dincin, J., and Witheridge, T. F. 1982. Psychiatric rehabilitation as a deterrent to recidivism. *Hospital and Community Psychiatry, 33,* 645–50.

Douzinas, N., and Carpenter, M. D. 1981. Predicting the community performance of vocational rehabilitation clients. *Hospital and Community Psychiatry, 32,* 409–13.

Dunham, C. 1982. Don't talk about your delusions on the job: An experience with competitive job placement in psychiatric rehabilitation. *Psychosocial Rehabilitation Journal, 5,* 41–46.

Dunn, D. J. 1981. Current placement trends. In *Annual review of rehabilitation,* ed. E. Pan, T. E. Backer, and C. L. Vash, 2:113–146). New York: Springer.

Early, D. F. 1975. Sheltered groups in open industry. *Lancet, 1,* 1370–73.

Ekdawi, M. Y. 1972. The Netherne Resettlement Unit: Results of ten years. *British Journal of Psychiatry, 121,* 417–24.

Estroff, S. E. 1981. *Making it crazy.* Berkeley and Los Angeles: University of California Press.

Evje, M. C.; Bellander, I.; Gibby, M.; and Palmer, I. S. 1972. Evaluating protected hospital employment of chronic psychiatric patients. *Hospital and Community Psychiatry, 23,* 204–8.

Fairweather, G. W., ed. 1980. *The Fairweather Lodge: A twenty-year retrospective.* New directions for mental health services, no. 7. San Francisco: Jossey-Bass.

Fairweather, G. W.; Sanders, D. H.; Maynard, H.; Cressler, D. L.; and Bleck, D. S. 1969. *Community life for the mentally ill.* Chicago: Aldine.

Faulkner, L. R.; McFarland, B. H.; Larch, B. B.; Harris, W. J.; and Yohe, C. D. 1986. Small-group work therapy for the chronic mentally ill. *Hospital and Community Psychiatry, 37,* 273–79.

Field, G.; Allness, D.; Knoedler, W.; and Test, M. A. n.d. *Employment training for chronic patients in the community.* PACT, Mendota Mental Health Institute, Madison, Wis. 53704.

Forman, J. D., and Hills-Cooper, D. 1986. *Sheltered employment outside the sheltered environment.* Paper presented at the annual conference of the International Association of Psychosocial Rehabilitation Services, Cleveland.

Fountain House. 1984. *Transitional employment.* Survey Memorandum 271 (Dec. 7). New York: Fountain House.

Gellman, W. 1957. Vocational evaluation of the emotionally handicapped. *Journal of Rehabilitation, 23,* 9–10, 13, 32.

Gold Award. 1980. Community support services for adult psychiatric outpatients. *Hospital and Community Psychiatry, 31,* 693–96.

Gray, J. 1980. A follow-up study of psychiatric patients in a sheltered workshop program. *Hospital and Community Psychiatry, 31,* 563–66.

Greenleigh Associates. 1975. *The role of sheltered workshops in the rehabilitation of the severely disabled.* New York: Department of Health, Education, and Welfare.

Griffiths, R. D. 1974. Rehabilitation of chronic psychotic patients. *Psychological Medicine, 4,* 316–25.

Growick, B. S. 1976. Effects of a work-adjustment program on emotionally handicapped individuals. *Journal of Applied Rehabilitation Counseling, 7,* 119–23.

Harding, C. M.; Brooks, G. W.; Ashikaga, T.; and Strauss, J. S. 1985. The Vermont story: A twenty-year follow-up of 269 rehabilitated psychiatric patients for their chronicity. Paper presented at the meeting of the International Association of Psychosocial Rehabilitation Services, Boston.

Hartlage, L. C. 1967. Hospitals' and patients' views of industrial therapy. *Psychiatric Quarterly, 41,* 264–67.

Hawryluk, A. 1972. Rehabilitation gain: A better indicator needed. *Journal of Rehabilitation, 84,* 22–25.

———. 1974. Rehabilitation gain: A new criterion for an old concept. *Rehabilitation Literature, 35,* 322–28, 341.

Hoffman, H. J. 1965. Paid employment as a rehabilitative technique in a state mental hospital: A demonstration. *Mental Hygiene, 49,* 193–207.

Hogarty, G. E.; Goldberg, S. C.; and Schooler, N. R. 1974. Drug and sociotherapy in the aftercare of schizophrenic patients. *Archives of General Psychiatry, 31,* 609–18.

Hursh, N. C., and Anthony, W. A. 1983. The vocational preparation of the chronic psychiatric patient in the community. In *The chronic psychiatric patient in the community: Principles of treatment,* ed. I. Barofsky and R. D. Budson. New York: Spectrum Publications.

Jacobs, H. E.; Donahoe, C. P.; and Falloon, I. 1985. Rehabilitation of the chronic schizophrenic: Areas of intervention. *Annual Review of Rehabilitation, 4.*

Jacobs, H. E.; Kardashian, S.; Kreinbring, R. K.; Ponder, R.; and Simpson, A. R. 1984. A skills-oriented model for facilitating employment among psychiatrically disabled persons. *Rehabilitation Counseling Bulletin, 28,* 87–96.

Johnson, R. F., and Lee, H. 1965. Rehabilitation of chronic schizophrenics. *Archives of General Psychiatry, 12,* 237–40.

Johnson, R. H., and Patterson, C. H. 1957. Vocational objectives for the emotionally disabled. *Journal of Counseling Psychology, 4,* 291–96.

Katz-Garris, L. 1982. Group-oriented therapy with psychiatrically disabled persons. In *Group psychotherapy and counseling with special populations,* ed. M. Seligman. Baltimore: University Park Press.

Katz-Garris, L.; McCue, M.; Garris, R. P.; and Herring, J. 1983. Psychiatric rehabilitation: An outcome study. *Rehabilitation Counseling Bulletin, 27,* 329–35.

Keith, R. D.; Engelkes, J. R.; and Winborn, B. B. 1977. Employment-seeking preparation and activity: An experimental job-placement training model for rehabilitation clients. *Rehabilitation Counseling Bulletin, 21,* 159–65.

Keys, L. M. 1982. Former patients as volunteers in community agencies: A model work rehabilitation program. *Hospital and Community Psychiatry, 33,* 1017–18.

Kiresuk, T. J., and Sherman, R. E. 1968. Goal attainment scaling: A general method for evaluating comprehensive community mental health programs. *Community Mental Health Journal, 4,* 443–53.

Klein, M. 1984. An annotated bibliography of the vocational rehabilitation literature. University of Medicine and Dentistry of New Jersey, Community Mental Health Center at Piscataway. Mimeograph.

Knoedler, W. 1986. Ohio DMH/DVR Cross-training workshop. Presented to the Ohio Department of Mental Health Cross-Training of Trainers Conference, Mohican Park, Ohio. Columbus, Ohio, February.

Kramer, L. W., and Beidel, D. C. 1982. Job-seeking skill groups: Review and application to a chronic psychiatric population. *Occupational Therapy in Mental Health, 2,* 37–44.

Kuldau, J. M., and Dirks, S. J. 1977. Controlled evaluation of a hospital-originated community transitional system. *Archives of General Psychiatry, 34,* 1331–40.

Kunce, J. T. 1970. Is work therapy really therapeutic? *Rehabilitation Literature, 31,* 297–99, 320.

Lamb, H. R., et al. 1971. *Rehabilitation in community mental health.* San Francisco: Jossey-Bass.

Lamb, H. R., and Goertzel, V. 1972. High expectations of long-term ex–state hospital patients. *American Journal of Psychiatry, 129,* 471–75.

Lang, E.; Richman, A.; and Trout, P. 1984. Project Outreach: Volunteer transitional employment. *The Psychiatric Hospital, 15,* 75–80.

Lanoil, J. 1982. An analysis of the psychiatric psychosocial rehabilitation center. *Psychosocial Rehabilitation Journal, 5,* 55–59.

Llorens, L. A.; Levy, R.; and Rubin, E. Z. 1964. Work adjustment program. *American Journal of Occupational Therapy, 18,* 15–19.

Lustig, P.; Lam, C.; and Leahy, M. 1986. A conceptual approach to job placement with psychiatric and mentally retarded clients. *Journal of Applied Rehabilitation Counseling, 17,* 20–23.

Malamud, T. J.; Horne, R.; Lee, L.; Davoli, A.; and Johnson, K. 1985. National clubhouse outcome evaluation study. Paper presented at the meeting of the International Association of Psychosocial Rehabilitation Services, Boston, June.

Marengo, J. 1983. The prognosis of thought-disordered schizophrenics: A follow-up study. Ph.D. diss., Counseling Psychology Program, Northwestern University.

Marx, A. J.; Test, M. A.; and Stein, L. I. 1973. Extrahospital management of severe mental illness. *Archives of General Psychiatry, 29,* 505–11.

Meltzoff, J., and Blumenthal, R. L. 1966. *The day treatment center: Principles, application, and evaluation.* Springfield, Ill.: Charles C. Thomas.

Mezquita, J. 1973. Four years of industrial therapy at Mapperley Hospital: A survey. *Acta Psychiatrica Scandinavica, 49,* 1–14.

Mezquita-Blanco, J. 1984. Work therapy in psychiatric rehabilitation. *International Journal of Rehabilitation Research, 7,* 3–10.

Miller, L. 1985. Community support program: Aggregated data of chronically mentally ill persons seen in the CMHCs. Indiana Department of Mental Health, Indianapolis. Mimeographed.

Miskimins, R. W.; Cole, C. W.; and Oetting, E. R. 1968. Success rates in the vocational rehabilitation of mental patients. *Personnel and Guidance Journal, 46,* 801–5.

Mosher, L. R., and Menn, A. Z. 1978. Community residential treatment for schizophrenia: Two-year follow-up. *Hospital and Community Psychiatry, 29,* 715–23.

Mulder, R. 1982. *Final evaluation of the Harbinger Program as a demonstration project.* Grand Rapids, Mich.: Harbinger.

Newman, L. 1970. Instant placement: A new model for providing rehabilitation services within a community mental health program. *Community Mental Health Journal, 6,* 401–10.

Olshansky, S. 1973. A five-year follow-up of psychiatrically disabled clients. *Rehabilitation Literature, 34,* 15–16.

Olshansky, S., and Beach, D. 1974. A five-year follow-up of mentally retarded clients. *Rehabilitation Literature, 35,* 48–49.

———. 1975. A five-year follow-up of physically disabled clients. *Rehabilitation Literature, 36,* 251–52, 258.

Pati, G. C., and Adkins, J. I. 1981. *Managing and employing the handicapped.* Lake Forest, Ill.: Brace-Park.

Pati, G. C., and Morrison, G. 1982. Enabling the disabled. *Harvard Business Review, 60,* 152–60.

Price, A.; Rance, C.; and Pribnow, J. 1979. A work-activity program for former mental patients. *Hospital and Community Psychiatry, 20,* 849–50.

Programs for patient-workers: Approaches, problems in four institutions. 1976. *Hospital and Community Psychiatry, 27,* 93–98.

Pumo, B.; Sehl, R.; and Cogan, F. 1966. Job readiness: Key to placement. *Journal of Rehabilitation, 32,* 18–19.

Purvis, S. A., and Miskimins, R. W. 1970. Effects of community follow-up on post-hospital adjustment of psychiatric patients. *Community Mental Health Journal, 6*, 374–82.

Reagles, K. W.; Wright, G. N.; and Butler, A. J. 1972. Toward a new criterion of vocational rehabilitation success. *Rehabilitation Counseling Bulletin, 15*, 233–41.

Richardson, N., and Krieger, N. 1976. An evaluation of vocational placement success at a comprehensive rehabilitation center. *Rehabilitation Literature, 37*, 237–41.

Roessler, R. T.; Hinman, S.; and Greenwood, R. 1985. Enhancing employability through skill training and placement interventions. Paper presented at the meeting of the International Association of Psychosocial Rehabilitation Services, Boston, June.

Roomy, D. J. 1984. Thereapia for the chronically mentally ill: The therapeutic program at PORTAL. *Psychosocial Rehabilitation Journal, 7*(4), 24–36.

Rose, M. 1984. Shift work: How does it affect you? *American Journal of Nursing*, April, pp. 442–47.

Rubin, S. E., and Roessler, R. T. 1978. Guidelines for successful vocational rehabilitation of the psychiatrically disabled. *Rehabilitation Literature, 39*, 70–74.

Rudrud, E. H.; Ziarnik, J. P.; Bernstein, G. S.; and Ferrara, J. M. 1984. *Proactive vocational habilitation.k* Baltimore: Paul H. Brookes.

Rutman, I. D. 1986. A comprehensive, national evaluation of transitional employment programs for the psychiatrically disabled. Paper presented at the annual meeting of the International Association of Psychosocial Rehabilitation Services, Cleveland, June.

Ryan, E. R., and Bell, M. D. 1985. Rehabilitation of chronic psychiatric patients: A randomized clinical study. Paper presented at the American Psychological Association Convention, Los Angeles.

Salkind, I. 1971a. The rehabilitation workshop. In Lamb et al. 1971, pp. 50–70.

———. 1971b. Economic problems of workshops. In Lamb et al. 1971, pp. 71–91.

Sands, H., and Radin, J. 1979. *The mentally disabled rehabilitant: Post-employment services.* Washington, D.C.: Department of Health, Education, and Welfare.

Schwartz, D. B. 1976. Expanding a sheltered workshop to replace nonpaying patient jobs. *Hospital and Community Psychiatry, 27*, 98–101.

A skills-training approach in psychiatric rehabilitation. 1980. *Rehabilitation Brief, 4*(1), 1–4.

Spooner, F.; Algozzine, B.; and Saxon, J. P. 1980. The efficacy of vocational rehabilitation with mentally ill persons. *Journal of Rehabilitation, 46*, 62–66.

Stein, L. I., and Test, M. A. 1980. An alternative to mental hospital treatment, I: Conceptual model, treatment program, and clinical evaluation. *Archives of General Psychiatry, 37*, 392–97.

Stevens, B. C. 1973. Evaluation of rehabilitation for psychotic patients in the community. *Acta Psychiatrica Scandinavica, 49*, 169–80.

Test, M. A.; Knoedler, W. H.; and Allness, D. J. 1985. The long-term treatment of young schizophrenics in a community support program. In *The training-in-community-living model: A decade of experience*, ed. L. I. Stein and M. A. Test. New directions for mental health services, no. 26. San Francisco: Jossey-Bass.

Turkat, D., and Buzzell, V. 1982. Psychosocial rehabilitation: A process evaluation. *Hospital and Community Psychiatry, 33*, 848–50.

Vitale, J. H., and Steinbach, M. 1965. The prevention of relapse of chronic mental patients. *International Journal of Social Psychiatry, 11*, 85–95.

Walker, R. and Asci, M. 1971. Evaluation of an experimental rehabilitation ward for chronic mental patients. *Rehabilitation of Literature, 32*, 40–41, 50.

Walker, R., and McCourt, J. 1965. Employment experience among two hundred schizophrenic patients in hospital and after discharge. *American Journal of Psychiatry, 122*, 316–19.

Walker, R.; Winick, W.; Frost, E. S.; and Lieberman, J. M. 1969. Social restoration of hospitalized psychiatric patients through a program of special employment in industry. *Rehabilitation Literature, 30,* 297–303.

Walls, R. T. 1982. Disincentives in vocational rehabilitation: Cash and in-kind benefits from other programs. *Rehabilitation Counseling Bulletin, 26,* 37–46.

Watson, C. G., and Maddigan, R. F. 1972. The effects of a paid work program on chronic and short-term patients. *Hospital and Community Psychiatry, 23,* 376–78.

Wehman, P. 1981. *Competitive employment.* Baltimore: Paul H. Brookes.

Weinberg, J. L., and Lustig, P. 1968. A workshop experience for post-hospitalized schizophrenics. In *Rehabilitation research,* ed. G. N. Wright and A. B. Trotter, pp. 72–78. Madison: University of Wisconsin.

Weisbrod, B. A.; Test, M. A.; and Stein, L. I. 1980. Alternative to mental hospital treatment, II: Economic-benefit cost analysis. *Archives of General Psychiatry, 37,* 400–405.

Whitehead, C. W. 1977. *Sheltered workshop study: A nationwide report on sheltered workshops and their employment of handicapped individuals.* Workshop Survey, Vol. 1, U.S. Department of Labor Service Publication. Washington, D.C.: U.S. Government Printing Office.

Wilder, J. F. 1976. The case for a flexible, long-term sheltered workshop for psychiatric patients. *Hospital and Community Psychiatry, 27,* 112–16.

Wilson, R. J., and Rasch, J. D. 1982. The relationship of job characteristics to successful placements for psychiatrically handicapped individuals. *Journal of Applied Rehabilitation Counseling, 13,* 30–33.

Wolkon, G. H.; Karmen, M.; and Tanaka, H. T. 1971. Evaluation of a social rehabilitation program for recently released psychiatric patients. *Community Mental Health Journal, 7,* 312–22.

17

Summary and Conclusion

JEAN A. CIARDIELLO

This book reflects the development of vocational rehabilitation in the United States during the thirty years after deinstitutionalization. Because persons with prolonged psychiatric disorders are no longer living predominantly in hospitals, effective vocational rehabilitation services for more than two million people have become vital to their success in the community. Psychotropic medication has gone a long way to relieve some of the major symptoms, but the lack of specific medical cures has put the onus on rehabilitation to help those afflicted with these disabilities to improve the quality of their lives. So, how well has vocational rehabilitation done since the 1950s? In 1979 the National Institute of Handicapped Research concluded that "although mentally disabled clients make up the largest number of cases eligible for vocational rehabilitation services, they have the least probability of success before *and after* rehabilitation." Several contributors to this volume have echoed similar sentiments concerning the efficacy of vocational rehabilitation. Neff, for instance, maintains that because of the lack of adequate community services and other reasons, the chronically mentally ill are worse off than they were a generation ago. Similarly, Anthony and his associates state that typical interventions have minimal impacts on employment outcomes. He goes so far as to say that we have done a better job of teaching those with prolonged psychiatric disabilities to be patients than of teaching them to be workers, since a person discharged from a psychiatric inpatient unit has a better chance of returning to the hospital than of returning to work. In their thorough evaluation of vocational rehabilitation programs from the research literature, Bond and Boyer reach the "general conclusion that *none* of the approaches discussed . . . have demonstrated efficacy in helping clients achieve and maintain competitive employment over any sustained period of time."

In many ways these conclusions should not be surprising. As Munich and Glinberg point out, there is a lack of consensus even just within the psychoanalytic school about what elements contribute to *any* person's capacity to work without even taking the level of personality organization into account. In addition, as Goldman and his associates note, when the clinical condition is taken into account, chronic mental illness is not easily definable even when using a multidimensional approach based on diagnosis, disability, and duration. The target population is difficult to determine because it includes persons whose clinical conditions are poorly understood and whose functional disabilities vary widely in time and change over time. If the variable nature of the disability makes determination difficult, how much more difficult will it make the task of rehabilitation.

Another major difficulty which surfaced repeatedly in these chapters and seems to contribute to the lack of greater success in vocational rehabilitation involves rehabilitation workers. According to McCrory, vocational rehabilitation workers need a variety of skills, including abilities in assessment, planning, counseling, and coordinating, combined with a knowledge of community resources and opportunities. She or he also needs to have an understanding of the world of work and of severe psychopathology. The rehabilitation worker must also, in Ryan's opinion, be able to form intensely personal and dedicated relationships with clients. However, vocational rehabilitation workers must be able to do this in the context of a system and a society which often undervalues and underpays them and, except in rare instances, without any formal training. It is no wonder that they are susceptible to "burnout"!

Examining the state of our conceptual base in vocational rehabilitation also makes some of our pessimistic conclusions more understandable. Strauss and his coauthors aptly describe the theoretical state of affairs as a "puzzle in pieces": the literature, training, and work setting of relevant disciplines are sequestered with very little consideration of cross-disciplinary issues which might help construct a firmer theoretical bridge between severe psychopathology and work. They point out the importance of identifying the functional characteristics directly influencing this association. For instance, which aspect of work might be crucial for which people with which mental disorders at which stage of the disorder? Like Strauss, we are able to put forth some of the pieces of the puzzle. We have explored the major issues so that they will be less segregated, offering others the opportunity of greater integration.

Despite these formidable obstacles, the past thirty years has taught us a great deal about vocational rehabilitation that can help persons with prolonged psychiatric disorders lead productive lives. As Bell states in the introduction, there is also a hopeful message conveyed by each of the contributors. It is captured in Goldman's definition of the chronically mentally ill when he says, "a significant proportion possess the capacity to live in relative independence *if* adequate community-based services, social supports, and life opportunities are provided."

Jansen elaborates this point in her discussion of the problems confronting vocational rehabilitation. She says: "Under ideal conditions, persons with chronic mental illness would be afforded a treatment in a rehabilitation system which met their needs and did so in an efficacious and cost-effective manner. Under such a system, treatment services designed to remedy ego deficits inherent in the illness would be provided and would be coordinated with other community-based services to remedy the social and vocational problems which result." Jansen offers a tremendous challenge to vocational rehabilitation, and it is this challenge that this volume addresses. What follows are highlights of some of the major advances and contributions to vocational rehabilitation over the past thirty years. These are presented in more detail in preceding chapters.

Turning first to the research literature and the empirical basis for vocational rehabilitation, it seems essential to summarize the 1984 landmark review of Anthony and Jansen. The following points are important guideposts which were cited by several authors:

1. Psychiatric symptomatology and diagnostic category are poor predictors of future work performance.

2. Intelligence, aptitude, and most personality tests are poor predictors of future work performance.

3. A person's ability to function in any given environment, (such as a home) is not predictive of his or her ability to function in a different setting (e.g., a job).

4. The best assessments of future work performance are ratings of past work performance, such as ratings of work adjustment made on the job or in a sheltered work setting.

5. The best demographic predictor of future work performance is an individual's previous employment history.

6. Social functioning is a significant predictor of work performance and of how well someone will "get along" on the job.

7. The best tests for predicting future vocational performance are those which measure a person's ego functioning and self-esteem with regard to work.

The research literature regarding the effectiveness of vocational rehabilitation programs looks more promising when paid employment is used as an outcome criterion and transitional and sheltered employment are included. In these cases, Bond and Boyer found that eight out of ten studies supported the effectiveness of these programs. They conclude: "When clients are given intensive support and are placed in jobs that are not too demanding, they often function at a level beyond usual expectations. Both intensive support and positive expectations that clients can succeed appear to be important elements. Given the additional finding that employment success is often not maintained after treatment ends, then supported work programs may be the best way to increase employment rates."

Turning to the contributions made by various approaches to vocational rehabilitation, the work done at the Research and Training Center of Boston University has received national attention. Applying the general theory used in psychiatric rehabilitation, Anthony and his associates give five important principles in their skill-building approach to vocational rehabilitation:

I. Effective vocational programming acknowledges each client's values and personal strengths.

II. Effective vocational rehabilitation programs have access to a network of learning and work environments.

III. Effective vocational programming provides the opportunity for clients to engage in activities designed to increase vocational maturity.

IV. Effective vocational programming provides for activities and environments which enhance self-esteem.

V. Effective vocational programming applies the psychiatric rehabilitation approach to diagnosis, planning and intervention.

While a social learning theory is implicit in many of Anthony's ideas, it is used more directly in Mueser and Liberman's skills-training model. The basic model is made up of a five-step process: (1) Identifying each patient's problems as to what, when, with whom, and where; (2) specifying the goals of training; (3) engaging the patient in a role play of the problem situation; (4) in a series of role plays, giving direct instructions, modeling, shaping, and gradually modifying the patient's behavior toward the goal; and (5) giving homework assignments to generalize the trained behavior to the natural environment. The attention-focusing and problem-solving models are variations on the basic model. Mueser uses vocational applications of these models in his training in job-seeking skills and in the job-finding club, which helps members obtain and sustain employment. Variations of the skills-training approaches of Anthony, Mueser, Liberman, and others are probably the most widely known and generally used approaches to vocational rehabilitation.

Since more than half of all persons with prolonged psychiatric disorders live with their families, Johnson emphasizes the importance of interventions designed to assist families and enhance their role in vocational rehabilitation. Anderson's psychoeducational model is particularly impressive. She uses the British expressed-emotion research to support her basic theoretical assumption that patients diagnosed schizophrenic have a "core psychological deficit" which results in difficulty in processing environmental stimuli. Therefore, very stressful and/or very stimulating environments often lead to relapse, and so she advocates deintensifying the family environment. Anderson's program provides "a variety of supportive and educational techniques to lower the emotional temperature of the family while maintaining sufficient pressure on patients to avoid the pitfalls of negative symptoms." It is a two-pronged approach. First, she decreases the level of expressed emotion in families through education about the illness, provision of support, expansion of social networks, and the establishment of clear boundaries and rules. Second, she helps the family to increase the social and vocational functioning of their ill relative in a slow and measured fashion. Johnson also describes the structural/strategic approach of Haley and Madanes, which focuses on correcting the problematic power hierarchies in families. It is only in the past decade that the positive influence of families in the vocational rehabilitation of persons with prolonged mental illness has been seriously considered. Use of the family context appears to be an important new advance warranting further attention and development.

The psychodynamic approach is the oldest approach to work and its inhibition with almost a hundred year history. It is presented by Munich and Glinberg in a general way; and then Ciardiello, Klein, and Sobkowski specifically focus on ego functioning and vocational rehabilitation. It is impossible to summarize Munich and Glinberg's work in a clear, concise way because of its complexity. They include developmental, drive, ego psychological, object-relations, and self-psychological points of view, as well as differences within each of these perspectives. In my view, these ideas are the most cogent in understanding vocational behavior. Having a psychodynamic understanding can be very important in dealing with the complicated intrapsychic issues involved in work inhibitions for those with prolonged psychiatric disorders. In particular, an ego-psychological approach has many theoretical and practical implications for vocational rehabilitation. Using Bellak's Ego Function Scale, Ciardiello, Klein, and Sobkowski found two ego functions to be empirically related to the vocational success of subjects diagnosed as schizophrenic: autonomous functioning (habit patterns, skills, routines, interests, intentionality, and motility) and regression in the service of the ego (essentially adaptability) are significantly related to work. They suggest ways in which ego strengths could be used to remedy deficits as well as ways in which ego function assessment can be used in determining work readiness and job placement.

An ego-function approach is combined with a vocational-psychology perspective in Bingham's chapter. He applies the developmental and structural theories which have been used with the general population for decades to those with prolonged psychiatric disorders. He describes the three major aspects of Super's theory of vocational psychology: the organization of vocational development into life stages; the formation, translation, and implementation of self-concepts in work; and the ways individuals progress through various work-related roles and manage transitions. Bingham recommends using Super's developmental theory to understand and intervene in the course of vocational development. He also recommends

Holland's structural orientation at certain points in the process in order to facilitate a more appropriate fit between client attributes and environmental demands. Four assumptions underlie Holland's formulation: (1) most persons can be characterized as one of six personality types—realistic, investigative, artistic, social, enterprising, and conventional; (2) environments can be characterized in parallel terms; (3) people seek out environments which permit them to exercise their personal attributes, fill compatible roles, and work on agreeable problems; and (4) behavior is determined by the interaction between personality and environment. For the most part, vocational psychology has been one of many important fields that has been functionally segregated from psychiatric rehabilitation. Bingham makes an important contribution toward theoretical integration.

The last approach described was transitional employment. As Malamud and McCrory note, transitional employment was started at Fountain House by Beard in 1958. There are now 135 rehabilitation facilities offering transitional employment opportunities. Most are modeled after Fountain House and combine supported, part-time work opportunities in the business community with a comprehensive psychosocial rehabilitation program. Workers are paid the normal wage by the employer. Rehabilitation staff work closely with the vocationally disabled member and the employer to maximize work adjustment. As Malamud and McCrory point out in their evaluation, transitional employment has been very effective in returning persons with prolonged psychiatric disabilities to the work force. These results have also been supported by Bond and Boyer in their evaluations of several similar programs.

The last section of the book focuses on several important aspects of the vocational rehabilitation process which each of the approaches have in common. The three aspects of process that I would like to highlight here are assessment, medication management, and the rehabilitation relationship.

Taking assessment first, Bolton emphasizes the importance of vocational assessment to successful work adjustment. He recommends a model assessing work personality, vocational abilities, interests, and temperamental traits which make up occupational capability. Because there is not sufficient evidence to the contrary, he assumes that vocational assessment techniques which have been found to be reliable and valid with a normal population are also valid, reliable, and useful with a severely disturbed psychiatric population. Although I have a great deal of respect for Dr. Bolton and his long history of excellent work in this area, my experience and research, as well as that of others, do not agree with this basic assumption. In addition to situational assessments, Bolton recommends the Work Personality Profile, the General Aptitude Test Battery, the U.S. Employment Services Interest Inventory, the Sixteen Personality Factor Questionnaire, and several others. In my opinion, more research needs to be done on the reliability and validity of these tests with persons with prolonged psychiatric disorders before they can be used with confidence in psychiatric vocational rehabilitation.

The role of psychotropic medication in the vocational rehabilitation process is rarely addressed. In his chapter Kane gives a lucid explanation of the ways in which drug treatment and vocational rehabilitation affect each other. He lists the most frequently used medications and their usual dosages, and describes their usefulness, as well as their adverse effects, limitations, and management difficulties. Kane's discussion of medication is in the context of a team approach to treatment which emphasizes working together to identify the early signs of relapse and sustain employment. Understanding the psychopharmacology of severe mental illness is essential for all those who work in psychiatric rehabilitation.

Lastly, both McCrory and Ryan discuss different aspects of the rehabilitation relationship. Ryan puts aside the technical "how-to" questions of vocational rehabilitation and asks "why"? He stresses that the whys of vocational rehabilitation need to be addressed in the context of a personal relationship between practitioner and client. A rehabilitation program which encourages the interest of staff members in the lives of clients is advocated. The five steps to develop this type of program are consideration, flexibility, creativity, opportunity, and curiosity. Staff burnout has been a major problem for both practitioner and client, and Ryan concludes that building and sustaining a personal relationship can help prevent burnout.

In a similar vein, McCrory describes building and maintaining a rehabilitation alliance. He emphasizes charting the course and identifying the crises along the way to achieving vocational goals. Having this long-term perspective, practitioners can better understand stress points and the difficulties involved.

I have summarized the problems, approaches, and aspects of the process which reflect some of the progress that we have made over the last thirty years in vocationally rehabilitating persons with prolonged psychiatric disorders. Given its short and fragmented history, psychiatric rehabilitation in the United States can point to substantial accomplishments. Before concluding I would like to cite some of the directions I think are important for the future. These recommendations can be divided into four categories: public-policy, research, training, and program development.

First, public-policy makers must recognize the need for a disability system which does not discourage work trials. In addition, resources must be made available to fund a well-coordinated system of rehabilitation and support services in the community. The costs of government and society for failing to vocationally rehabilitate persons with prolonged psychiatric disorders are well documented.,

The need for more and better research is clear. Questions about the rehabilitation process are crucial. For instance: who can benefit most, by what type of intervention, and at which stage of recovery? A conceptual bridge needs to be built between severe psychopathology and work. This type of bridge-building requires that the pieces of the vocational rehabilitation puzzle be brought together in more cross-disciplinary study. It also requires that outcome studies be done more frequently and more thoroughly so that the effects of programs which are already in place can be better understood.

In terms of training, the wide range of demands placed on vocational rehabilitation workers make formal training and better salaries imperative. Rehabilitation workers are an unusually dedicated group, but we cannot depend on dedication alone to attract and keep the kind of people needed to do this challenging work.

Although recommendations for program development are the most tentative of the four categories discussed, there are some directions that seem very promising. First, intensive and long-term program support is very important. For many chronically mentally ill individuals, vocational rehabilitation is a lifelong endeavor. Programs which recognize and address this need have been found to be more effective than those which do not. Transitional employment programs that combine positive expectations, social support, and job opportunities which are not too demanding have been found to be particularly successful. Enhancing self-esteem and ego functioning through graduated success experiences has also been found to be particularly helpful.

Addressing these challenges to vocational rehabilitation in the areas of public policy, research, training, and program development will determine the future of vocational rehabilitation in the United States, as well as the futures of over two million persons with prolonged psychiatric disorders.

Contributors

WILLIAM A. ANTHONY, PH.D., is director of the Center for Psychiatric Rehabilitation, and professor in the Department of Rehabilitation Counseling of Boston University. He has written more than fifty articles and a dozen chapters and books on the topic of psychiatric rehabilitation. He is co-editor of *Psychosocial Rehabilitation Journal.*

MORRIS D. BELL, PH.D., is associate clinical professor of psychology in the Department of Psychiatry at Yale University School of Medicine. He is also the assistant chief of the Veterans Resource Program at the Veterans Administration Medical Center, West Haven, Connecticut.

WILLIAM C. BINGHAM, ED.D., was, until his recent retirement, professor and coordinator of the Counseling Psychology Program of the Graduate School of Education, Rutgers University. He is a past president of the National Career Development Asssociation and is currently president of the International Association for Education and Vocational Guidance.

BRIAN BOLTON, PH.D., is professor at the Arkansas Research and Training Center in Vocational Rehabilitation, University of Arkansas, Fayetteville. He is the editor of *Handbook of Measurement and Evaluation in Rehabilitation,* the former editor of *Rehabilitation Counseling Bulletin,* and has published extensively in rehabilitation psychology.

GARY R. BOND, PH.D., is an associate professor in the Department of Psychology and director of the Doctoral Program in Rehabilitation Psychology at Indiana University—Purdue University. He was formerly director of research at Thresholds, a psychosocial rehabilitation program in Chicago.

SARA L. BOYER is a doctoral candidate in the Rehabilitation Psychology Program of Indiana University—Purdue University.

JEAN A. CIARDIELLO, ED.D., is adjunct assistant professor in the Department of Psychiatry at the University of Medicine and Dentistry of New Jersey and formerly directed the Research and Evaluation Unit at the Community Mental Health Center at Piscataway. Presently she is a psychoanalyst in private practice in Highland Park and Lawrenceville, New Jersey.

MIKAL R. COHEN, PH.D. is director of training, at the Center for Psychiatric Rehabilitation and research associate professor in the Department of Rehabilitation Counseling at Boston University. She has written seven training books, developed videotapes, and published numerous chapters, articles, and monographs. She is currently a director of a project producing a series of multimedia training packages in psychiatric rehabilitation.

KAREN S. DANLEY, PH.D., is assistant research professor in the Department of Rehabilitation Counseling, Sargent College, Boston University. She is also a senior training associate at the Center for Psychiatric Rehabilitation, where she is involved in research and training related to vocational applications of the psychiatric rehabilitation approach.

ANITA EICHLER, M.A., is a social science analyst for the Office of Special Populations, Office of the Director, National Institute of Mental Health. She was formerly a public health advisor in the Center for Prevention Research, NIMH.

TSILIA GLINBERG, M.D., is assistant unit chief of the Extended Treatment Services, New York Hospital—Cornell Medical Center, Westchester Division, and an assistant professor in the Department of Psychiatry, Cornell University Medical College.

HOWARD GOLDMAN, M.D., PH.D., is associate professor of Psychiatry and director of Mental Health Policy Studies at the University of Maryland School of Medicine.

COURTENAY M. HARDING, PH.D., is an assistant professor in the Department of Psychiatry, Yale University School of Medicine.

MARY A. JANSEN, PH.D., is consultant and temporary advisor for the Program in Chronic Mental Illness, World Health Organization, Geneva, Switzerland. She has been involved in the recent reform of the Social Security disability system in the United States and is an expert on European rehabilitation practices and policies.

THOMAS W. JOHNSON A.C.S.W., is a clinician and administrator at the University of Medicine and Dentistry of New Jersey—Community Mental Health Center at Piscataway. He has had extensive experience with chronically mentally ill patients and their families and has presented numerous papers on the family approach to rehabilitation at national conferences.

JOHN M. KANE, M.D., is director of Psychiatric Research at Hillside Hospital (a division of Long Island Jewish Medical Center) and professor of psychiatry at the State University of New York at Stony Brook School of Medicine. He has conducted an extensive series of investigations into the treatment of schizophrenia, with particular emphasis on the role of medication. He has written more than one hundred articles on psychiatry.

MYRA E. KLEIN, ED.D., is a clinician at Wayne Township Counseling Center, Wayne, New Jersey. She was formerly a researcher in the Program Planning and Evaluation Unit of the University of Medicine and Dentistry of New Jersey, Communtiy Mental Health Center at Piscataway. She is currently pursuing training at the New York Center for Psychoanalytic Training.

ROBERT PAUL LIBERMAN, M.D., is a professor in the Department of Psychiatry, UCLA School of Medicine, and director of the Clinical Research Unit at Camarillo State Hospital. He has directed the Clinical Research Center for Schizophrenia and Psychiatric Rehabilitation at UCLA since 1977. He is also chief of the Rehabilitation Service at the Brentwood Psychiatric Division of the West Los Angeles Veterans Administration Medical Center.

MAURY LIEBERMAN M.U.R.P., M.A., is program director for the State Comprehensive Mental Health Planning Program, State Planning and Human Resources Development Branch, Division of Education and Service Systems Liaison, National Institute of Mental Health. He was formerly head of the Work and Mental Health Section, Center for Prevention Research, NIMH.

DENNIS J. McCRORY, M.D., is chief psychiatric consultant for the Massachusetts Rehabilitation Commission. He is a member of the Fountain House Council for Education and Research and a staff psychiatrist at South Shore Mental Health Center.

THOMAS J. MALAMUD is research director at Fountain House, New York City.

RONALD W. MANDERSCHIED, PH.D., is chief of the Survey and Reports Branch, National Institute of Mental Health. He has been engaged in the evaluation of the Community Support Program for the chronically mentally ill for the past six years and has published extensively in this area.

KIM T. MUESER, PH.D., is an assistant professor of psychiatry at the Medical College of Pennsylvania, Eastern Pennsylvania Psychiatric Institute. He is also coordinator of the Schizophrenia Treatment Program and director of family therapy training in the Behavior Therapy Clinic, EPI.

RICHARD L. MUNICH, M.D., is division head of Extended Treatment Services, New York Hospital—Cornell Medical Center, Westchester Division, and associate professor of clinical psychiatry at Cornell University Medical College.

WALTER S. NEFF, PH.D., is professor emeritus in the Department of Psychology, New York University. He is the author of many publications about work, including the seminal book *Work and Human Behavior*.

He is a pioneer in vocational rehabilitation and was the developer and director of the doctoral program in community psychology at New York University.

JACQUELINE ROSENBERG is associate chief for policy in the Office of Policy Analysis, National Institute of Mental Health. She was formerly an assistant director of the Office of State and Community Liaison at NIMH, where she served as co–staff director of the National Plan for the Chronically Mentally Ill and coordinated a service systems research program on the chronically mentally ill for the NIMH Community Support Program.

EDWARD R. RYAN, PH.D., is associate chief of Psychology Service at the West Haven, Connecticut, Veterans Administration Medical Center, and associate clinical professor of psychology at Yale University School of Medicine. He has developed several treatment and rehabilitation programs for patients with prolonged psychiatric disorders and has directed funded research projects evaluating the effects of these programs. He has also made contributions in the areas of the psychotherapeutic outcome, the therapeutic community, and therapeutic relationships.

MORTON SILVERMAN, PH.D., is associate administrator for the Prevention, Alcohol, Drug Abuse, and Mental Health Administration. He was formerly chief of the Center for Prevention Research and chief of the Center for Work and Mental Health at NIMH.

SHAWN SOBKOWSKI, ED.D., is a clinician at the University of Medicine and Dentistry of New Jersey—Community Mental Health Center at Piscataway, Metuchen Office. She is a member in training at the National Psychological Association for Psychoanalysis.

JOHN S. STRAUSS, M.D., is professor of psychiatry in the Yale University School of Medicine.

Index

**Vocational Rehabilitation of Persons with
Prolonged Psychiatric Disorders**

Designed by Ann Walston.

Composed by Brushwood Graphics Inc.
in Sabon with Optima Bold display.

Printed by Edwards Brothers, Incorporated
on 50-lb. Glatfelter Offset
and bound in Holliston Roxite B.